Fighting Back with Fat

Fighting Back with Fat

A Parent's Guide to Battling Epilepsy through the Ketogenic Diet and Modified Atkins Diet

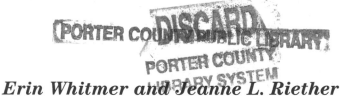

Erin Whitmer and Jeanne L. Riether

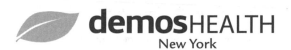

demosHEALTH

New York

Visit our website at www.demoshealth.com

ISBN: 978-1-936303-45-8
e-book ISBN: 978-1-617051-44-9

Acquisitions Editor: Noreen Henson
Compositor: diacriTech

Photos of Erin Whitmer Courtesy of Dara Nicely.

Photo of Jeanne L. Riether Courtesy of Hao Feng Bo.

Medical information provided by Demos Health, in the absence of a visit with a health care professional, must be considered as an educational service only. This book is not designed to replace a physician's independent judgment about the appropriateness or risks of a procedure or therapy for a given patient. Our purpose is to provide you with information that will help you make your own health care decisions.

The information and opinions provided here are believed to be accurate and sound, based on the best judgment available to the authors, editors, and publisher, but readers who fail to consult appropriate health authorities assume the risk of injuries. The publisher is not responsible for errors or omissions. The editors and publisher welcome any reader to report to the publisher any discrepancies or inaccuracies noticed.

Library of Congress Cataloging-in-Publication Data

Whitmer, Erin.
  Fighting back with fat : a parent's guide to battling epilepsy through the ketogenic diet and modified Atkins diet / by Erin Whitmer and Jeanne L. Riether.
    pages cm
  Includes bibliographical references.
  ISBN 978-1-936303-45-8
  1. Epilepsy—Diet therapy. 2. Ketogenic diet. 3. Low-carbohydrate diet.
I. Riether, Jeanne L. II. Title.
  RC374.K46W45 2013
  616.85'30654–dc23

                    2012035143

Special discounts on bulk quantities of Demos Health books are available to corporations, professional associations, pharmaceutical companies, health care organizations, and other qualifying groups. For details, please contact:

Special Sales Department
Demos Medical Publishing, LLC
11 West 42nd Street, 15th Floor
New York, NY 10036
Phone: 800-532-8663 or 212-683-0072
Fax: 212-941-7842
E-mail: rsantana@demosmedpub.com

Printed in the United States of America by Hamilton Printing.
12 13 14 15 16 / 5 4 3 2 1

Contents

Foreword

"Another ketogenic diet book? Really?" Yes, I'll admit it, when Jeanne L. Riether and Erin Whitmer, two of my "Keto mothers" approached me in August 2011 about the idea of writing a ketogenic diet book, my first reaction was skepticism. Besides my book, there are *Keto Kid* and *The Keto Cookbook*, so why do we need a fourth book? Jeanne and Erin, as firm and forthright as ever (which you'll determine are their styles rather quickly as you read this book...), told me that although these three books were great, they weren't enough. In Jeanne's original thoughts about the book relayed to me by e-mail, this would be "from the parents' perspective...it would go into our experiences cooking, shopping, getting child compliance, travel tips...." Erin added a month later after she and Jeanne had started to collaborate, "this will also be a sort of handbook that encompasses the emotional preparation of these diets and survival tricks of the trade." Aha! now I got it! At the time I thought this was a great idea and certainly unique. After seeing the final project, it exceeds my expectations!

What makes this book different? First, this is the first ketogenic diet book to have literally dozens of parents, patients, and caregivers express their thoughts and tips about this amazing treatment from the "trenches," so to speak. *Keto Kid* has one family's journey, *Ketogenic Diets* has several brief family stories, but *Fighting Back with Fat* has direct, first-person accounts. In many situations, these parents are brutally honest: Ketogenic diets are not simple and do involve a change in lifestyle, especially the first few weeks. Hearing these families' stories, and how they dealt with and solved some initial difficulties getting started on the diet, will be extremely helpful to new families. At Johns Hopkins Hospital, we have a parent support group that comes on the Wednesday of our monthly admission week to chat with new families starting the Ketogenic diet. This book is essentially that support group's manual.

The second major difference is the broad, all-encompassing nature of this book. You will hear from adults, adolescents, and parents of formula-fed infants and gastrostomy-tube-fed children. Some of the children in this book are completely normal, others are disabled. Many families are from outside the United States, including one of the co-authors (Jeanne). Large sections are devoted to practical tips and advice for families on the modified Atkins diet. Practical tips are given for interacting with your ketogenic diet team, other family members, school representatives, and anyone else who may join you on this ketogenic journey. Throughout all this, the medical advice is sound and reasonable. Erin and Jeanne e-mailed me very frequently through this process to double check their facts, but also to know when to avoid going into medical details best left to ketogenic diet teams and information in *Ketogenic Diets*. I truly do respect them for doing this and keeping *Fighting Back with Fat* accurate and focused on parent-based tips.

So did we need another Ketogenic diet book? I believe we did, and *Fighting Back with Fat* is a worthy and unique supplement to the other ketogenic diet books available. Although written for parents, I think any neurologist or dietitian from a ketogenic diet team would find it a valuable insight into what our families deal with in order to use dietary treatments successfully. I was honored to be included and sincerely hope new Keto parents read this book and subsequently contribute their own tips and ideas to Jeanne and Erin to be included in a second edition!

Eric H. Kossoff, MD
Associate Professor, Pediatrics and Neurology
Medical Director, Ketogenic Diet Program
Johns Hopkins Hospital
Baltimore, Maryland

Acknowledgments

Erin Whitmer: Writing this book has been a great labor of love, and it wouldn't have been possible without the warriors in my life: my family. To my husband, Mike, thank you for providing me with the resources to pursue my dream of becoming an advocate for the Ketogenic diet and of becoming a writer—a long journey in every way. You have endured my exhausting passion for taking on too much, and you have loved me and supported me through my greatest and hardest moments. I'd like to thank my father, Paul Bauer, for his unending faith in my talents and for giving me a detail-oriented personality, without which we never would have been able to keep track of more than 70 contributors to this book. My mother, Susan Bauer, continues to show me that the trials in life don't define us unless we let them; she is the reason I am a mother warrior. And to my always enthusiastic parents-in-law, John and April Whitmer, thank you for dropping everything to watch my tireless toddlers while I locked myself away to write or catch up on everything else I had neglected while writing. A thank you wouldn't be complete without telling my boys, Noah and Avry, that you are my everything, and I have learned life's greatest lessons and most profound joy since you came into my life.

Jeanne L. Riether: This book is the fulfillment of a dream and an answer to a prayer, and I would like to thank my family and friends for their inexhaustible patience and unfailing support that made it all happen. To my son Jordan, a seizure warrior and hero who now uses his experiences to encourage others; to Chris and Sparrow, his amazing brother and sister who helped me cook, shop, and care for Jordan during the 2 years he was on the diet; and to his other sisters, Shalimar, Angela, and Maya, who loved and encouraged their brother from the other side of the globe. You all put up with a parent who was temporarily "missing in action" while immersed in the preparation of this manuscript. Please know that you, my children, are my greatest treasures.

I would also like to thank my dear friends and colleagues, Hugues and Anna de Gaalon, and Liu Xu, for being my rocks of support during the rough times and encouraging me to tackle this project in the first place. Many thanks to Dr. Eric Kossoff, for having the faith to answer the e-mail of this desperate mother in China and guide us through 2 years on the diet; you are incredible. And last but not least, my dear friends on the *Healing Young Hearts* Modified Atkins for Seizures Yahoo Group: the stories and experiences you contributed make up such a great part of this book, and you have become like a part of my family. Thank you, each and every one!

We would also like to thank the following list of wonderful individuals who contributed to the making of this book. The list is long and includes our dedicated researcher; medical doctors; nurses; dietitians; teachers; a psychologist; parents of children on the diet; as well as children, teenagers and adults who are personally using diet therapy themselves. Each one graciously shared their time and unique experience to help create the collective wisdom found on these pages.

Researcher

Kira Bolton

Contributing Medical Professionals

Claire M. Chee, RN, Children's Hospital of Philadelphia, Philadelphia, PA; Liao Jianxiang, MD, Shenzhen Children's Hospital, PRC; Eric H. Kossoff, MD, Johns Hopkins Hospital, Baltimore, MD; Christiana Liu, MSc, RD, CHES, The Hospital for Sick Children, Toronto, Canada; Janak Nathan, MD, Shushrusha Hospital, Mumbai, India; Elizabeth G. Neal, RD, PhD, Matthew's Friends Charity and Clinics, Lingfield, and UCL Institute of Child Health, London, UK; Zahava Turner, RD, Johns Hopkins Hospital, Baltimore, MD; Deng Yuhong, MD, 2nd Affiliated Medical University Hospital, Guangzhou, PRC; Beth Zupec-Kania, RD, CD, The Charlie Foundation, Santa Monica, CA.

Reading Panel and Consultants

Talia Berger, Oliver's Magic Diet; Marilyn Dixon; Heather Ewing; Gerry Harris, The Carson Harris Foundation; Kathryn Hively Lane; Dawn Martenz; Laurie Myers; Heather Pereira.

Contributors

John Ballas; Dorene Bankester; Ann Barczewski; Eli Berger; Oliver Berger; Chris Carmody; Kevin Carmody; Liam Carmody; Randlyn Clemons; Rebecca Crosby; Mike Dancer; Georgia Denby; Lynette Dergen; Jennifer DiMartino; Abbie Ewing; Heather Fleming; Wanda Flores; Rose-Marie Gallagher; Shannon Graham; Maridali Gonzalez; Ashley Hamilton; Karolina Ivankovic; Stephanie Jutras; Jennifer Katz; Tiffany Kim; Machell Wesley Klee; Teri M.; Michael McHugh; Carol Moran; Phil Morris; Lori O'Keefe; Wendy Ormsby; Amy Palmer; Heidi Pask; Patricia Perry; Samantha Raftery; Jordan Riether; Heath Robbins Photography; Orlando Rodriguez; Maria Roemer; April Runge; Amy Sauer; Michael Sauer; Bethany Saxton; Lisa Schneider; Laura Sharpe; Holly Skillen; April Smith; Pam Smith; Debbie Sprang; Kendra Stewart; Kay Summers; Jenna Teeson; Emma Williams, Matthew's Friends; Krista Williams; Ashlee Yuskis; Dana; Jenny; Joanna; Sam; Sabira; Lynn.

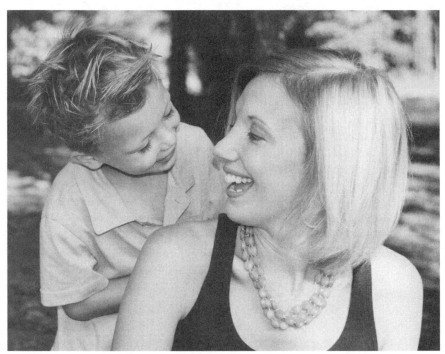

Erin and Noah

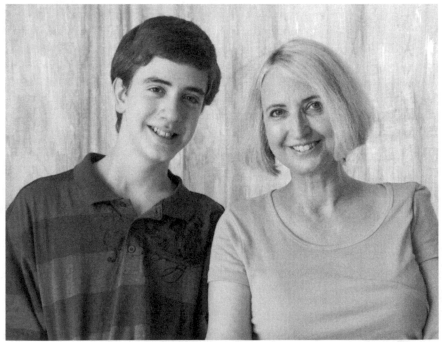

Jeanne and Jordan

How to Use This Book

Every parent of a child with seizures understands that epilepsy can be a complex and difficult journey through uncharted territory. The first frightening seizure thrusts us into a world of unfamiliar tests and mysterious medical terminology that we may need a dictionary to decipher. It's challenging enough to navigate these waters, but when seizures prove difficult to control we may feel like we're sailing off the edge of the map entirely. When we enter the realm of the diet therapy, we desperately need clear information and the comfort of hearing the experiences of those who've traveled this route before us.

Fighting Back with Fat was written by two mothers, one with a child on the Ketogenic diet, the other with a child on the Modified Atkins Diet (MAD), who each went looking for a book that would tell them how to plan, shop, cook, deal with travel, school, parties, and holidays, and manage all the emotional minefields of parenting a child on diet therapy for epilepsy—only to discover that such a book hadn't yet been written. If you are on a quest seeking an informative practical resource written from a parent's perspective that details the management of these diets in day-to-day life, *Fighting Back with Fat* is what you need. You will get the most from these pages when using this book as a supplement to resources written by medical professionals. This book does not fully explain the dynamics of the various ketogenic diets, how they are initiated, or how they work. If you are looking for an easy-to-understand resource written by an expert we whole-heartedly recommend the book, *Ketogenic Diets* (5th edition) by Dr. Eric Kossoff, et al. In fact, we like to think of our book as a practical companion to Dr. Kossoff's book. While some topics in *Fighting Back with Fat* might overlap the topics in the *Ketogenic Diets* book, please do not rely on our book to replace the advice of a medical team. You should be under the care of a qualified physician when following these diets, and cannot use this book as a substitute for proper medical supervision.

Here are a few helpful tips for the reader to remember:

■ **Dietary Definitions**: This book is about all of the ketogenic diets. When we say *the Ketogenic diet*, or *Keto*, we mean the classic Ketogenic diet that is initiated in a hospital and uses a gram scale and ratios. When we say *a ketogenic diet, dietary therapy*, or *the diet* we are referring to any of the ketogenic diets for epilepsy, whether it be the classic Ketogenic diet, MAD, Low Glycemic Index Treatment diet (LGIT) or the Medium Chain Triglyceride (MCT) diet.

■ **Adults, Teens, and Children**: This is a book written for people of all ages who are considering diet therapy, but because we are addressing such a large audience and the majority of readers are likely parents of children with epilepsy, we often default to addressing parents as a group. However, adults on the diet will benefit from the information in these pages equally as much, and we devoted an entire section to adult stories in Chapter 9, "Warriors of All Shapes and Sizes."

We hope the advice and stories in these pages will provide a shortcut to learning and make your entire experience with these diets as easy as possible. If you use it as a companion to relevant medical resources, it will serve you well. We wish you all the best on your journey, and hope that diet therapy proves as wonderfully successful for your family as it did for ours.

Erin Whitmer and Jeanne L. Riether

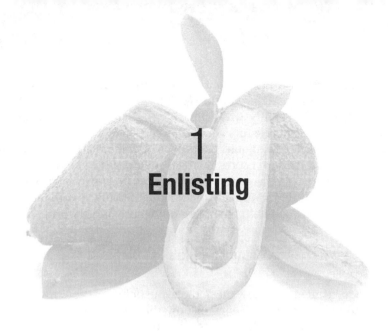

1
Enlisting

As the parent of a child with epilepsy, or perhaps as an individual with epilepsy yourself, you are acutely aware that seizures will hold your life captive. For the 30% of people whose seizures aren't controlled by anticonvulsants, there's no such thing as waving a white flag in the hope of peace. Epilepsy is a unique enemy that is still greatly misunderstood, and it continues to take prisoner after prisoner while loved ones grapple with feelings of frustration, heartache, helplessness, and fear. Those of us who continue to struggle with the havoc epilepsy wreaks in our lives can feel guilty, overwhelmed, emotionally numb—or for some, emotionally super-charged; we feel anxious or hopeless about the future, having trouble concentrating on some of the smaller aspects of our lives, and at some point perhaps isolating ourselves from the world around us.

These emotional symptoms are also characteristic of people who are suffering from Post-Traumatic Stress Disorder (PTSD). While we don't have PTSD (at least not most of us), we are suffering in some of the same ways—because we have been thrust into our own war, and we are fighting battle after battle. Thankfully, epilepsy's little white flag is flying closer than you might think, and it's not at all where you would expect to find it: in mayonnaise and butter and in every glorious fat that we have never allowed ourselves to indulge in. Until now.

Fighting Back with Fat is not only the name of this book, it's become a mantra for many, and believe it or not, it's been a utilized battle tactic against seizures since the beginning of the twentieth century, before anticonvulsants were at the forefront of seizure management. In this book we will show you how you, too, can fight back with fat using a ketogenic diet, including the classic Ketogenic diet (Keto), the Modified Atkins Diet (MAD),

1

and we will spend some time on the Low Gylcemic Index Treatment (LGIT) and the Medium Chain Triglyceride (MCT) ketogenic diets as well. The Ketogenic diet, until recently, was primarily used on children, but research has shown it can be successful even in adults. Thanks to the introduction of MAD only a decade ago, dietary therapy is now more approachable than ever, and many of those who try it, from toddlers to adults, are finding seizure improvement. As we write this book, advances in dictary therapy are rapidly changing and improving, making fighting back with fat a viable option for almost anyone with epilepsy—anywhere in the world.

The Skinny on High Fat Diets

In order to have an idea of how these diets can help cure you or your child, you need to understand the basics of how they work. We will try to give you the skinny on these high fat diets without making you wish you had a medical degree.

Ketogenic diets trick the body into thinking it's fasting by switching from the body's primary metabolism of burning glucose for energy to a fat-based energy source. Our body only maintains a 24 to 36 hour supply of glucose, so when carbohydrates, which are converted to glucose, are limited, the body begins to burn fat instead. Once your body runs out of glucose it will naturally begin to burn stored body fat. By feeding your body a diet that is high in fat, while restricting the carb intake, your body continues to burn fat, creating a never-ending fasting-like state.

When the body converts fat into energy it leaves behind a residue in the form of ketone bodies, which in turn build up in the blood; the body is now using a ketone metabolism instead of a glucose metabolism. These metabolized ketones are released into the bloodstream and can be excreted in the urine, which is why it's standard practice for both the Ketogenic diet and MAD to test ketones by checking urine (some Keto Clinics also measure ketone bodies by blood test). When ketones in the urine are large, as indicated by the test strip, the body is officially in a state of ketosis. *Not to worry, this is a good thing*! It is not known (and highly debated) whether ketosis is why the diets work, with most studies saying it's possibly necessary but not the actual reason. Ketosis is the first of many goals of the high-fat diet therapies we mention in this book. The biggest goal, of course, is the elusive white flag, or seizure control.

The classic Ketogenic diet, first created in the early 20th century, has evolved and become far more user friendly in the last couple decades, though it is still a strict diet that is initiated in a hospital and is continued under direct medical supervision. Though not all Keto Clinics begin the diet with the recommended 24-hour fast (some clinics don't begin with a fast at all), the diet is always begun under the watchful eye of a neurologist and dietitian as well as a full team of medical staff, such as nurses and technicians. Please note that the Ketogenic diet is not a diet that should ever be tried without medical supervision, as it could put your child at very serious risk for health issues and even death, but with a medical team's supervision the diet is safe.

The Ketogenic diet is 80% to 90% fat and is calculated in ratios. The most common ratio, sometimes called the "true ratio" is 4:1, meaning four times as much fat as protein and carbohydrates combined. Ratios range from 1:1, which is similar to MAD, to 2:1, 3:1, and up to 4:1. Some clinics will do up to a 5:1, but rarely. Keto Clinics don't always start children off at the 4:1 ratio, which used to be common practice. Now, some clinics believe that it's possible to try a lower ratio first, such as 2:1 or 3:1, moving up in ratio over time to gain seizure control. Infants are typically started at a 3:1 ratio because they require more carbohydrates and protein than other ages due to their rapid growth and brain development. Adolescents are also often placed at a lower ratio because of the intense period of development that accompanies the teen years.

In order to accomplish this exact ratio on a scientific level, all food is weighed on a gram scale. While weighing every food down to the gram is time-consuming, for many Keto parents, thinking of foods and recipes in terms of grams becomes more second nature than the previous method of measuring with cups and teaspoons. A great benefit to this exact measurement system is that it's accessible on an international scale, since forms of measurement aren't hindered by cultural differences.

The popularity of the Ketogenic diet has exploded in the last decade, thanks in part to Jim Abrahams, a movie director and writer whose personal fight to heal his child's catastrophic epilepsy catapulted this near-forgotten form of treatment back into the forefront of most neurologists' treatment plans. In 1993 Jim Abrahams, who founded The Charlie Foundation, a fantastic resource for the Ketogenic diet, took his son Charlie to Johns Hopkins Hospital in Baltimore, where the Ketogenic diet had been used as a seizure treatment for decades. Charlie quickly became seizure free on the diet, and after continuing diet therapy for several years with a few ups and downs, he is now a normal adult. *First Do No Harm*, a film that promotes the Ketogenic diet and was directed by Jim Abrahams, officially put the diet on the map—and offered hope for parents who had all but given up.

The MAD was created at Johns Hopkins Hospital in the early part of the new millennium. It began as a way to offer a less-restrictive version of the Ketogenic diet and is approximately a 2:1 ratio in the beginning, especially if utilizing KetoCal, a pre-made formula high in fat that has proven to improve seizure control when first beginning MAD. After the first month or so, the diet is more like a 1:1 ratio. Carbohydrates are limited to 10 to 20 net grams a day in the beginning, though that number can be adjusted in time, depending on the success of the diet and the individual's dietary needs. Unlike the Ketogenic diet, protein and calories are not limited, and fats are used liberally, though not formally measured. No food is weighed; instead, carbs are counted using standard USDA food guidelines as outlined in carb-counting books and online programs. There are even apps for counting carbs now. Chapter 4, "The Mess Hall," has a useful list of carb-counting books and online resources.

As both MAD and the Ketogenic diet gather momentum in popularity, we continue to learn that these diets, while different in their execution, are really quite similar. Both hinge on the diet's ability to burn fat instead of glucose, effectively tricking the body into thinking it's fasting. Both diets are low carb and high fat, and each of these diets requires an entirely new perspective on what's "healthy" for your child. There's less focus on the more popular concepts of healthy eating such as whole grains, organic, low fat and high protein; instead, fat is the focus: oils, nuts, avocados, and heavy whipping cream. Both these diets require strict adherence, though the method of measurement for MAD is less time-consuming than weighing each food by the gram. In many respects MAD is easier due to the lack of limitations and the less formulated approach, but for some people the Ketogenic diet is easier because it lacks the guesswork. With MAD people wonder, How much fat is enough? When do you know your child is getting too many calories? Your personality as the caregiver will have a large role in which diet therapy you choose, whether it's the classic Ketogenic diet, MAD, or even LGIT or the MCT diet. One of the goals of this chapter is to introduce you to these diets on a more intimate level so that you can learn which diet might suit you or your child. Choosing your personal diet therapy journey is a tough decision. We hope this chapter helps break down some of those big decision points.

Choosing to Enlist

Parents often write in to the online support forums of which both authors are members and ask whether or not they should pursue diet therapy, be it the Ketogenic diet or MAD. People on the forums jump at the opportunity to share their personal stories of success with these diets, sharing with searing honesty their heartache and trials before the diet, and how diet therapy has changed their child's life, and their own. Keep in mind: these are people in the epilepsy community. If nothing else, we are realists who have been handed one challenge after another. We know disappointment. We know fear. And those who have tried a ketogenic diet know that the spatulas we carry are silver lined, and we'll tell that to anyone willing to listen. In the several years combined that Jeanne and Erin have been a part of these forums and in a ketogenic community, we have yet to see someone steered away from trying one of these diets. Sure, we've seen a few quit when the diet didn't offer what they had hoped for, but had they not tried the diet they never would have known it wouldn't work—just as we never would have known that our children would become seizure free on the diet had we *not* tried it.

Our approach to the big question of "Should I try dietary therapy?" is this: unless you or your child has a metabolic condition that makes the diet unsafe, and you've tried more than two anticonvulsants without success (frankly, we wish we could skip the drugs and go straight to the diet), put on your apron, get out the mayonnaise, and start cooking. We'll be surprised if you say it wasn't worth it. Yes, following a diet is harder than popping a pill. But for so many who found that pills did not deliver as hoped, these diets can be life changing. Many parents eventually find themselves asking, "Why in the world didn't we try this sooner?"

If our enthusiasm for these diets isn't enough to convince you, or if you're like a lot of parents out there and want some hard evidence, here are a few statistics. 50% of children on the Ketogenic diet will have at least a 50% seizure improvement after six months. 10% to 15% of children on the diet after six months will become seizure free. Children who fall into that 10% to 15% range are considered "super responders." Luckily for both of the authors of this book, our boys were both super responders, with Noah, Erin's son, going seizure free after 17 days on the Ketogenic diet and Jordan, Jeanne's son, becoming seizure free on the morning of day four. A study by Johns Hopkins, published in the April 2012 issue of the *Journal of Child Neurology*, showed that overall long-term statistics of children who have done MAD are similar to those of the Ketogenic diet, with a 40% seizure improvement after six months. This is great news for MAD, a diet that is still not supported everywhere, but certainly should be.

What's also significant to mention, in addition to improved seizure control on these diets, are the other potential positive side effects. A vast majority of parents say their child became more "bright," often as though a haze had been lifted or a light had been turned on. Anecdotal evidence also shows that many children make better developmental gains on these diets, and children also seem to have more energy than pre-diet. One of the greatest benefits of these diets, especially when seizures are controlled, is the ability to wean off some or all anticonvulsants. In fact, many parents come to diet therapy with the ultimate goal of getting the drugs out of the picture, which is not always a fair expectation, but certainly a commendable one. Later in this chapter we will discuss expectations, and how they can ultimately affect your experience administering these diets.

Now, let's imagine you've donned your apron and you're armed with a spatula. You're ready to move forward with diet therapy. How do you know which diet is best for you or your child?

Picking Your Battle

At some point in this book you might decide to go back and count how many times we tell you that a decision you make is personal and depends wholly on your own unique variety of factors. We will tell you often. This is not our way of avoiding the tough questions, but because epilepsy is such a complex topic on its own, coupled with each individual's fluctuating variables such as cognition, dietary restrictions, sensory issues, food intolerance, or pickiness, we can only provide you with a big chunk of the puzzle. You'll have to arrange the rest of the pieces using *Ketogenic Diets* (5th edition) by Dr. Eric Kossoff, et al., where you can learn further about these diets from the medical perspective—how they work, the differences in the diets, medical research and statistics, and how to initiate them—and ultimately you'll do a little soul-searching too.

For some people picking the best diet for their family is as simple as 1-2-3. For others the decision becomes a complex problem in which they need to learn what factors are vital to calculating their decisions and what factors are less significant. The age of a child is often a big factor that parents need to consider, as is the type of epilepsy. A child's cognition, his ability to understand the limitations of the diet, as well as his ability to adhere to the diet are crucial to its success. On the flip side, children who are developmentally delayed and less aware of food are great candidates for a stricter version of the diet because they are likely to have an easier time adapting to their new foods.

In this section we hope to present some guidance on which diet might suit your family's needs, while giving you first-person accounts from parents who have been in your boots before. We will highlight the similarities and differences in these diets from our perspective as moms who have been in the trenches getting our hands oily. While we present the pros and cons of each—and whether or not the pros and cons feel equal in weight or not—we are not advocating one diet over the other.

Understanding the Differences in the Ketogenic Diet and the Modified Atkins Diet

The Ketogenic diet is like a ballet, an art that can be perfected and precise. Imagine MAD as hip hop, full of the freedom to improvise. Not surprising to anyone who finds they can relate to one type of dance over another, the restrictiveness of the Ketogenic diet and the freedom of MAD are two of the biggest factors people take into consideration when trying to choose which diet will be best for their child, and for them. You might be a person who needs control, who needs fewer variables. If this is the case, the Ketogenic diet might be a good choice for you. The biggest complaint of parents who tried MAD before moving onto the Ketogenic diet was that MAD overwhelmed them due to the lack of restrictions.

Conversely, some parents need the flexibility of MAD because they find restrictions and exact rules too rigid for their lifestyle. Jeanne Riether, co-author of this book, admits she hates numbers, and the more she learns about the Ketogenic diet, the more aware she is that MAD was the best choice for her. Co-author Erin Whitmer, on the other hand, loves the exact-science nature of weighing food to the gram. It's predictable, and after an unpredictable life with seizures, she finds peace in that.

The Ketogenic Diet

The most exacerbating element of the Ketogenic diet, the scale, is also one of the greatest benefits, and a real relief to some parents. When beginning these diets, even though a medical team guides us, there is still a great deal of learning on your behalf. Creating recipes based on this foreign concept of food can be daunting. The scale and the exact calculation of food for the Ketogenic diet take out some of the guesswork. There's no question about how much fat, carbohydrates, and protein to use, as the dietitian provides all of those requirements, including calorie counts. Using the KetoCalculator, an online program that allows you to create ketogenic meals without any longhand math, you can make meals according to the exact requirements your dietitian has outlined for your child's meal plan. (We will discuss the KetoCalculator further in Chapter 4.) When you are overwhelmed with this new diet, and your family is going through the emotional adjustment, just going about the simple task of weighing food can be a relief. Yes, it is tedious. But in time you will become efficient and confident, and weighing food on a scale will become second nature.

In addition to the requirement of weighing foods on the gram scale, in order to always achieve the perfect ratio, food must be eaten in its entirety. There's no option to eat half the meal and save the rest for later, which is why you'll read of parents scraping the bowls with rubber spatulas to make sure their little warrior gets all the protein, carbohydrates, and fat of the meal. Every time a gram of food is lost to a spill or un-scraped bowl, the ratio is compromised. While not all Keto Clinics push this now, it was once common practice to have a very strict time schedule at which time all meals needed to be consumed. For some children, setting an eating schedule and sticking to it is essential for their seizure control; for other children, it doesn't make a difference—just another small example of the great variety in how individuals react to the diet.

The greater challenge of the Ketogenic diet is not the scale, but creating recipes at the higher ratios that are appealing to children and adults. Most kids are used to foods like chicken nuggets, pizza, and milk, and even if you are a strict healthy whole-food kind of parent, your children pre-diet will have had the luxury of eating far more fresh fruit and vegetables than they will be able to consume once on the Ketogenic diet. Factoring in upwards of 36 grams of fat with only about 4 grams of protein and 4 grams of carbohydrates (just as an example of a high-ratio meal) can require imagination and a commitment to experimentation. The real time-consuming factor is brainstorming, calculating, and then experimenting with new recipe ideas, especially anything between 4:1 and 3:1 ratios. 2:1 ratios and below become much easier, as the carb and protein amounts make it easier to have tasty food. The potential fresh fruit servings at these lower ratios will be enough to make you, and likely your child, giddy.

While recipe creation is a challenge, you are considering these diets at a great time. Because they are more popular and with the increase of mom bloggers, Facebook, and other online support groups, it's far easier than even two years ago (when Erin Whitmer's son started the Ketogenic diet) to find recipes. *The Keto Cookbook* is a great resource and all its recipes are at the 4:1 ratio; in addition, the author of *The Keto Cookbook* has started a new website dedicated to recipe sharing and practical advice for every facet of the Ketogenic diet, www.ketocook.com.

When the Ketogenic diet might be a good choice:

- **Infants:** Infants and toddlers below the age of two should be placed on the Ketogenic diet instead of MAD because of their need for additional carbohydrates. They also require supervised care because they are in a significant state of brain growth and development.

- **G-tube fed:** Mixing a ketogenic formula for those with g-tubes is relatively simple and there are no pre-made formulas for MAD.

- **Infantile spasms:** Infants with infantile spasms respond so well to the Ketogenic diet that it's becoming common practice to use the diet as a front-line course of action.

- **Children with developmental delays:** One of the greatest challenges of dietary therapy is helping your child adapt to new foods while eliminating foods she used to love. Children with mild to severe developmental delays are often less concerned with how their food compares to those around them. While they will still have to adjust to food on the Ketogenic diet, it is easier to shelter them.

- **Parents who need additional support and guidance:** Many parents choose the Ketogenic diet over another dietary therapy because they found the restrictions of the diet helpful. These people often find more anxiety than freedom in a less restrictive diet therapy.

The Modified Atkins Diet

For those who cherish flexibility, an attractive benefit of MAD is that while it is also effective in improving seizure control, it is less restricted than the Ketogenic diet. Here's something that might surprise you however: you actually get less grams of carbohydrates on MAD than on the Ketogenic diet, especially at lower ratios of the Ketogenic diet, 2:1 and below. A low-ratio meal on the Ketogenic diet might give you upwards of 8 to 10 grams of carbohydrates per meal, while on MAD you are overall limited to about 10 to 20 carbohydrates a day. If you have a child who loves his higher-carb fruits and isn't as interested in cheeses and meats, the Ketogenic diet might be a better choice. However, if your child—or you—loves to eat cheese, chicken, steak, eggs, bacon, and any other protein out there, and enjoys salads and vegetables topped with dressings or butter, MAD might be a choice that won't seem overwhelmingly difficult. Small amounts of fruits (mostly berries) are used, along with low-carb foods such as nut flours. MAD has no limit on protein consumption but moderation is encouraged. Your biggest challenge is finding all the hidden carbohydrates that lurk in foods you wouldn't expect, picking the best carbs for your daily allowance and learning how to efficiently measure them.

In the beginning, approaching food from a mathematical perspective can take some getting used to. However, don't panic. In reality you only need to be able to count to 10 in order to add up the 10 net grams of carbohydrates in the foods your child will eat in a day. (Older children and adults usually start the diet at 15 or 20 net grams.) You don't need to weigh anything or measure proteins. After the initial few months on MAD, you will learn to eyeball measurements of food and you will have the carbohydrate content for every major ingredient you frequently use memorized. Just remember to add lots of fats to foods and drinks. You can also easily take MAD with you; it just becomes a matter of learning what foods you can select from the world around you.

With endless options, however, it can be overwhelming to know which road to take. This is why the personality of the parent needs to be considered. For some parents, including Erin Whitmer, MAD was frustrating without the exact science. The flexibility in MAD forced her to make the diet into something it wasn't. Before officially starting her son, Noah, on the Ketogenic diet she put Noah on MAD. She created food charts that outlined every gram of carbs, making sure that Noah had at least 30 grams of fat per meal, and if Noah didn't meet his 10 carbs in a day, she'd panic, trying to find a higher-carb food to give him to round out his carb allowance. When Noah was initiated on the Ketogenic diet and Erin told Dr. Kossoff, Noah's neurologist at Johns Hopkins Hospital, how she'd been orchestrating MAD, Dr. Kossoff chuckled and told her that she was really doing something like a modified Keto. MAD is much simpler than she had made it out to be. It was a testament to the fact that Erin's personality as an individual and a mom made her a more ideal candidate for the Ketogenic diet.

But for a mom like Jeanne, who admittedly hates numbers—don't even bother asking her what her apartment number is!—MAD gave her the freedom she craves. She kept a short list on the fridge door of the carb values of various vegetables, fruits, and other foods she routinely used. By glancing at the list, she eventually learned how to whip together a meal. She liked the fact that if she wasn't sure she'd given her son enough fat that day, she could just make him an extra snack of a cream shake, or a bowl of homemade ice cream or butter chocolate candies. It took time and experimentation before she learned to slip into a routine, but once she mastered the basics and knew which foods to use, the diet became easy to follow.

When the MAD might be a good choice:

■ **Parents who prefer simple, free-style ways of preparing foods:** If you are not going to agonize over exactly how much fat to use when told to "use very, very generous amounts" and are willing to do some tweaking to find out what works best for your child, then MAD will probably be a good fit.

■ **Adults, teenagers, and older children:** The choices and options of food that MAD provides can sometimes make the diet easier to adapt to and to stick with over the long haul.

■ **Kids who need a less restricted system of eating:** If your child has behavioral issues that make following a restricted way of eating difficult, MAD may be a better option. The flexibility of MAD may defer tantrums in your child and help avoid frustration for kids and parents both.

■ **You don't have a Keto Clinic nearby where you can initiate and closely follow-up the classic Ketogenic diet:** Traveling isn't an easy option for some, and MAD does not require hospital admission in order to begin the diet. MAD typically has fewer side effects than the Ketogenic diet, so progress can usually be monitored by a local pediatrician or neurologist even without the benefit of a full-fledged Keto Team. (We will discuss all the potential side effects of these diets in Chapter 5.)

■ **You intend to eat out at restaurants, family events, and social functions often:** It is easier to adapt MAD to food-centered social occasions, so if these types of events are a regular and important part of your life, MAD may be a better fit.

■ **There is a long wait for hospital admission to begin Ketogenic diet therapy:** The admission list for the Ketogenic diet at many clinics is long; it may be months before you can start. Studies show that the sooner the diet is started the better the outcome, so time is of the essence. Starting a child on MAD while waiting to be admitted for Keto can be a first treatment step, even if only as a stop-gap until the child later switches to Keto.

■ **When parents or adults want to try diet therapy before anticonvulsants:** In most cases patients who turn to diet therapy have previously tried and failed medications. However, a small but growing number of patients are turning the tables and wish to explore diet as a first-line therapy. They are reluctant to start anticonvulsants for various reasons (whether valid or not). Most who opt to try the diet before meds feel that if the results are not satisfactory, after three to six months they will move on to medication. Be aware, though, that trying MAD before meds has raised the hackles of some in the medical community. Choose a doctor to work with who understands that you are not an ignorant fanatic who is opposed to modern medicine, and be prepared to take some flack.

A Closer Look at These Diets

We understand that you could potentially view dozens of pie charts with the ratio of fats, carbs, and proteins colorfully illustrated without really knowing how that food might look on a plate. For many parents on these diets, the amount of fat can be hard to conceptualize, especially because we live in a society that views fat as a food that should be consumed in extreme moderation. In order to show you how ketogenic ratios can differ from each other and how MAD generously allows for more protein, we have created bar graphs with simple foods that can be found in everyone's home, or in a restaurant if you choose to eat out on one of these diets.

With a 4:1 ratio, it is clear how the cream, butter, and avocado—that is, the fats—are the majority of the meal. Broccoli and chicken breast account for very little, and without some creative ingenuity, this meal would be wholly unappealing to most children. For this reason, we will teach you how to be creative with meals, and how to use a variety of fats and carbohydrates in order to whip up high fat, yet delicious meals.

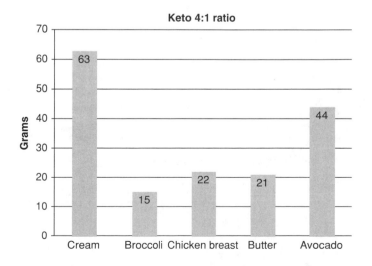

While the 3:1 ratio has virtually the same amount of fat at the 4:1 ratio, the protein and broccoli allotment are considerably higher, which will increase the palatability of the meal. Still, this is a high ratio and figuring out how to sneak fats into the meal in an appealing way is something learned, not necessarily inherent in any of us.

With a much higher allowance of chicken and broccoli, the ketogenic 2:1 ratio has a much more appealing ratio of carbohydrates and protein to fat. The fat numbers are still quite high, but there's a lot of freedom to play around with recipes on this low ratio. In fact, a 2:1 ratio is very similar to MAD, especially in the beginning of MAD, when a good deal of the fat could come from KetoCal, which gives the diet a boost.

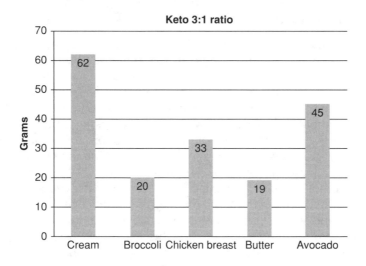

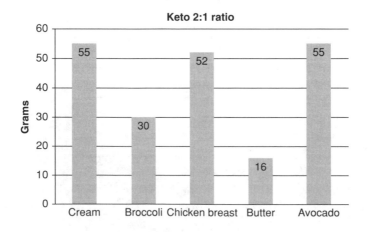

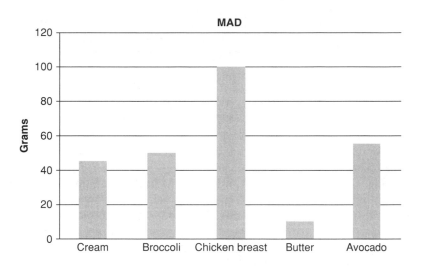

MAD

As you can see, the protein takes the lead in most MAD meals. Fats are still much higher than the average portion size, but the protein can glisten with fat instead of being saturated in it, as in a higher ketogenic ratio. While we used grams to help reference the difference between MAD and the other ketogenic ratios, it is important to remember that MAD is not weighed on the gram scale, nor are its measurements nearly this precise. There is a great deal of flexibility on MAD, allowing for a large variety of foods.

Additional Variations of the Ketogenic diet: LGIT and MCT

LGIT

The Low Glycemic Index Treatment diet (LGIT) is a relatively new diet that was created by Dr. Elizabeth Thiele and dietitian Heidi Pfeifer at Massachusetts General Hospital about ten years ago. While it is still considered a high fat diet, it allows for greater freedom with 40 to 60 grams of carbohydrates, using only carbohydrates that are low on the glycemic index (GI) (<50). The GI is a measure of the effect of carbohydrates on blood sugar levels. The lower the number, the less the carbohydrate will alter your blood sugar level. When you hear the term "sugar rush," that is often due to the rise of glucose in your bloodstream after consuming a sugar-rich food; foods that are high on the glycemic index raise the blood sugar levels in your body, and because all that goes up must come down, eventually the blood sugars will descend, causing the classic "crash" we've all felt hours after indulging in sweets. By choosing foods low on the glycemic index, the body doesn't have such dramatic ups and downs of glucose in the bloodstream. The steadying of glucose levels in the blood (and therefore the brain) has had a positive impact on seizure control, though the reason why isn't exactly known. The body does produce ketones but very small ones, and ketones aren't at all important to the maintenance of the LGIT diet, and therefore aren't checked.

The LGIT diet is monitored under the strict supervision of a dietitian and neurologist, just like the Ketogenic diet and MAD, and it is done as an outpatient, with no need for fasting. Like the Ketogenic diet, the calories are restricted and nutritional goals are set for carbohydrates, proteins, and fats. Because the amount of carbs is higher than MAD or the Ketogenic diet, there is more flexibility with LGIT. Foods such as low glycemic pasta or bread are actually possible on this diet; they just need to be balanced with a protein and fat.

There are two main challenges of this diet. First, it is not offered at many clinics around the United States, though it is gaining popularity in Europe. If you can't commute to the Massachusetts General Hospital, then you'll have to find a dietitian and neurologist willing to learn how to administer this diet and who can guide your family through the experience. Second, because there is currently very little published material about LGIT, it is harder to understand exactly how to create meals using the recommended portions since there are no hard and fast rules. And while this diet was designed to be less rigid than the Ketogenic diet, some parents consider it too difficult to follow long term. Parents who need a strong support system and who find creating meal plans intimidating might also consider the lack of resources and recipes to be another hindrance, though most lower ratio ketogenic or MAD recipes could be altered to allow for more carbohydrates, therefore becoming more LGIT friendly.

MCT

Dr. Peter Huttenlocher, who wanted to create a diet that would more closely resemble normal food, created the MCT ketogenic diet in the early 90s. Like the classic Ketogenic diet, the MCT diet still requires food to be weighed on a gram scale. Foods and fats are calculated based on percentages of daily calories. The classic Ketogenic diet has about 90% of its calories coming from fat, and as some of you might recall from a science class ages ago—or maybe not so long ago—a calorie is basically a measurement of energy.

The key ingredient of this diet is MCT oil. The body absorbs a medium chain fat or MCT much quicker than long chain fats such as butter. Because MCTs metabolize so quickly in the body, the body's ketogenic potential is increased, making the body more efficient in producing higher ketones with less overall fat. It's the basic "more bang for your buck" kind of theory: the MCT oil is so great at helping the body produce high ketones, less overall fat is needed.

The big perk to the introduction of MCT oil into the diet is the possibility for higher carbohydrate foods such as rice, pasta, and potatoes—major no-no's on both the classic Ketogenic diet and on MAD. The challenge then lies in calculating the diet and the calorie amount, and creating meals where the MCT oil can be cleverly incorporated. The MCT oil must be distributed throughout the day to fill the overall MCT daily goal, and it should be included in all meals and snacks.

> The MCT ketogenic diet is calculated based on energy. About 70% of total daily energy comes from fat, with the remaining energy (calories) coming from proteins and carbohydrates. Of that 70% of total fat, about 10% to 40% of it will come from long-chain fat and the rest of the fat will come from medium-chain fat (MCT oil).

The MCT diet is equally effective as the classic Ketogenic diet and seems to be more suited for people who require additional carbohydrates—teens, for example. Like the other diets, the total time on the diet averages two years.

Joaquin is at the age now where he is starting to go over to friend's houses and to birthday parties where of course, food is a big part. For example, if Joaquin is going to a birthday party where they are serving pizza, we will make him his own pizza to take with him so that he can eat the same as everyone. The MCT diet gives us the flexibility to do this. —Kendra

Emma Williams, the creator of Matthew's Friends in the UK, shares her experience using the MCT diet for her son Matthew:

My son Matthew had been on the classic Ketogenic diet for three years and had done very well on it. As he was growing older and reaching puberty, his carbohydrate level was going down to minuscule amounts because we needed to allow for his protein. If we dropped the ratio too low the ketones would go down. The only way to get adequate protein in, get a good level of carbohydrates and keep ketones at Matthew's optimum level was to switch

*him over to the MCT diet, which we did, when he was 11. He
responded very well. His ketones stabilized, control was regained
and Matthew thought his birthday had come early because all of
a sudden his tiny meals had turned into a lot larger ones than
those he had been having previously on the classical version.
Also, pasta, rice, and potatoes were back on his menu. Matthew
never really went above 50% of his energy coming from MCT oil,
which was really easy to lose in his food, and he was on about
60 grams of net carbohydrates a day. Matthew was on the MCT
ketogenic diet for nearly three years before I was brave enough to
wean him off diet therapy altogether. I am delighted to report that
even though Matthew is not on diet therapy, the benefits of six
years on the diets are still with us.* —Emma

Below is Stephanie's story of why she chose the MCT Diet for her son
Cobey:

*At the age of four, after a tonic clonic that left Cobey in a code
blue, epilepsy exploded into our lives. Over the next five years,
our family life changed dramatically and we became familiar
with the incredible team of doctors and supportive staff at the
Hospital for Sick Children in Toronto. I had never seen someone
have a seizure before, but have now seen more seizures than
I thought possible and more seizure types than I thought even
existed. Cobey was diagnosed with a severe seizure disorder,
then intractable epilepsy when medication proved unsuccessful.
When discussing the different types of ketogenic diets the MCT
oil ketogenic diet seemed to be best suited for Cobey. This diet
includes fruit and veggies and more food options than that of
the classic Ketogenic diet, which is more strict and limited
to higher amounts of butter and cream, also having a higher
risk of side effects such as kidney stones. Being seizure
free is something I had begun to doubt Cobey would ever
experience, but seizure freedom has been the biggest benefit from all the commitment and determination of sticking
with the MCT oil Ketogenic diet through the Hospital for Sick
Children.* —Stephanie

How We Picked Our Battle: First-Person Accounts from Parents

As we mentioned earlier, some parents' decisions to put their children on
MAD or the Ketogenic diet were determined by several complex decision
points and other decisions were easier, based upon the age or medical

needs of the child. In this section we have included several first-person stories detailing how families came to their personal decision to choose one diet therapy over another. Just as every child is unique, so are these stories.

My daughter Devyn has Angelman, which is a rare genetic disorder that is similar to having autism and epilepsy. Angels have profound developmental delays, significant motor issues (some never walking), often have little speech (seizures often wipe out the words they do have), and severe sleep disturbances are common. When Devyn's seizures became more and more frequent and the effects of the seizures became more devastating, I knew we had to do something different. I had heard of the Ketogenic diet during our visit to Cleveland Clinic and it sounded like it could be the magic bullet we were looking for, but it was so incredibly restrictive. I couldn't imagine how I could get her to eat such a delicate balance of this and that. Then I learned about MAD and I thought, "We can do this." Little by little we replaced things and when she had her last big cluster of seizures at the beginning of December, we knew it was time to go all the way. Luckily Devyn loves meat, always has, so she is enjoying eating large quantities of chicken and steak. —Heather P.

Heather chose MAD over the Ketogenic diet because she wanted to try a therapy that was less restrictive than the Ketogenic diet, as she knew feeding her daughter was likely to be a challenge because of her developmental delays. Heather carefully weighed her daughter's needs with her own concerns as the adult preparing the diet. MAD was the clear choice, and fortunately, a successful choice.

My son was ten when we started the Ketogenic diet, and we researched MAD first due to his age, thinking it may be easier for him to do. The closest dietitian who could work with us doing MAD was three hours away, and our local Keto dietitian is very experienced. In addition we would have had to change neurologists to do MAD, while our son's neuro is a firm believer in Keto and very experienced with administering it so we knew we would be in good hands. We also chose Keto because I needed the rules and guidelines to follow as a parent; it made me feel organized and disciplined and in "control" of a situation I had been stumbling through for two years. —Laura

For Laura, her decision to pursue the Ketogenic diet instead of MAD was due largely in part to the resources she had available. As we will discuss later in this chapter, traveling across the state or across state lines for dietary support can be a tremendous challenge for some parents. Having a convenient resource should be an important factor in choosing your therapy, especially since some Keto Clinics don't always provide support on MAD.

Our son was diagnosed with Doose Syndrome at age two and a half and after averaging approximately 40 seizures a day. We wanted to try the option with the greatest chance of immediate success. We figured it would be easier to start with a very strict Ketogenic diet with a 4:1 ratio and then ease off the diet if all went well. Our son was young enough that we were able to control everything he ate. He started preschool taking his own snack with him. He was on Keto for almost three years. My husband and I like the precise nature of the Keto diet at opposed to the looser MAD diet. From a scientific perspective it was much easier for us to figure out what foods and calorie levels worked for our son. He became seizure free within a month of starting Keto. He was weaned off all medications within another year and is currently seizure free, drug free, and diet free. —Lisa

The Ketogenic diet was the only thing offered after many meds failed Luke. I did not know about MAD until later. As we wean Keto now, I am happy to switch to MAD and I am very thankful that we did Keto first. I feel it disciplined me, since Keto is much more strict. —April

Our clinic gave us a choice: MAD or Keto. I knew we needed straightforward parameters on how to go forward with a diet so we chose the Ketogenic diet. We had a lot on our plate, and without definite guidelines we were afraid it wouldn't be successful. I just couldn't imagine Kay's dad counting carbs for her or keeping track of what she ate. It was easier for us to imagine knowing what and when she needed to eat. Voila! Two and a half years later, we are weaning the diet. I don't know if it was the "right" choice, but it was successful for her. —Randlyn

As the previous three stories from Lisa, April, and Randlyn show, the scientific nature of the precise Ketogenic diet actually gives frightened and overwhelmed parents a chance to do something "by the book." Each of these mothers didn't think the freedom of MAD would work for their family at the time that they began their journeys. However, this intense requirement to follow the rules and to live by numbers and calculations can prove to increase some parents' anxiety instead of alleviate it, and those parents will likely choose MAD over the Ketogenic diet.

If you aren't sure which diet to choose, remember that there is no one-size-fits-all right-or-wrong answer to the question. It depends wholly on what drives you, what services you have available, and a good understanding of your own limitations and challenges. Weigh your options, trust your gut, and make the choice that feels right for you.

Preparing for Battle

Once you've cast your lot in the diet therapy camp, you'll need to start preparation, and not surprisingly, much of the initial battle prep is mental rather than physical. We explore this more fully in Chapter 2, "Boot Camp," but it is important to know from the start that your attitude will largely influence whether you succeed or fail. It's normal to be nervous, but if you honestly dread starting the diet and view it more as a punishment rather than an opportunity, you're going to find the going very tough. If you agonize that your poor child, already suffering from seizures, is now going to have to "suffer" on this diet, take note of what one parent had to say:

> *Most important: do not feel bad for your child because they cannot have certain foods. There are plenty of delicious recipes and sweets your child can have. You are not taking food away from them. You are giving them their life back.* —Teri

Weighing up the option of being able to freely eat mashed potatoes against possibly becoming seizure-free may seem like an easy choice, yet we can still be haunted by the fear that ultimately a ketogenic diet—whether it is the Ketogenic diet, MAD, or another diet—will prove to be too hard. What will get you through the rough patches is conditioning your mind for success. Remember the title of this book, *Fighting Back with Fat?* Surprise! You're under attack and you've joined the army! Pull out some mental weapons to defend yourself. Work at cultivating a positive mental attitude and an I-can-do-this style of resilience. Read this book from cover-to-cover and study what people who once felt exactly as you feel now have gone on to accomplish. Realize that though many of the battles in this war are going to take place between your two ears, you don't have to go it alone. Learning from the experiences of others will help you manage the skirmishes you face with the enemy.

Managing Expectations

History tells us that during the American Civil War large numbers of soldiers enlisted on both sides of the conflict, fully expecting the war to be over in a very short time, perhaps after only one brief battle. Such unrealistic expectations greatly contributed to morale problems that plagued troops as the fighting dragged out. If you don't want to make the same mistake in your dietary war against seizures, give yourself a reality check about how long all this might take, and just what the outcome might be. Whether you find yourself here after several years and several failed medications or whether you are new to battling seizures, most people hope to soon be watching epilepsy wave its little white flag. Remember, however, that while total seizure freedom is a very valid wish, it isn't always a realistic goal. We don't write this to discourage you or frighten you. This diet can be a miracle, as evidenced by each of the author's sons, but it's good to clearly understand that not all children are super responders, and total seizure freedom might remain elusive.

We all have different goals and reasons for attempting diet therapy, and those are what determine how satisfied we are with the outcome. What might be wonderful news for one parent may prove to be a bitter disappointment for another. Find out what your personal deal breakers are before you even start, and it will help you determine if diet therapy is right for you or not.

> *After starting my son on diet therapy, a mother who heard about what we were doing excitedly approached to ask if MAD might be a possibility for her son. She had learned that my child's seizures stopped soon after starting the diet and she carefully asked question after question about seizure freedom, how long it would take to attain it, and how long we expected it to last. I explained to her that research shows 50% of people see a 50% improvement in seizures when doing diet therapy. Her face fell. Her son was on medication and about once every month or two he had a brief seizure in his sleep. In her mind, nothing short of guaranteed seizure freedom was acceptable. She decided the diet was not for her because without the promise of seizure freedom, it just wasn't worth the trouble.* —Jeanne Riether

If you set an inflexible goal of complete seizure freedom and a completely normal childhood for your child, you may be setting yourself up for heartache and disappointment. However, if you clearly understand that there are other important gains that this diet can accomplish, when diet therapy doesn't end up being all sunshine and buttercups—it isn't—you will not be crushed by the weight of your initial expectations.

Let's face it, if your child has refractory seizures you are likely already accustomed to being disappointed. You've tried drug after drug. You've watched your child go through EEGs, MRIs, and you've likely seen more than one neurologist, desperately seeking answers. Rather than trying to protect yourself from further disappointment by grimly expecting that diet therapy "probably won't work either," instead we suggest you make a wish list. Approach it from a positive angle. Even if seizure freedom might not be attainable for everyone, what else would be worthwhile to gain from this? Write down your expectations while looking through a positive lens rather than the perspective that comes from never-ending disappointment. This journey will definitely be a challenge, but there are hundreds of potential rewards to be earned along the way, from breakthroughs in cognition that result in a tiny new smile on your baby's face, to watching your child run for the first time, to being able to reduce or even eliminate medication. Believing that something great is always about to happen will keep hope alive, and help you remember that "something great" can sometimes be something small. Keep your eyes open for the little miracles. They can add up to a wonderfully changed life.

> *My son Landon had been seizure free for nine months, but the night before his fifth birthday, he experienced his first break-through myoclonic seizure. For the first time Landon verbalized that the seizure scared him, and that was hard to stomach. Yet it was a moment that made me realize how far he has come cognitively. I think about the gains that the diet has given us and I refuse to give up hope. I will take the cognitive, verbal, and physical gains and rest in the fact that Landon has come so far.* —Sam

Even if you occasionally lose a few skirmishes, it is still very possible that you are winning the war. Understanding that there are goals to be reached other than total seizure freedom will buoy your spirits when you encounter setbacks and aid you in accessing your progress along the way. Below is a list of ideas to help you create your own wish list, the expectations of what you hope you or your child and your family might gain from diet therapy.

Determining Realistic Expectations

■ **Seizure improvement:** Instead of looking for seizure freedom, adjust your mindset to seek seizure improvement. About 50% of children will have a 50% or greater reduction in seizures. This is a fantastic number for a group of children who are already among a small percentage of people with intractable epilepsy. Many children and adults also comment that the duration and strength of their seizures lessen on these diets, and the recovery time can also be decreased. By choosing to hope for seizure improvement instead of total freedom, you will give yourself the mental momentum necessary to stay on the road of diet therapy even if seizures still persist several months in.

- **Improvement in cognition:** Our children are often fogged over with drugs, especially when they are on more than one medication. This can result in excessive sleepiness, slower thinking and decreased cognition. Children on these diets often have a new surge of mental energy and brightness on a ketogenic diet. Should you be able to wean some of the medications, the mental alertness only improves further—that is, if a decrease in medication doesn't increase the seizures.

- **Reducing medication:** While many are able to eliminate meds, it is wise to remember that the point of diet therapy is to achieve better seizure control; many times this is attained in partnership with medication. There may be a period of adjustment working out which type of medication works best in combination with the diet, and there may be tweaking of dosages. If you can achieve good seizure control, with or without medication, you can consider it a glorious battle won.

- **Increased energy:** Just as medications and seizures can affect cognition, they can also deplete energy. After the body's initial adjustment to changing from a glucose metabolism to burning ketones, and the first few days of lethargy that usually accompany it, many parents comment on the increase in energy their child experiences. Can your child now make it through an afternoon play date with ease, when before he just didn't have the strength to keep up with his peers?

- **Improved quality of life:** This is a broad category that can lend itself to anyone's personal experience. Maybe your child has been missing out on school activities because of her seizures. Is the diet helping make that goal possible? If your child has developmental delays, is diet therapy making it possible for him to reach the next milestone? You, as a parent, are in the position to observe and assess how the diet is impacting your child's quality of life in ways other people cannot. Acknowledge each small improvement, as they can collectively add up to big victories that make life better.

- **A happier kid:** Your child might end up complaining about the amount of heavy whipping cream he has to drink, but take a step back and look at your child's overall emotional state. How is his own unique "happiness meter" reading since starting diet therapy? If your warrior has learned to smile and laugh through the hours that might have previously been riddled with seizures, you have already won a momentous battle.

A Challenging Experience That's Worth the Work

As far as expectations go, we'd be remiss if we didn't prepare you for an experience that will be altogether challenging as well as rewarding. You should *expect* to be challenged. You should *expect* trials. But you should also expect rewards, and should *any* of the above expectations of improvement come your way, you've most likely already figured out that they're worth every bit of trouble to get there.

Remember, however, that seizure improvement is not the same thing as Nirvana. If your child is fortunate enough to be a super responder, congratulations, you are extremely lucky. If your child has shown measurable improvement in seizure control, you're also most likely happy and excited. While you've gained valuable territory in this war, don't be surprised to find that simply holding your position after gaining control can also bring its fair share of stress and challenges. Life suddenly won't be transformed into a utopian paradise just because the seizures are gone. Worry about seizures returning, battles about food, shopping, cooking, making sure your child complies with the diet, and just coping with the mechanics of living are things that each of us has to deal with whether we get full control or not.

While hitting the seizure control jackpot may not solve all of life's problems, it's still a reason to celebrate. And if you are still waiting for your winning number to turn up, find reasons to celebrate along the way. Take positive steps to cope with the stress in your life and count your blessings. A life with epilepsy is not perfect, just as a life without epilepsy is not perfect, yet life is still a perfectly wonderful gift.

Endurance Training

If you're like most people, as soon as you start this diet you'll find yourself wrapped in suspense, trying to figure out how it's all going to turn out—for you or your child. From day one you'll likely be watching your child like a hawk, analyzing every small movement, making note of everything from how sleepy he is to how much he eats, what his energy level is, and of course how many seizures you observe. Was that a twitch or a seizure? Counting it would at least give you something to record that might someday disappear...

Welcome to the waiting game. Your anxiety will rise and your excitement may get the better of you, even when you are bracing yourself for possibly seeing no change at all. Ultimately, no matter how realistic and steadfast you are in your very grounded expectations, you're going to be eyeing your kid and hoping he'll become a super responder. We wouldn't be human if we didn't want our child to be within that elusive 10% to 15% of children who go seizure-free quickly. But at the same time, we have to try and reign in our anxiety and report back to that common-sense list of expectations we created before starting the diet.

It can be as little as a week, but usually around two to four weeks along, parents generally begin actually voicing the big question: is the diet working? Maybe the seizures have even increased in the beginning, which can be frustratingly common. The brain can do strange things sometimes, and may try to get away with something comparable to a last ditch toddler-style hissy fit of renewed seizure activity before settling down and complying with this new seizure control program. Maybe you're experiencing some of the side effects that are common with the diet (discussed in depth in Chapter 5). Or maybe your child found immediate relief on the diet, but then all of a sudden the seizures returned. When that happens, the bewildered parents usually frantically search their food records and consciences, wondering what in the world they changed or did wrong. A couple bad days like that can drive you up the wall, desperate for reassurance that sometimes, in the course of seizure activity, hiccups just happen.

But the question on everybody's mind, regardless of their experience and the things they observe, is always the same: Is the diet working? Don't be discouraged if the road is bumpy. It doesn't necessarily mean the diet *isn't* working. Take it step-by-step and be prepared that it might take a while to get the results you want.

> *One of the things I wish people knew about the diet is that if it doesn't work right off the bat it doesn't mean it won't! We've had very slow progress but it was worth the wait overall. I also wish someone had told me more honestly how hard it was— so that when I came home and it felt impossible, I didn't feel like a failure, but rather like I was just doing something really hard.* —Keto mom

Waiting can be hard on everybody. This diet is not usually an overnight wonder. It probably took time for your child's occasional seizure to turn into epilepsy, and it probably will take time for the diet to do its healing work. The diet may be working behind the scenes in ways you can't observe, so stop tugging its elbow and give it time to work.

Once you're a month or so in you can refer back to the list you created not so long ago. What are your goals and expectations? If you aren't seeing seizure improvement, have you noticed other changes? Has your child improved cognitively or does he have more energy? Wait and watch for the smaller changes that can get easily lost in the shuffle. You might be surprised to see that, yes, the diet is working, just perhaps on a smaller scale than you had originally hoped.

For many families however, when the "big question" comes around, it's usually the beginning of the sleuthing and tweaking phase, which we discuss in Chapter 5, "In the Trenches." Discovering children's sensitivities and potential seizure triggers, or fine-tuning the calories and ratios of the Ketogenic diet are all part of a lengthy process that, for many people, make the difference between a lack of seizure control and seizure freedom. For some, the results are seen quickly; for others it's a journey that can vary anywhere from weeks to months, and even years. Sometimes the search for a solution is exhausting and all consuming, while at other times it can be as simple as making a switch in a particular food that is causing your child trouble. Below is a story that shows how seizure freedom can sometimes come late in the game, so late in fact that other people might have already given up. This family decided to persevere, and they gave their child the greatest gift she could ever hope for: seizure freedom.

Our daughter was diagnosed with generalized epilepsy before she was four years old, and a sleep study determined she'd been having hundreds of petite mal seizures a day in addition to the occasional grand mal. Eventually she was having myoclonic jerks that coincided with the petite mals. No medication helped. At about age eight and after trying almost all the meds, we were able to get into Dr. Kossoff's Modified Atkins Diet study at Johns Hopkins. We could choose to start at ten or twenty net carbs, and we chose ten. When we began, we were given the Atkins book to read; it was so overwhelming and scary for me, but my husband was determined this would work. She went into deep ketosis right away, and we even saw improvement, but it was followed by seizures again. We started to see partial seizures, then one day three grand mals.

We didn't know what to do. I think we expected the diet to work right away. As Dr. Kossoff told us, you can expect bumps along the road, so we kept on it. When she had a setback we would try to see what she had eaten. At almost a year's time of being on the diet the store ran out of the one thing she was eating since the start of the diet: the Atkins bread that we sliced and served with peanut butter. After about two weeks we noticed we weren't seeing any seizures. When the store got the bread back we didn't buy it. Coincidence or not, I really can't say. That was the start of her seizure freedom. With the exception of a grand mal a couple of months later that was short and stress related, our daughter has been seizure free for about six and a half years now. We are so thankful and we don't take a day for granted. The healing power of food is amazing. —Teri

Teri's story reminds us that it's our ability to keep trudging forward in spite of the challenges that has the potential to give us the greatest rewards. On days when your feet feel heavy and you're so tired you can hardly take another step, keep on believing that something wonderful is about to happen. For so many of us, it already has.

Choosing Your Keto Clinic

After deciding to pursue diet therapy as a treatment for your child, and after you've re-trained yourself to appreciate the glories of oils and mayonnaise—while fearing, perhaps for the first time, the menace of high carbohydrates—you are ready for your next assignment: finding the best medical team to guide you through this journey. While MAD, LGIT, and the MCT diet aren't always initiated in a hospital like the Ketogenic diet, they do require a Keto Clinic and its dietary experts. Just as the decision to pursue dietary therapy was intensely personal, so is choosing the right Keto Clinic. For most, the decision often comes down to geography, picking the clinic that is the most convenient. This is not only logical, but a decision that *might* make the next couple years of your life a little easier. Continue reading to see why we emphasize "might."

When initiating the Ketogenic diet, most clinics require a three to four day hospital stay in order for the child to be closely monitored while fasting, becoming ketotic, and beginning the early stages of eating ketogenic food. During this time parents also learn how the diet works, how to calculate the diet, and how to best care for their child during this new endeavor. Being close to home is not only more cost effective, as you will not have to pay for airfare, cab fare, hotels, and the other expenses accrued when traveling for several days, but it will ultimately save you time and energy. In the two or more years that your child will be on the diet, he will have checkups every three months in the beginning, and then every six months. Choosing a Keto Clinic across the country or even across the state will prove to be costly, and sometimes quite stressful.

However, as parents of a child with epilepsy you've likely given up on the idea of ease and convenience in your life, so it shouldn't be a surprise that convenience won't necessarily be the deciding factor when choosing a Keto Clinic. Each clinic has its own specialties, flaws, and nuances. For instance, some Keto Clinics allow parents to use the KetoCalculator, the online program that allows easy calculation of meals to the perfect ratio, while others do not. If you are a parent who is excited to experiment with recipes for your child, you will run into unending frustration if you don't have control over your child's meals, which the KetoCalculator can easily give you.

There is no "right" Keto Clinic just as there is no "right" answer when deciding whether to do Keto or MAD, but there are several topics you should consider when making this decision. Both writers of this book have had tremendously different experiences in beginning these diets, but what we have in common is a desire to help our readers learn from our own experiences as well as the many friends and acquaintances traveling these rocky roads with us. Besides the advice we will give you here, it is essential to do your homework: scour the Internet, check out books from the library, seek out others who have tried diet therapy and pummel them with questions. You will not regret it in the end.

Decision Factors

Below is a bulleted list of some of the topics to consider when looking into different Keto Clinics that apply to those starting the Ketogenic diet, MAD, the LGIT diet, or the MCT diet.

- **Proximity to your home:** Traveling for medical attention can be extremely costly. When looking into clinics out of state, remember that you will not only have to pay for airfare, hotels, and food, but you will have to arrange for childcare for your other children in your absence. If your child has a waiver through Medicaid, remember that Medicaid is not always accepted across state lines, which could increase your out-of-pocket expenses.

- **Insurance:** Make certain that the Keto Clinics you are considering accept your insurance. The initiation cost without insurance could be monumental; couple that expense with the fees for lab work and check-ups and you're dealing with another costly sum. It can be a hard call for any parent, but financial realities have to be factored into the equation.

- **Ketogenic diet, MAD, LGIT, or MCT diet?:** The diet you choose to pursue can also impact your decision towards a Keto Clinic. Some clinics—though this is becoming increasingly rare—only offer the Ketogenic diet, while others have numerous clients on both the Ketogenic and MAD. Also consider that your child might switch from one diet to the next over the course of several years. Some children begin on MAD and switch to Keto, while other children find more success on MAD after switching from Keto. Ideally, you want to find a clinic that is well versed in both therapies, with a nutritionist who can monitor either diet. Your choices of Keto Clinics dwindle considerably when you choose to do LGIT or the MCT diet. However, if these are diets you would like to pursue, talk to your local Keto Clinic about their willingness to learn about these diets and assist you in implementing them.

- **The Keto Team:** Most Keto Teams consist of at least a neurologist and a dietitian. Others have nurses and social workers as well. How does the Keto Team interact with one another, and how will your challenges as a parent be addressed? The manner in which they communicate can be essential to the success of your child's diet, and ultimately to your sanity. Some Keto Teams won't allow your current neurologist to continue managing your child's care, and for some parents that will be a deal breaker, while other parents are relieved to have fewer cooks in the Keto kitchen.

■ **Ease of communication:** When looking into Keto Clinics, there's a pretty simple way to determine how you will likely be treated as a patient: try to get in touch with them and then gauge how long it takes someone to answer the phone, how long it takes an individual to call you back, or how courteous the staff is when you call. If they consistently score high on all these points, they will likely also score high in availability when your child is a patient in their care. It is essential, especially in the early days of these diets, that you have easy access to nurses, the dietitian and the neurologist. You may encounter situations that require urgent attention, such as when you are weaning drugs, when your child is sick and vomiting all his meals, or when your child has a new seizure type, and you will need access to your team. Granted, many Keto Clinics are busy and possibly overloaded with patients, but you don't want to feel that your child is just another e-mail or phone call that will go unanswered.

Note: You'll notice we talk a lot about peace of mind and sanity in this book. Now that you're embarking on this journey, learning to find peace in your decisions is an important strategy that will help you survive and thrive when the going gets rough. Listen to your gut and don't get pressured into doing anything you don't want to do. Consider your decisions slowly and carefully. Though it may seem counterintuitive, you'll get where you really want to go on this journey more quickly if you don't rush.

A Professional's Perspective

Claire Chee is a bit of a living legend in the world of families and diet therapy. She is a nurse specialist at CHOP (Children's Hospital of Philadelphia). Claire's work is so highly regarded among the neurological community that in 2006 the Association of Child Neurology Nurses renamed its annual service award to the "Claire Chee Award for Excellence." Claire tells us,

> I have a passion for dietary treatment of epilepsy. I have witnessed so many miracles over the years and I continue to do so. The diet is not a lifetime treatment, but may give lifetime benefit. A positive attitude is most important when dealing with dietary treatment. Over the years, I have helped families deal with an array of dietary treatments; dietary treatment of epilepsy certainly is the most demanding of all. Not only family and friends need to be supportive, the professional world does as well. The "professional team" implementing the diet needs to be readily available for questions/concerns/support. Again, I put "professional team" in quotes, as soon, the expert is the family. I often call us the "hospital based team."

Switching Keto Clinics

One of the last things you want to discover, months into the diet, is that you're facing the need to switch teams because your Keto Clinic doesn't prioritize its care in the way you had hoped. By that we mean: is your Keto Team unwilling to tweak your child's diet, despite hundreds of stories to the success of tweaking? Have you learned that your neurologist is more content to increase anticonvulsants than to alter the ratio? Are you stuck waiting behind your computer for an e-mail on how to address the tonic clonic—a new seizure type—that your daughter had in school this morning? While every parent will likely become frustrated with their Keto Clinic and Keto Team at some point (it is a deeply personal relationship with incredibly high stakes so emotions can run high), determining whether or not to switch Keto Clinics is a big decision. We advocate that you learn what you're signing on for before picking your team, but if you're already in and you find out down the road that something is fundamentally wrong with your child's care, by all means, get out. Below is a story of Lynette's experience with her Keto Clinic and why she ultimately packed her bags and found someplace new:

We live in Omaha, NE and when Zach, then three, had his first TC in November 2009, we were told it was fairly common and chances are it wouldn't happen again. Then two days after Christmas, he had two more. After an MRI and EEG both came back normal, Zach was prescribed Trileptal. Overall, things were calm until March and that's when we started noticing the jerks and drops. They progressed to 100's a day, his speech took a hit, and there was little he could do but watch TV. Even after two more EEGs, and me videotaping my son, I wasn't getting any solid answers. They tried different meds and that seemed to make him worse. At one point, we were giving him Diastat daily. The child I knew was slipping away and no one could tell me why.

I couldn't accept that no one could tell me why or what was happening to my son. I made an appointment in July of 2010, and the neurologist was able to give Zach his Doose diagnosis, and we began the blood work for the Ketogenic diet. While waiting, I asked about alternative treatments, such as steroids, but the epileptologist said they were not used for Doose, so we continued to adjust meds, but nothing was working. Zach started the Ketogenic diet in October 2010. At our four month check, they deemed the diet was not working, and told us it wasn't healthy for Zach to stay on the diet. While Zach's seizures had not consistently decreased, in my journals I had documented how much his personality had come back and his speech was clearing up. I was not about to give up. I begged the doctor to let us continue. She gave us three months.

At the suggestion of many Doose parents, I begged the dietitian to adjust calories, ratios, etc., but she refused, citing all his blood work indicated things were fine. In March 2010, Zach had one allergy test come back that he was severely allergic to dairy and mildly allergic to eggs and soy. After speaking with Beth from the Charlie foundation about how hard this was going to be, she suggested we go to 2:1 (we were currently at 4:1 where we started) and add MCT oil. Our dietitian did not agree, so this did not happen. I knew if we went back to Zach's current Keto Clinic that they would wean Zach off the diet. I just wasn't ready to give up.

Again, we turned to the Doose board and found many people having success with another team a couple states away. In June of 2011, we met the treating neurologist at that center, and she gave us so much hope. She wanted us to continue with the diet. She said he was overmedicated. There was also a dietitian who believed in tweaking the diet! We tweaked all we could with some decrease in seizures, but nothing that would stick. We switched meds and had the same pattern. It was then that his new neurologist suggested steroids. That has been the best decision we've ever made. Zach is still not 100% seizure free, but we are getting there.

The biggest obstacle (outside of fighting physically, mentally and verbally for your child) is the financial burden. It is SO expensive to travel for his care. The Keto meal preps, the hotel and gas bills, and the out-of-network expenses I pay just to see his doctor are huge. We will be in debt for a while. However, all these monetary things are nothing compared to having my boy back, hearing his funny jokes, watching him run and play. Priceless. —Lynette

Lynette and Zach's experience really drives home the necessity of researching all the Keto Clinics you are considering for your child. Had Lynette known ahead of time that her previous Keto Team wasn't willing to tweak the diet, she might have chosen a different clinic. It's important to be up-front with your Keto Team and talk about your expectations—and theirs. Will they suggest your child quit the diet if, after four months, he hasn't improved as significantly as they expect? In the *Ketogenic Diets* (5th edition) by Dr. Eric Kossoff, et al., they are very specific about the importance of both the parent and the Keto Team outlining clear goals before beginning.

Lynette is also very clear about wishing she had joined the Doose online forum earlier. Forums provide valuable networking resources. Had

Charitable Assistance for Medical Transport and Accommodations

If you are in a situation like Lynette describes above, and carrying a heavy financial burden from traveling to receive care at a distant Ketogenic Clinic, you may want to investigate whether or not you are eligible for free or discounted programs that will help cover costs.

Travel for Treatment: For information about free or low-cost medical transport for children, a good place to look is on the **Bridges4Kids** website that has contact information for various programs: www.bridges4kids.org/Disabilities/Transport.html

Accommodations Near Hospitals: Ronald McDonald House Charities have a wonderful program that offers accommodations, meals, and services in family-friendly facilities located near major hospitals to assist eligible families of children who must travel to receive hospital treatment. Many of their houses accommodate families of those receiving both in-patient and out-patient care. Families either stay at no cost or are asked for make a donation of up to $25 per day per family, depending on the house. However, no one is turned away, and if it's not possible to pay, the fee is waived. For information on Ronald McDonald Houses in 57 countries around the world, visit their site at: http://rmhc.org/

it not been for her membership in the forum, she never would have known about thew other more suitable Keto Clinic several states away. Research options and educate yourself! Doing so may make all the difference in your child's treatment.

While you may need to make a change if you are genuinely concerned about your child's care, keep in mind that switching Keto Clinics is not always easy. For various reasons, not all clinics accept patients that have been initiated elsewhere, and the process of obtaining and transferring medical records can be time consuming and sometimes costly. One way to possibly circumvent this is to seek a second opinion at the new clinic you want to try. When Lynette initially wanted to switch Keto Clinics, she found the obstacles to be too overwhelming. Instead, she found that arranging to get a second opinion in the new clinic was enough to get her in the door, and she had an opportunity to present her case to a doctor there.

Solo Mission—Doing MAD with Limited Support Resources

While Lynette had a trying time with her first Keto Clinic, and her son Zach likely suffered to some extent because of it, she was fortunate to find another clinic that provided exactly the kind of care that Zach needed. However, not everyone who endeavors to take on diet therapy has access to a Keto Clinic. This is mostly true of people in countries where dietary therapy is still very much in its infancy. Jeanne Riether, the co-author of this book, had to tackle the task of educating herself, and persevere despite numerous obstacles, before her son found his miraculous answer through diet therapy. Below is her story of initiating the MAD across a vast ocean, far from any support team.

Jeanne's MAD Solo Journey in China

I am an American living in China, and we did not have the benefit of working with a ketogenic diet center when my 12-year-old son Jordan started the Modified Atkins Diet in 2009. Though MAD was virtually unknown in mainland China at the time, the Internet bridged the gap for us. Thankfully our MAD journey proved to be a successful one, but going it solo was not an easy experience and the learning curve was definitely steep when we started.

I first discovered MAD on a late night internet foray, searching for answers for my son. I was comparing treatment options in China with those at Johns Hopkins, when I did a double take. Dietary therapy to treat seizures? Nobody had mentioned anything like that at the hospital here! I read into the wee hours of the morning until my eyes blurred about the latest research and clinical trials being conducted on kids using MAD to treat difficult seizures.

Oddly, our discovery of MAD occurred almost simultaneously with a sudden drastic change in Jordan's seizure pattern. His adolescent hormones were bursting into bloom and without warning he experienced a frightening series of tonic clonics (grand mals) involving hallucinations, as well as the routine atonic drops that had been sending him crashing to the floor over the preceding months. In the emergency room I talked to the neurologist about what I'd just read about the Modified Atkins Diet and whether it would be a worthwhile therapy to consider. His reaction was anything but supportive; he smiled, gave a patronizing shake of his head, and explained that diet therapy was "difficult, unreliable, and old-fashioned" and that "no modern neurologist would advise it."

Finding yourself stranded in what I call the "desert of misinformation" is a frightening place to be when your child is

*seriously ill. You long for straight talk and clear facts, yet are
so caught up in the pathos of your child's illness that you can
barely sort fact from fiction. Realizing, however, that what we
were hearing from this physician did not jibe with what we'd
read from Johns Hopkins, we gathered our things and left. The
ensuing game of hide and seek, searching for a neurologist
familiar with MAD in our area, was a brief but nerve wracking
time. Armed with print-outs from the Johns Hopkins site and
the clinical study results I downloaded, I made the rounds to
various hospitals. No doctor we talked with had any experience
with dietary therapy, however they were universally in agreement that we shouldn't try it.*

*Finally, I found an angel of a doctor who, though reluctant,
consented to supervise us in our attempt to try MAD. She made
it clear, however, that the ball was in our court to research the
how-to; her role was to be our safety net in case we encountered a medical emergency. We were on our own, but at least
we had back-up. My resources when starting MAD were limited
but I pieced together all the information I could find and had
a somewhat sketchy idea of how to proceed. I followed the diet
protocol from a published Korean clinical trial of MAD from
2006, starting at 10 grams of net carbohydrates per day and
liberally using butter, oils, and fats. However, at the time, I
didn't yet know what a "net carbohydrate" was or how to calculate it. I looked up various carbohydrate values of foods online
and mapped out a simple, though admittedly Spartan, menu.
I found out later my menus were a bit lower in carbs than
necessary, so I readjusted things once I learned how to subtract
grams of fiber from grams of carbohydrates, to calculate net
carb values. Because everything was new and unfamiliar our
initial meals were plain and seemed to take me forever to prepare, but I was determined to give it my best shot.*

*Even harder than the diet itself, however, was the stress, uncer-
tainly and constant second guessing that comes with going it
alone. I believe working with a team greatly alleviates this type
of pressure. At times my hands literally shook as I measured
out my son's food, as I feared I would make a mistake that
might make things worse.*

*Despite our less-than-flawless entry into the MAD world, the
diet proved to be a miracle for our family. To our amazement,
Jordan turned out to be in the lucky percentage of children
on the diet who are regarded as "super responders," those*

who show immediate marked improvement and gain rapid seizure freedom within days. Almost from the moment he started ingesting high fat, low-carb food, I could see a change in him. He became calmer and his seizures grew shorter and less frequent. After three days passed, to our astonishment, his seizures simply melted away.

Yet, despite such dramatic success, I couldn't shake the feeling that I was in over my head. I worried that it was all going to unravel if I slipped up, or what might happen if we encountered an unexpected complication. I contacted Dr. Eric Kossoff at Johns Hopkins Hospital when we were about a month into the diet, describing our experience and pleading for advice. Considering the unique circumstances and the lack of ketogenic resources in China, Dr. Kossoff graciously agreed to work with us from a distance, providing we continue with the oversight of a local neurologist or pediatrician to monitor my son.

Dr. Kossoff sent me the material used at Johns Hopkins to initiate patients on MAD including a few sample menus, suggested blood lab work, advice on how to calculate net carbs, and tips on reading product labels to look for hidden carbs. Apparently we were already doing it right, but it was an enormous relief just to hear him say so. As I began to feel more comfortable with the diet and trusted that our miracle wasn't about to fall apart at the seams, I started experimenting with recipes, searching online low-carb diet forums for dishes that I could adapt to MAD. I also joined an online Yahoo support group for parents of children on MAD, and I found it to be a haven of warmth and encouragement. Having contact with other parents online helped me feel I wasn't alone, and proved to be a place where I could get advice and talk about shared experiences.

After two years of seizure freedom and a clear 24-hour EEG, in September 2011 Dr. Kossoff gave us the go-ahead to attempt a diet wean, a process that took almost two months. Our last MAD meal was the day before Thanksgiving that year, and Jordan has remained seizure free ever since. He eats what he wants with the exception of avoiding highly refined, concentrated sugars (we decided to wait at least a year before trying them) and thankfully he is happy, healthy, and living an active normal life.

The bottom line is, it may be rough, but doing MAD solo can be done. If you can get the assistance of a qualified ketogenic support team, by all means use it. If not, with the supervision of your local neurologist, you can use the Internet, relevant books, and online support groups to widen your knowledge base in order to make MAD work.

Hearing about the necessity of going it alone in China, you might wonder if something similar could ever happen in the United States? There are now numerous Keto Clinics in many cities throughout the country, and if you are willing to travel you can find the help you need from a specialized team. Many neurologists who do not work with Keto Clinics are also very supportive of the diet, and encourage their patients to try out MAD after reading about its success in published clinical studies. But just because your doctor may be supportive, doesn't necessarily mean he knows all that much about it. Unless you travel, you may find yourself in the position of having to learn how to do the diet along with your doctor or dietitian. Pam, like Jeanne, shares a similar story about attempting MAD without a Keto Team in the United States, while under her local doctor's care.

Pam's MAD Solo Journey in the US

Desperation and frustration would be the two best words to describe how we ended up putting our son on MAD. Our son also has autism, so looking at unconventional treatments was not new to us. We have always been cautious, never buying into any potentially harmful treatments for his autism. For his seizures though, we had always been "by the book": medication after medication, VNS, possible brain surgery—you name it—our neurologist offered it, and we tried it. Our son still lived with daily, multiple seizures and the side effects of numerous medications.

Our neurologist pointed me in the direction of MAD, giving me a website to begin my research. It sounded promising, so I made the call to the neurologist, expecting her to lead the way. Since we travel four hours to see her, she suggested we contact a local dietitian to get started. That is where our MAD journey began and most medical/professional help ended. Knowing that our community would most likely not have a nutritionist (or anyone, for that matter) familiar with MAD, I spent hours and

*hours reading anything I could get my hands on, enlisting the
help of the local epilepsy support group as well as our primary
care physician. After spending an hour educating the dietitian
who knew about the Ketogenic diet (translation—she had read
about it), I knew we were on our own.*

*I spent two months reading whatever I could get my hands on,
specifically focusing on Dr. Atkins, book and the fifth edition of*
Ketogenic Diets. *Hands down the best thing I did was to join
the Yahoo! support group where I am sure I drove everyone nuts
with my constant questions—ha!*

*We still needed the baseline labs to be done first. The neurolo-
gist said the dietitian could handle that. The dietitian said
the primary care physician would order it. The primary care
physician thankfully said to just give him a list. I actually
just copied the pages out of the* Ketogenic Diets *book and away
we went. The primary care physician was not comfortable
interpreting the results so we were responsible for faxing the
results to the neurologist and following up with a phone call
(or two or three!).*

*We finally started the diet and quickly learned that actually
implementing the diet was the easy part! And when we saw our
son improve before our eyes, it was so easy to handle any more
bumps in the road. He is not seizure free, but he is enjoying
life again. The frequency, intensity, and length of his seizures
have all decreased drastically and the quality of his life has
improved by leaps and bounds.* —Pam

Obviously both Pam and Jeanne would have benefited from a professional Keto Team if they had access to one. However, if professional help
is limited or non-existent and you are forced to go it alone on MAD, at the
very least, you will need to have:

■ **Proper medical supervision, including a neurologist who is aware
   that you will start MAD and is willing to provide you with medical assistance:** While you might not have a neurologist who is familiar enough with MAD to guide you, you should still be under his care.
   You should be provided with baseline blood work that includes a full
   metabolic profile, and follow up blood work every few months to monitor cholesterol, blood fats, and liver function. There are definitely cases
   when MAD therapy is not recommended, such as when a child's liver

cannot handle a high fat diet, or in certain types of metabolic syndromes. For that reason, the diet should not be attempted without a doctor's guidance. Failing to have the support of a medical team, whether or not that team is officially part of a Keto Clinic, can result in extreme dangers for you or your child.

■ **A good working knowledge of how MAD works, what you can eat or not eat, and how to cook and shop for the diet:** Be aware that the learning curve is steep when you begin, but it can be done. Besides this book, we strongly recommend reading *Ketogenic Diets* (5th edition) by Dr. Eric Kossoff, et al. If possible, get your neurologist or dietitian to read it also, so you are all on the same page.

■ **Your child's willing participation, or consistent supervision of your child in order to monitor all food intake:** Children with poor impulse control, who are not cooperative or who cannot be under a parent or caregiver's close supervision, would not be good candidates for MAD. If you are not emotionally prepared to become the "food police" in your child's life, it might be a diet deal breaker.

After finishing this chapter, you may feel a bit overwhelmed by all the decisions that are now before you. Our advice is to take things one step at a time, do your research, and learn all you can until you've mapped out a plan that feels right for you. As we said before, many of the challenges you will face are going to be fought in the ultimate battleground, your mind, so having the right attitude about diet therapy is a key that makes decision making easier. In our next chapter, "Boot Camp," we talk about how to prepare yourself, your child, and your family, mentally and emotionally, for the battle that lies ahead.

2
Boot Camp, i.e., Retraining Your Brain

Boot camp is a place where people leave their comfort zones behind and learn new skills, techniques, and weapons. When the conventional anti-seizure medications don't do the trick and it is time for a weapons upgrade, often the big guns—ketogenic diets—are pulled out. A common sense approach to diet therapy should include assessing how you've fared so far in this war against epilepsy. If you're one of those rare people who have run the gauntlet of difficult-to-control seizures and emerged emotionally unscathed, then go ahead and skip this part of the training. (We personally doubt such super heroes exist, but we'll make allowances.) If you're like the rest of us and suffered some emotional battle wounds from your experiences, then read on.

It was five months and several unsuccessful drug trials after Noah's seizures began that his neurologist casually mentioned a low-carb diet as a potential course of action. I was pacing in my bedroom on the phone with him, nine months pregnant— my second son would be born less than two weeks later—and utterly overwhelmed by this life we were living. Noah was about 14 months old then. He was smiley and snuggly and hadn't yet been dimmed by all the drugs we would eventually end up try- ing because, in those early months of epilepsy, depriving my beautiful boy of one more thing in this world, carbs included, seemed cruel. It wasn't until several months later, when Noah's eyes would roll into the back of his head a moment after walking up to me, or when he lost use of his legs for a couple days due to a drug side effect, that I chose to let go of my personal love *of food and see where diet therapy could take us. By then I had nearly lost my son, and the emotional heft of daily life with seizures was dizzying. A friend once told me that when Noah was first initiated on the Ketogenic diet I was clearly broken, that I had lost all hope. I don't remember life that bleak in those moments when seizures controlled our every thought, but now, with Noah nearly two years seizure free on the diet, I realize we weren't living at all; we were struggling to survive, powerless, exhausted, and moving through life as though it were a never-ending nightmare. And yet, it was my attachment to food that prevented my son from starting the diet sooner.* —Erin Whitmer*

Each one of you, like us, has a story to tell that at some point has been marred by the common denominators of fear, disappointment, and heartbreak. We human beings are complicated creatures, and psychologists tell us that the thoughts we think often dictate our emotions, while our emotions strongly influence our behavior and choices. The attitudes we embrace play a large part in determining how effectively we resolve and overcome difficult experiences. We may put on a brave face and attempt to soldier on, but if we find ourselves picking our way through a mental landscape dotted with dysfunctional attitudes, like undetonated landmines, we naturally will be very cautious and hesitant about moving forward.

Before you start the physical preparation needed to journey deep into ketogenic territory, you may want to perform a "mine sweeping operation" by taking a long hard look at what may be buried in your own backyard. We are not intending this chapter to be a psychological self-help manual by any means, but hope it will function as a tool to help you recognize some possible emotional roadblocks to diet therapy success. If you feel stuck and need help to work through these issues, then by all means seek it out. You deserve as smooth a journey as possible and every chance at success.

Know Your Enemy: Targeting Dysfunctional Attitudes

"Whether you think you can or think you can't, you are usually right." —Henry Ford

You may find yourself doing battle with the voices in your head before you even start a ketogenic program. *"You've tried so many things before and they never worked, don't risk any more disappointment....No way can you pull this off! You're not organized and methodical enough. You can hardly keep the checking account balanced let alone balance carbs and fat grams!...Your poor child already has to deal with seizures, and now you will heartlessly deprive him of one of his few remaining pleasures—food!"*

Recognizing and targeting dysfunctional attitudes is probably one of the most important skills you can develop in this mental war of attrition. Neuropsychologist Dr. Robert Mittan, founder of the Seizure and Epilepsy Education Program, organizes seminars for epilepsy patients, families, and caregivers on the emotional and practical aspects of managing seizures successfully. His research has found that many families gradually allow epilepsy to overshadow and control their lives in response to feelings of fear, guilt, and stigma. Fear of the next seizure can paralyze normal family function, guilt can cause parents to live under a condemning cloud, and the perceived stigma of being "different" can cause people with epilepsy to withdraw. While Dr. Mittan's research did not specifically examine the effect of ketogenic diets on families coping with epilepsy, it is safe to assume that those doing diet therapy are not immune to problems.

So how do you rid yourself of dysfunctional attitudes? The first step is to know your enemy. Find and identify the thoughts and attitudes that will work against you if you attempt diet therapy. We'll "round up the usual suspects" below; look them over and see if you recognize any of them loitering in your neighborhood.

Coping with the Fear Factor

Mark Twain once observed that he was an old man and had known many troubles, but most of them never happened. Anticipation of a fearful experience can be as terrifying and stressful as the dreaded event itself. (It is interesting to note that Mark Twain's daughter, Jean Clemons, suffered from epilepsy brought on by a head injury long before the days of anti-seizure medications.) Most of us already have had a few genuinely petrifying experiences to contend with; helplessly watching a child's first seizure is probably as frightening as living through a major earthquake. We survive, but the experience leaves us shaken.

The Ketogenic diet, and its less complex cousin, the Modified Atkins Diet (MAD), seem to strike a particularly fearful chord in the hearts of parents who first consider them. Why? Perhaps for several reasons: in the not-so-distant past, neurologists tended to reserve the diet as a worst-case-scenario treatment, a sort of "extreme unction" given after every available anti-seizure medication had failed. Currently, Ketogenic diet specialists recommend trying the diet after only two medication failures and in certain cases (infantile spasms, for one) neurologists might recommend it as a first-line-therapy; still, the negative "last chance" stereotype lingers in some epilepsy centers. Thankfully this seems to be becoming less of a problem over the past few years.

Additionally, the diet is sometimes presented in a very unappealing light, described as "unpalatable" and "disagreeable." Many parents conjure up visions of a Ketogenic Corner in Dante's *Inferno*, endlessly preparing and weighing revolting food to force down their gagging child's throat. For those of us who've spent several years cooking for a child on the Ketogenic diet or Modified Atkins Diet, we can confidently say that with some creative effort and an organized schedule, you can prepare very pleasant, enjoyable meals. True, most kids would probably prefer a burger and fries to a low-carb, high-fat menu, but most kids would also honestly prefer a life without seizures. This diet gives them a shot at that. How miraculous that food—common ordinary fare like butter, cream, and oil—can cause seizures to simply melt away. With patience, planning, and probably a few rough starts, most families eventually settle into a familiar routine. You will certainly be very busy, and initially the learning curve will be quite steep, but for some, the results are remarkable. In addition, a large number of children now are receiving the Ketogenic diet as a formula only: hard to argue that it's not palatable when all your doctor is doing is changing the formula.

But let's get back to those discomforting voices in your head: "What if it doesn't work? What if you go to all that effort and trouble and it's just as ineffective as all the other treatments you've tried!" If your heart is aching from all the past disappointments you've suffered, remind yourself that some risks are simply worth taking. It might not work, but then again, it might prove to be the answer you've been seeking all along. Ask your doctor about your specific situation, because the odds may be in your favor for a positive outcome; 50% to 60% of children on the diet show considerable improvement. And if it doesn't work, you won't be any worse off than you are now.

You'll find those voices don't give up easily, however: "What if all that fat hurts your child? What if it stunts his growth and makes him sick?...you aren't a dietitian, you can't do this alone!" Knowledge is power, so go for the facts. Published evidence shows that many, many children on every continent thrive on these diets—a quick visit to websites dedicated to the Ketogenic diet and MAD—we mention several of these sites in Chapter 3—will arm you with photos and success stories from young and old around the world. Side effects are manageable and once the diet stops, there doesn't appear to be any long-term negative problems. And remember, nobody expects you to go this route alone; you will have professional medical supervision and can also benefit from online support groups where parents doing ketogenic diets with their children are more than happy to guide you along the way. It takes time to learn the skills necessary to follow these diets successfully, so don't expect to have it all down pat in one day. But as Charlie Brown of "Peanuts" fame says, "I've developed a new philosophy…I only dread one day at a time." Focus on today. Once you get through it, you will realize you have the power to get through tomorrow, and the next day, and the next day as well.

Lifting the Burden of Guilt

As parents we can deceive ourselves into believing the myth that if we were really, truly, good parents and worthwhile human beings we would somehow intuitively know how to protect our child from all possible harm. The truth is, this myth is simply just that, a myth, and it's a harmful one at that. When life hands our child a difficult-to-treat seizure disorder, sometimes this myth kicks into overdrive. We experience feelings of hyper-responsibility; it must somehow be our fault when the meds fail, the diet needs tweaking, and the seizures are difficult to control.

Putting my daughter on medication has been a very difficult decision for me. I felt like I had failed her somehow, I wanted so badly for the diet to be a cure. I thought motherhood was hard but you don't realize how hard until one of your children gets sick and no matter what you do you just can't wish it away. —Jennifer

It is a natural and healthy thing for parents to desire the best possible seizure control for their child, and any normal parent is saddened and discouraged when it is hard to achieve. However, carrying the burden of guilt when things do not go as we sincerely wish is overstepping the boundaries of parental responsibility. We all tend to do it, but we pay for it dearly as this guilt gnaws away at our peace of mind, our family harmony, and our child's developing sense that they are, somehow, responsible for everyone else's misery.

It is wise to learn to catch ourselves when we are falling into this dys-functional attitude trap. Upholding this pattern of self-imposed guilt and blame while attempting a ketogenic diet can become an enormous cross to bear. If your worth as a parent depends on whether or not you can get the seizures to stop, life can quickly descend into a type of tortured hell. Every break-through seizure is perceived as a value statement; once again, you've failed. For some parents, even the news that someone else's son or daughter is responding more rapidly to the diet than their own can be devastating. Why? There is a very different sense of control with the diet versus meds.

Compared to doling out anti-seizure meds, a ketogenic diet is a hands-on parental affair that you administer and prepare, so it is easy to falsely assume it's your fault if things aren't going as hoped. You are no longer dealing with the abstract failure of a medication, but rather, a personal perceived failure if the diet isn't working. Even when parents are closely following the diet, nevertheless, it is easy to take it very personally if setbacks occur. Our minds may understand that it is humanly impossible to control every outcome, but our hearts still want us to be the exception to the rule so we can help our child.

Similarly, when break-through seizures occur, the burden of control may cause parents to push for immediate dietary changes, fearing the therapy has failed and they must quickly do something to remedy the situation. It's wise to remember that these diets are medical therapies that work in ways similar to medication. When a child is on medication and a single seizure occurs, the standard procedure is to wait and see if it is just a temporary hiccup in an otherwise beneficial therapy. Likewise, if a seizure occurs when a child is on the diet, patience is needed. Occasionally, for reasons we don't yet understand, the brain seems to remember that seizing was once the default setting, and decides to act up again in the old unwelcome pattern. If that happens, your doctor will usually advise to wait out the storm before making a drastic change. Keep pushing the fats, and bide your time so you can honestly see just what the diet can do. Sometimes healing just takes time and patience.

Whether or not a ketogenic diet therapy proves to be the answer for your child, recognizing the pattern of guilt and blame, and making the deci-sion to stop the vicious cycle, can be one of the most healthy, liberating choices you will ever make. One of our favorite reminders to parents is that you are the good guys in this story. You bought this book because you are obviously motivated to try to make this diet work, otherwise you wouldn't be reading it! Stop beating yourself up, lift the burden of guilt from your shoulders, and don't ever allow yourself, or anyone else, to place it there again for it never belonged there in the first place.

Healthy Grief and Moving Forward

So much of life genuinely seems unfair at times. None of us had a choice about whether or not our child would get epilepsy. None of us voted that some kids could take pills to control their seizures and experience no side effects, while others would have to be put on a ketogenic diet. Some achieve seizure control in days on the diet, while others struggle for months sleuthing and tweaking before gaining any noticeable improvement. Some try their best to make the diet work, only to find that it didn't help as much as they'd desperately hoped.

We aren't in control of the difficult circumstances life hands us and when the ravages of epilepsy leave us shaken, vulnerable, and confused, it is necessary and healthy to grieve our losses.

The day we had to put Jordan in a wheelchair and helmet because he was battering his head so badly from falling when he had seizures, my heart ached so much I felt I'd gone under a surgical knife without anesthesia. My son had been a laughing, normal child with wide and trusting eyes, and then suddenly it was all ripped away from him, from all of us, without warning. I had worked for years in humanitarian projects and had witnessed disaster and suffering on a massive scale in Asia. And yes, I knew the textbook answers—this isn't anyone's fault, it's not a punishment, we're experiencing normal reactions to frightening abnormal circumstances. Somehow I'd assumed that knowing all that would have helped me cope better, but still, when my child and I became the refugees fleeing from this devastating natural disaster, seizures, the pain was raw, debilitating. When it is your child, no matter what your head knows, your grieving heart can't help but respond in astonishment, "How could this happen to us?" —Jeanne Riether

We usually associate grieving with death, but grief is experienced with all kinds of loss. The loss of health, dreams, finances, security; the loss of what we expected life to be, the loss or normalcy, all need to be acknowledged in order to heal. Studies suggest that there are states of grief and acceptance and that we tend to move in and out of them as we journey along the path of healing. At different times we may experience denial (*"He can't have epilepsy!"*), bartering (*"I promise I'll be a better parent if these seizures will only go away"*), anger (*"Why don't these meds help!"*), depression (*"Things will never be the same again..."*) and finally, acceptance (*"Our life is different, but we're coping"*). Moving through this cycle according to our own sequence and time frame allows us to come to terms with the changed circumstances of our lives. For some, these stages seem short or even non-existent, for others they can take much longer to navigate. According to psychologist Heather Pereira,

> *"We might accept what life has thrown our way today, but tomorrow we find ourselves back in the bargaining phase, trying to find a way to fix everything. It is perfectly normal to revisit states of acceptance. How healed we are shows in how quickly we can snap from sad or angry, back to hopeful."*

Problems occur when we get stuck in any of the stages and can't move forward. Anger, for example, can be a healthy emotion as it helps us establish boundaries where we need them, or helps us fight for our child when necessary. But ongoing, unresolved anger is debilitating and threatens our physical and mental health, our happiness, and our supportive relationships.

Perhaps the most important question to ask ourselves is not whether or not all we've experienced in our war against seizures is "fair" for it will likely never seem to be so, but rather, will we remain stuck in a place where epilepsy is allowed to overshadow, control, and define us? As frightening as it can be to have no idea what lies ahead, we are not powerless. The turning point for most of us isn't the meltdown we may experience on the kitchen floor at midnight when we feel we just can't deal with it all anymore, that epilepsy, seizures, a ketogenic diet therapy, and all they entail are so miserably unfair. But rather, it is the moment afterwards, when we wipe our nose on our sleeve, pick ourselves up, and take the next shaky step forward. When you've had your cry, but then choose to go back to the stove, the carpool, the playground, your job, or the doctor's office, and just keep on keeping on, then your courage, not epilepsy, defines you.

If you are in pain and are having trouble coming to terms with all you've experienced getting to this point, seek out help. Find a therapist, a religious counselor, or a wise and trusted friend who will encourage you to steadily move forward at your own pace. You deserve all the support and help available, so don't hesitate to reach out and receive it.

Allied Forces: Preparing Your Family and Friends to Fight by Your Side

They say it takes a village to raise a child, and when your child goes on a ketogenic diet you may sometimes feel like it requires that just to feed one. Without a doubt, it's easier to make it work if you have the support and cooperation of your immediate family, as well as others who have regular contact with your child. Families usually take the first hit when dealing with the stress of chronic medical conditions, and starting diet therapy comes with its own unique set of stressors:

- One parent may be more willing or enthusiastic than the other to attempt the diet. Additionally they must negotiate and assign the practical duties of preparing ketogenic meals and shopping.

- Single parents may feel overwhelmed at the thought of shouldering the bulk of the responsibility alone. Those who share parenting responsibilities with a former spouse must solicit their ex's support to keep the child on the dietary straight and narrow while away from home on sleepovers, visits, or outings.

- Grandparents or other relatives may not initially be supportive of the decision to attempt the diet, yet the family may be dependent on them for caregiving or other help.

- Spouses who are not the main caregiver must contend with the fact that a good deal of their partner's time will now be invested in cooking, shopping, and learning the ropes of diet therapy. There will most likely be a period of adjustment as both partners strive to find a new "normal."

- The child who will be going on the diet may initially strongly resist the thought of a life without their favorite foods.

- Sometimes resentment from siblings can arise if favorite forbidden foods are no longer allowed to be eaten in front of the child on the diet, or in some cases are completely banned from the home (not all households go to this extreme, but for some children with very poor impulse control it becomes necessary).

- Holidays and festive celebrations where food has always previously been the focus can become awkward. This may mean creating new family traditions that are no so longer so food-centric.

- In some countries and cultures where food sharing at meals is commonplace, the sudden lack of sharing foods for one particular child can be stigmatizing.

- Some find it stressful to tackle the task of educating family, friends, teachers, classmates, and peers about the diet and why your child (or you, if you are an adult on the diet) must follow it rigidly.

Bracing for Impact: Ketogenic Diets and Your Cushion of Support

Perhaps the best way to understand what you're going to be getting yourself into if you opt for diet therapy is to listen to stories from those who've done it. The following accounts offer candid views about the ways diet therapy can impact close relationships and the emotional climate at home. Some recall their experiences with satisfaction and gratefulness, others with anger and frustration. A recurring theme throughout all the stories is that caregivers who had the benefit of sufficient emotional support and physical assistance from family and friends carried a considerably lighter load. Knowing this can help you plan effective strategies together, and create the supportive "band of brothers" that you need.

> *This is a difficult journey for the whole family and I can easily see how stressful something like this can be on a marriage without the support of a partner. The most important part of Jason's (my husband's) contribution is that he fully understands how difficult it is to think of, calculate, and prepare meals for Oliver. So he supports the efforts fully whether by prepping food, weighing items, baking meals, or taking the kids out of the house so I can play loud music and cook un-interrupted. While I do 95% of the cooking for our son, I know that at any moment I could turn to my husband and ask him to take over and he would happily do it. —Bethany, married mother of a child of the Ketogenic diet.*

> *Watching your child have seizures gives a parent a profound feeling of helplessness. I have always found that starting something new to control seizures (like changing or adding meds) is very emotional because having hope can cause a painful free-fall if things don't work. I have found controlling my "hope*

bank" to be very difficult and challenging. [Doing this diet] gave me hope that I had lost many years ago. For the first time, I felt like I was doing something tangible and worthwhile for my daughter. That's a powerful feeling.

The responsibility of nurturing the diet and tracking food, seizures, behaviors, etc., can feel overwhelming. To mitigate this, I was vigilant about making changes very, very slowly. I had to feel I had complete control over every step we took. We embraced the diet as a family, including my college-aged son. My husband was on board with the diet as much as me. We totally understood each other's need to try this as a last resort to control my 21-year-old daughter's seizures. My husband and I enjoy cooking and so our shared focus on the diet brought us together as a team. I have been very private about my daughter's disability. It's a lonely place to be. When starting the MAD diet, I decided to be more open with family and friends. I received an abundance of support from everyone. I have a small inner circle of close relationships. I felt supported by everyone. —Wendy, mother of a daughter on MAD

I felt totally broken hearted initially, I couldn't even eat my meals; the diet was really tough to start. We are carb lovers so cutting down all this was, and is, sooo hard. She keeps asking me whether she can eat some rice or macaroni n' cheese, and I tell her to please give it some more time, and assure her that this diet is for her own good. My daughter is a wonderful child, and she understands and doesn't fuss in any way.

My relationship with my husband is really strong, by God's grace, so it hasn't impacted our relationship in any negative way...we are in this together. Our relationship did feel the impact, as we hardly have time for each other, we always watch our daughter, either me or my husband, and never let her out of our sight. We feel as though our hopes and dreams for her are totally crushed at times...but we try to stay positive.

We keep our socializing to a minimum due to our daughter's health. We do feel alone in this situation. We have kept our daughter's health issue a secret so far to avoid all the social stigma; nobody knows that my daughter has seizures up until now, except for my family and a couple of very close friends, and of course my daughter's school. —"Patricia," married, mother of child on MAD (Name changed for privacy)

By the time we started MAD I was already overwhelmed dealing with his seizures, so in some ways being able to actually do something constructive to help seemed like a relief. It's kind of like childbirth and being in labor for a very long time, then finally being told you can push—it's not a comfortable place to be, but at least things are finally moving forward.

I am not naturally a systematic or organized person in the kitchen, so learning to be exact and precise added pressure. Also, I feared I would make a mistake that could potentially harm my son. About two weeks in, I remember someone asked a well-meaning but badly timed question, "How are you going to cope if your son is on this diet for years?" And I wanted to burst into tears at the thought of it, even though we already had seen great results in seizure control. However, in many ways the whole experience drew us closer as a family, rallying around helping my son. His older brother and sister were very helpful and learned how to help prepare at least some MAD meals, even though I did the cooking most of the time. As a single parent, having their help meant a lot. I slowly gained confidence preparing meals, things became more routine, the tension lessened, and the results were very exciting. After getting the swing of it, I felt intense pride in the fact that we were actually pulling this off, maybe the kind of pride you must feel after completing something difficult like basic training in the army. The whole journey has become part of us, shaped us, and changed us in ways nothing else could have done. For us, MAD was an answer to prayer. —Jeanne Riether, single, mother of child on MAD

The diet added extra tension to our marriage. Whenever you have a child with a chronic illness I believe there is extra tension, but when only one person is doing the brunt of the work to help the child, well, there is some resentment. My husband did not help prepare the food nor did he play a big role when my son was initiated on the diet. We both brought our son into this world, but why am I the only one trying to save him?

*I felt a tremendous amount of pressure and it was scary.
I didn't want to fail my son. I was exhausted, mentally and
physically. He is a very picky eater and getting him to eat
Keto food was quite the challenge. I felt very lonely. Even
though I talked to many Keto parents on a regular basis, it
just wasn't the same as when I walked out the door and had to
face the rest of the world. Many people didn't understand the
diet. It became just easier to pull away than have to deal with
others. I wish I had turned to my close friends more for help
with preparing food. I should have gone out more too. I would
just stay home a lot during the day and night, and work on
recipes or do research. I feel a tremendous weight has been
lifted now that he is off the diet and seizure free. The relationship with my son is incredible! Many friends and I are closer
too. They say they admire what I did and gave up for my son.
I made some wonderful new friends as well, Keto families
I will forever be grateful for and keep in touch with. They have
become family to me. —Amy, married, mother of child on the
Ketogenic diet*

*In the beginning my wife and I had a few fights because she
did not want to start the diet as soon as I, and also it was
a bit overwhelming for both of us, so it was very stressful.
I was more under pressure than her. I was pushing for the
diet harder, although she was on board also. Our relationship
is a very good one so luckily it was not too hard. —Orlando,
married, father of child on MAD*

*The improvements I was seeing when I started Kim on MAD
were motivating and empowering to me. In the beginning,
I wanted to have hope but I was afraid to get too excited about
this diet, as we had seen so many things help Kim a little or
work for a while and then stop. The initial learning curve was a
struggle, but once I understood the diet better, I gained confidence that I could do this.*

*I am blessed to have a very supportive husband. He doesn't do
the cooking for Kim himself unless I am away, but he helps
clean up my messes. I am also blessed to be part of a wonderful church family. During times when Kim was in the hospital
with intractable seizures, they provided meals for our family.*

My friends are so accepting of Kim and will often ask what Kim can eat when they invite us over. We also have some wonderful caregivers who help out with Kim during the day so I can get things done or get a break.

Of course, the best thing that has come out of doing this diet is that Kimberly's seizure control is much better. Finally, it feels like all we have been through with Kimberly has not been for naught. Though some of the things Kim has suffered throughout her life have been terrible and so hard to go through at the time, I can now see how sharing our struggles and some answers we've found are helping others. That makes me feel like there was some purpose in the pain. —Marilyn, married, mother of adult daughter on MAD

There were a lot of ups and downs. I think I spent the first two weeks crying because of the cravings I had, but to me that was a positive step, because I was grieving a loss. My best friends were extremely supportive. One of them came over the day I started the diet and we cleaned out my cupboards and refrigerator of anything that wasn't acceptable for the diet. She helped me figure out where to donate that food, so I didn't feel like I was wasting it, and then took me shopping for what I needed. She and her husband always make sure they have acceptable foods for me on hand so I can visit whenever and not feel like food is an issue. I'm not married and have dated two different men during the time since I started the diet and both of them have been extremely supportive, understanding that there are certain restaurants that don't work for me and being willing to sacrifice their favorite foods when they are with me. They also seem to love my home cooking and are more than willing to eat food from the diet. So much so I usually get left without leftovers!

The most important coping mechanism I have is my faith; without God, I would be lost. At times I felt alone at church dinners when everyone else had something to eat and I felt like it was too much of a hassle to bring something different (and for the people who don't already know, to answer their questions) so I would just be there not eating, surrounded by all this food. That is an extremely lonely feeling. It's hard to even talk to people when they are eating and you aren't because you can't, but would like to be.

*For a while I felt protective of my food, like I had to not let any-
one else touch it or prepare it for me so that I knew it would
work. Now after almost 18 months on the diet, I trust people to
cook for me. The best thing that came out of doing the diet is
the best seizure control I have ever had. It has reduced my seizures by over 50%, taking my daily grand mals away to every
other week or even less. As far as my relationships go, it has
brought me closer to some people. I never before realized that I
had people in my life who were so kind, caring, thoughtful, and
amazingly giving to think of me at every meal we would share,
that they could remember every dietary restriction I have, and
prepare food that meets the needs I have and not feel burdened
by it. —Heidi, single, adult with epilepsy on MAD*

Foxhole Strategies: Creating an Effective and Emotionally Safe Circle of Support

The army acknowledges that three-man foxholes have advantages to one
or two-man defensive fighting positions. One soldier can provide security,
another can do priority work, and the third can eat, rest, and do maintenance. You can use this strategy when creating your own family "foxhole"
in the Ketogenic war. Though you may initially feel very busy when starting
out, it's wise to remember we come out ahead when we keep the people
we depend on high on our list of personal priorities. Investing time and
communication is important, because the emotional support that healthy
relationships and friendships provide can give us the endurance we need
when the ketogenic road seems like a long and lonely haul. To cultivate
needed personal support you can:

- Affirm your close relationships, and take time to strengthen and invest in
  them.

- Acknowledge that caring for a child's needs, dealing with seizures, and
  scheduling time to manage the diet is an intense workload.

- Have an honest discussion with your family to work out a fair and equi-
  table division of duties.

- Find practical ways to recruit a "third man in the foxhole," by reaching out to friends, relatives, or paid assistance when your tasks are
  overwhelming.

Try to step away from your all your ketogenic duties long enough to accomplish one worthwhile goal: take the time to tell those who are most important to you how much they are valued and loved. It may be your husband, wife, a significant other, your kids, parents, best friend, the family dog, or all of the above; the important thing is, you're making an investment in those who matter to you. It may seem like an insignificant achievement, but verbally affirming those you care about will go a long way in sustaining a healthy emotional climate at home, and help cultivate the emotional support network you will need to fall back on.

Take Care of the Caregiver—You!
Survival Strategies 101

If you have ever flown, you've undoubtedly watched the flight attendants demonstrate routine safety procedures: in case the oxygen masks drop, passengers traveling with children are to place the mask over their own face first before assisting the children in their care. Why? It's simple logic. If you don't take care of yourself, you won't be able to protect and care for your child.

While it seems reasonable to follow those instructions if the plane is going down, it goes against all our parental instincts when our child is chronically ill. We neglect our own needs and forfeit sleep, meals, relationships, exercise, and personal hygiene—we cut back on anything and everything we possibly can and then wonder why we're at the edge of physical and emotional collapse. Family circumstances, time constraints, and financial limitations all converge and, more often than not, we end up finding ways to make do with less than we really need. Continuing this over the long haul, however, makes it difficult to sustain something as demanding as diet therapy.

Dana has mothered seven children, and is now a single parent caring for two children with disabilities, one of whom is deaf, blind, and autistic and on MAD. She comments:

> *A whole book could be devoted to the spiritual journey of caregiving. Unfortunately, most families who end up with a child with special needs do not realize what a spiritual journey this is going to be, and those who do may often wind up feeling that they did not ask for this or volunteer for this path.*

> *Getting from the place where one feels that one has been somehow robbed of the life one was promised to the place where one can embrace the beauty of the life one has been given is more than can be handled in a chapter.*

Determine what supports one's own growth and happiness.
Make time to care for oneself. To keep sane, I have a huge read-
ing list of novels I want to enjoy. I grow a gorgeous garden
complete with 16 fruit trees. I paint or write fiction for fun.
I am part of online parent support groups. I am not religious,
but prayer is an essential part of each day. When I am stressed,
I take my own medicine, hot baths with epsom salts. If the kids
are on supplements, I am, too, because I have to live to 100 so
that I can care for them. No one else is perfect and no one has
the right to expect you to be either. Learn to forgive. As you can
see, there is a lot to getting to that particular place where one
can live in gratitude with this many challenges.

Heather, a school psychologist and mother of a child with Angelman Syndrome who is on MAD sums up our thoughts on the subject:

I think it is very important for parents to be passionate about
their children but to also take care of themselves. I do my best to
find "me time" and not feel guilty about it. Without the chance to
rest and regroup, I am less capable of doing what needs to be done.

Here are six strategies to consider while pondering how to care for yourself, along with your child, on this journey:

1. **Safeguard your own health by getting adequate sleep, eating nutritious meals, and getting regular exercise:** Your body needs proper maintenance and getting sick yourself is only going to complicate your situation further. Proper nutrition, good sleep, and vigorous exercise boosts your immune system, and relieves stress. Sounds great, but is it unrealistic? Try going to bed a little earlier each night, take turns with your spouse listening for the seizure monitor, borrow a workout video from the library and do 25 minutes of cardio in the living room, drink less caffeine, take supplements, and eat those greens! Sometimes small changes collectively add up to better health.

2. **Enlist help from others so you can step away from your caregiver role when needed:** (And it is needed.) This one is never easy to manage, but until you realize it is a necessity and not a luxury, it won't happen. Even if the only practical solution you can muster is to pay a sitter so you can go grocery shopping, make it count by combining

work with pleasure: take a friend along for company, visit a café for a quick bite to eat, or park the car in a shady spot for a short break to unwind. Stepping away briefly from your responsibilities allows you to come back refreshed and recharged.

3. **Join an online support group of parents doing the Ketogenic diet, MAD, Low Glycemic Index Treatment (LGIT) diet, or the Medium Chain Triglyceride (MCT) diet:** This can be a wonderful resource of strength, encouragement, and counsel. There are some welcoming ones out there where you will find people who have been where you are now, and who understand the frustrations and challenges you are facing. (Chapter 3 will tell you more about the importance of support groups.)

4. **Find one fun thing:** Yes, you heard right. When you are fully involved in something like a ketogenic diet, it is easy to get so preoccupied with the mechanics of living that joy and normalcy are slowly edged out. Inviting fun into your life is one way to refuse to let epilepsy control you. Combat drudgery by finding at least one thing you love to do (within the bounds of reason and legality of course) and then do it without guilt or hesitation. It doesn't have to be time consuming or expensive and can be something as simple as taking up a relaxing craft a couple hours each week (knitting, macramé, water color painting, fix-it projects, woodworking, etc.); creating a special corner to retreat to in your home (think Hawaiian island beach poster, potted plants, comfy chair, and a cool talk drink); or an enjoyable activity (early morning run, leisurely walk, game night, bubble bath, mystery novel, dinner by candlelight after the kids are in bed, or even just renting a movie). When you make time for fun and enjoyment, you will find you are a caregiver who has more to give.

5. **Practice gratitude:** As "Pollyanna-like" as this may sound, studies by Dr. Robert Emmons of UC Davis show that there is a measurable connection between gratitude, emotional wellbeing, and even physical wellbeing. Volunteers participating in studies were asked to keep track of their experiences of gratitude by journaling on a weekly basis. Compared to control groups instructed to journal about hassles or neutral life events, those who kept gratitude journals tended to exercise more regularly, report fewer physical symptoms, were more optimistic and felt better about their lives, and made more progress towards important personal goals. Being grateful for a child's kiss, one less seizure, or even that last box of sugar-free whipping cream on the supermarket shelf, can do much for our own health and wellbeing.

6. **Find someone who has it tougher than you do:** It is very easy to feel alone and overwhelmed by our struggles. Reading about someone who

faces an even more challenging situation can add needed perspective. Life can be worthwhile and meaningful despite the difficult challenges we face, a fact that is sometimes lost in our personal day-to-day struggle.

Preparing Your Child for Battle (and Sometimes Preparing to Battle with Your Child)

When it comes time to break the news of the Ketogenic diet or MAD to your child, you might do well to consider the old folk tale of the aging king who began to fret about growing old. He called upon the royal soothsayers to predict how the final years of his life would be. One sour-faced courtier sadly stepped forward to give his prophecy: "Sire, I am sorry to say that over the course of many years, one by one, all the members of your family will die before you. At long last, you will be left to reign utterly alone!" The king was furious with such a gloomy prediction and angrily ordered the man into exile. The next counselor to come forward tried a more enticing approach. "Wonderful news, your Majesty!" he beamed. "I see a long reign with abundant years ahead of you! In fact, you will outlive the rest of your family by many, many years!" The jubilant king thanked the man for the good report and heaped wealth and riches on him, even though the bottom line of both messages was essentially the same.

Your child, like the king, will be interested in learning "what's in it for me" when told about the diet. A well thought out presentation can help even young children see that while there are disadvantages, there are also some interesting perks. After all, you've discovered wonderful news! There is a special magic diet that has helped many other kids' seizures go away, and you want to find out if it can help him too. And guess what! Instead of adding another new kind of pill, the new medicine is going to be bacon, whipped cream, and berries!

It is important to also break the news that the "magic" in this diet only works when you don't cheat, but letting your child have choices of acceptable foods and some say-so in what he will be eating goes a long way in securing cooperation. Ice cream for breakfast? Why not? As long as it's made with heavy whipping cream and an allowed sweetener, it's an acceptable food. A wonderful free online book that you can read with your child and family is *Grace's Magic Diet*, written by a mother and illustrated by the siblings of a child on the Ketogenic diet describing their journey from hospital stay to daily life. You will be delighted by the story and can find it at www.epilepsy.com/epilepsy/gracesmagicdiet. Another fantastic book for young readers that will help them understand the power of their new diet is *Gordy and the Magic Diet*, available now at bookstores and online.

Recruiting Child Soldiers

Your child may resist the diet when he realizes many of his favorite foods are now on the nix list, but if he is a preschooler you can usually ride out this storm with patience; eventually most small children eat what's set before them once they get hungry enough, and since they usually have no other way to bootleg contraband, time is on your side. If they are older, however, they can easily engineer all sorts of ingenious schemes to sneak forbidden food at school, while out with friends, or even beneath your very nose at home. With big kids it becomes important to ensure that their will is on your side from the get-go.

Some children quickly warm to the idea of being an "amazing kid on an amazing diet" and tend to own it from the start. Other kids make it clear they are not volunteers in this war but have been drafted against their will; they are only doing it because they "have to." Sometimes all the whining is simply the noise kids make when they are grieving their losses. Acknowledge their struggle and let them know you understand that it isn't easy. But when it seems they would practically sell their soul for a double dip chocolate cone, you can sympathize without caving in to their demands. You will probably shed a tear or two along with your child at times, but remember, this is a medical therapy meant to improve the quality of your child's life. Your child will suffer if he is:

- Pitied and treated as if he is a "victim" of the diet.

- Expected to be "tough" and unaffected emotionally by the difficulties he will face in sticking with the diet.

Though sticking to a restrictive diet can be hard for a child, and there are bound to be times of tears, frustration, and anger, challenging experiences also offer opportunities for positive emotional growth. A child who perceives himself as an overcomer who fights seizures through diet therapy develops a healthy self-image. The struggle to stick to the diet should be acknowledged, and the child should be praised and encouraged as he makes good daily choices. Regularly tell your child how proud you are of him, and work out a reward system in advance to recognize and celebrate success. Knowing that he can rack up valuable points to redeem for a prize, or that he will receive acceptable treats and other small rewards for his sacrifices can go a long way to control the impulse to cheat. Keep in mind, however, that young children aren't usually very good at delayed gratification. You may have to keep some acceptable treats, toys, or other small enticements on hand to quickly reward them when they must forego favorite foods.

The Empowerment of Choice

It can be enormously frustrating for any child, let alone a preteen or teenager, to feel he has no control over meals and snacks, for food is often associated with fun, affection, and reward. The diet can easily be perceived as a power struggle if your child isn't able to make any decisions whatsoever over what he gets to eat. If he is balking at the prospect of the diet, let him grieve his losses—favorite foods, being "different," or missing treats—and then get him involved in the process of finding new favorites. Presenting a child with options is empowering.

> *Jordan went through "rice withdrawal" at first, and it was terrible. He had grown up in Asia and really was shocked and appalled at the idea of going without rice and noodles when he started the diet. But he became seizure free quickly after he went on MAD, so I wasn't about to give in without a fight when he begged to quit. It took some tough love to say "no" and insist we stick with it at least for a few months, but I knew we'd never make it over the long haul without his willing cooperation. What ultimately pulled us through, besides a lot of reasoning and negotiation, was giving him a range of acceptable choices and getting him involved in planning meals. I had to accommodate his choices, and once I discovered he liked shirataki noodle curry, faux fried cauliflower "rice," buttered sweet oopsie rolls, and MAD-friendly pizza, I bent over backwards to fix things he enjoyed. They seemed "starchy" enough to satisfy his initial carb cravings, but mostly he liked the normalcy of being able to make choices and decide what he wanted to eat. Eventually he became very satisfied with the diet and was able to stay on it successfully for two years without difficulty, even though his initial carb cravings were hard on both of us. Amazingly, he never cheated the whole time, even though I am sure he was greatly tempted. —Jeanne Riether*

There are many different tricks of the trade you can learn to use to make the diet seem exciting and special to your child, which helps encourage compliance. Sometimes simply serving whipped cream in a parfait glass with a long spoon does the trick. The great restaurants of the world charge high prices for delivering top-notch presentations because they know a little flair makes even an ordinary meal enjoyable and interesting. (See Chapter 9, "Warriors of all Shapes and Sizes," for more ideas on how to interest your child in acceptable foods.)

Schooltime Strategies

School and group settings present challenges for children on the diet, but most can manage it with a well-packed lunch bag and some coaching from home. Depending on their age, children should be prepped on how to answer questions if they are offered forbidden food. A simple, "Sorry, I can't eat that or I'll get sick," or "No, I'm on a special diet" will usually suffice. You can also arrange to be informed in advance about classroom celebrations involving food, such as birthdays, and can send your child armed with his own ketogenic- or MAD-friendly treat to enjoy when the other kids have forbidden cake, cookies, or candy. The teacher and nurse should know your child is on the diet, a subject we cover more fully in Chapter 7, "Sending Your Warrior to School."

If you find your child is being teased about either the diet or epilepsy (or if you are looking for a preventative strategy to avoid that from happening) talk to the teacher to see if peer education is an option. Simple explanations can demystify epilepsy, dispel ignorance, and go a long way to educate students about the challenges people with epilepsy face. Many local chapters of the Epilepsy Foundation, as well as programs run through the Anita Kaufmann Foundation, will gladly come into schools and do age-appropriate, anonymous (about the patient) presentations to inform the other kids about how they can actively support others who struggle with seizures. You can also campaign to involve your local school in Global Purple Day for Epilepsy activities, where children participate in events to show support for people with epilepsy.

I am a strong believer in promoting change through kids! I do a lot of peer education at Devyn's preschool. All the children at her school know about her seizures, her special diet, and her medical alert dog. At the tender ages of four and five they seem more accepting of it all than their parents who try, but often fumble over the right words to say. —Heather P.

Teenage Recruits

Many people wonder if it is possible for an active teen to do MAD or the Ketogenic diet and the answer is a resounding yes; however, there are some points to carefully consider. Some of the difficulties in getting a teen to comply with diet therapy may have more to do with adolescent hormones than ketones, for this is an age when kids become very conscious of not standing out socially in an undesirable way. Even without seizures, teenagers typically struggle with issues of peer image and self-identity. The vagaries of social acceptance and the "what will my friends think" issue, along with differences in temperament, varying levels of impulse control and some kids' inherent resistance to structured oversight, all need to be factored in. Some kids are just at a stage in life where they don't want to be told what to do, period, and until they change their tune the diet may not be a viable option. However, if your teen is struggling with seizures, the prospect of controlling them can be a powerful incentive to give the diet a fair shot. You will have to discuss all this frankly and openly with your teenager, and make the decision together.

Presenting diet therapy as a challenge often resonates, because overcoming challenges is one of the ways we boost self-image and confidence. While sticking to a rigid diet is a tough assignment, the upside is that people who face such challenges may be better equipped to later tackle other difficulties life throws their way. Kids can develop resilience in even the most challenging situations if they are surrounded by supportive relationships and can form a positive image of themselves in their struggle.

Your teen is most likely going to have a lot of questions when considering the diet. Some teens, for instance, worry that eating so much fat will make them fat. The more they learn about the diet, the more their fears will likely vanish. Consuming more calories than your body needs, not eating fat per se, is what causes weight gain (unless there is fluid retention or other underlying problems that can be detected by your doctor with lab work). If there is a problem, it is a simple thing to slightly adjust calorie intake to slow unwanted weight gain.

When I first heard about the Modified Atkins Diet it seemed to me to be the most ridiculous diet that someone could recommend. High fat, low-carbohydrate, and low-glycemic foods were supposed to control my seizures? I can still remember the day when my dear mother told me how much fat I was going to be eating! Although for my whole I life I had been something of a skinny squirt, I began to imagine myself joining a sumo wrestling club within the next month. Thankfully, that didn't happen. With MAD, your body will burn fat instead of carbo- hydrates, so although I gained needed weight and muscle when going MAD (no pun intended), my worst nightmare of becom- ing a sumo wrestler never came to pass. —Jordan Riether, age 15, on MAD from age 12 to 14

If they do opt for diet therapy, some more flamboyant teen person- alities manage to embrace it and almost flaunt it to their peers. They turn down offers of chips and candy with righteous zeal and design T-shirts that proclaim, "Ketogenic Warrior!" Others prefer to stay under the social radar and avoid disclosing their diet therapy, or their epilepsy, to most people until they feel comfortable doing so. They simply explain they're "allergic" to certain foods, decline them when offered, and leave it at that.

If your teen has decided that discretion is the better part of valor, keep- ing a low profile is very possible when doing MAD. The diet can be managed easily in many restaurants once you learn to navigate a menu and scout out hidden carbs. You can show your young person how to look online for lists of acceptable choices at restaurants likely to be frequented with friends. Roast meat, chicken, or fish, or even a double cheeseburger with a side order of salad, will often work, (hold the bun, watch out for sauces, and check beforehand that the restaurant uses no high carb fillers to stretch the meat). (For more information on eating out while on a ketogenic diet, see Chapter 6, "On the Move.")

Keeping your teen well fueled and happy with the menu at home plays a big part in helping them avoid cheating while at school or out with friends. Think low-carb pizza, fried chicken, turnip fries, heavy cream smoothies, cheesecake, and other goodies. And if your teen is active in sports or other high calorie-burning activities you are going to have to provide regular snacks to grab when needed, because like all teenagers, they are likely to be hungry.

My teen son is in a fencing club and burns a lot of energy in his classes and competitions. While he was on MAD I had to keep his furnace really stoked with high fat and calorie-dense food. He couldn't grab a quick-fix snack of junk food like the other kids when hungry, but honestly, who wants that for their child, anyway? He tends to get woozy when hungry—once he keeled over after running laps when he hadn't had a good snack before class. So I kept a bag packed for him with some high energy

food like nuts, cheese, and tuna packed in oil in case of an
emergency hunger attack at the gym. —Jeanne Riether

March a Mile in *Their* Boots: Try Out Atkins Yourself

If you are being pummeled with fears that low-carb eating is tantamount
to condemning your child to purgatory, one eye-opening strategy is to try
going on the Atkins diet yourself for a time. There are numerous websites
dedicated to low-carb lifestyles, offering scads of recipes, strategies, chat
rooms, and support. Most of the people on these sites have chosen low-
carb eating to try to shed a few pounds and maintain a healthy weight, but
others do it to control blood sugar issues, and some do it just because they
feel better eating that way. The Atkins weight loss diet doesn't provide
anywhere near the amount of fat needed on the Ketogenic diet or MAD,
but the low-carb aspect of it will at least familiarize you with the basic
mechanics of it all. Realizing that many people without epilepsy choose
to live a low-carb lifestyle adds perspective. And if you don't particularly
like low-carb eating, then you can honestly tell your child what parents
have been telling their offspring for millennia, "This hurts me more than
it hurts you."

Eating Low Carb as a Family

If I could have done one thing differently when starting out,
it would have been to first go on the Atkins diet myself before
starting my son on MAD. When I switched to a low-carb diet,
it rather took me by surprise that I experienced what is com-
monly known as the "Atkins Flu." I never was a great fan of
sugars and starches and didn't think cutting them from my diet
would have much effect on me. Nevertheless, I still experienced
the mild complaints so many low-carb dieters initially report
for the first week or two. I felt lethargic, cranky, head-achy and
an all-around unhappy camper for a couple of weeks until my
body adjusted to ketosis. The same thing happened to my son,
but of course at the time I worried and fretted until he pulled
out of it. Doing it myself first would have helped me realize it
isn't the end of the world when our kids experience some physi-
cal adjustment when starting out on these types of diets, but we
should make allowances for them when they do.

*Also before I switched to low-carb eating myself, I nearly
wore myself out preparing different kinds of meals for each
member of my family. My 12-year-old son Jordan was doing
MAD, Jordan's older teenage brother was a "carbivore" who
needed his daily fix of starches, and I was trying to lose
weight, so was preparing low-calorie meals for myself.
It simplified things enormously when I started centering
family meals on Jordan's menu—meats, fish, eggs, salads,
and vegetable dishes for lunch and dinner. Of course I added
lots of extra fat to Jordan's meals, and adding a side dish
of potatoes, rice, noodles, or bread for his older brother who
wasn't eating low carb was easy enough to make and plan.
Doing Atkins together as a family eventually made the diet
feel more "normal" for us all, and I recommend it for those
starting their kids on MAD. —Jeanne Riether*

Courage under Fire

Sometimes, despite the best of your intentions to make the diet work, you
hit a rough patch. Maybe your child is cranky and sick, maybe you're sick
yourself, maybe you just dropped the new expensive blender on the floor
and cracked it, or maybe you're exhausted and discover your spouse ate
your child's dinner by mistake. Whatever the reason, today you are feeling the hit. The accumulated stress and the continuous tasks of cooking,
measuring, shopping, label reading, and coaxing your child to eat suddenly
seem overwhelming. Or maybe you are a teen or adult with epilepsy on the
diet and you feel you just cannot keep on eating this way one more day.
You break down and partake of some "forbidden fruit" even though you
know a one-time cheat may result in more than a one day loss of seizure
control. If this happens to you, take heart, for you aren't the only one who's
been there.

*One time, my son was on one of his "starvation" kicks. He
would do this frequently on the diet, eat the bare minimum.
When he would do this he would be an emotional wreck as he
was hungry but yet, not eat the food I would give him. I lost it. I
was in tears and wanted to give up the diet. We ended up lowering his ratio and things got better for a while. —Amy, mother of
child on the Ketogenic diet*

One day when I just didn't have the willpower, a friend gave in and bought me a hamburger, french fries, and apple pie from McDonald's. I was begging for it and in the mindset that if I was going to screw up I was going to do it big (it was within a month of starting the diet). I had horrible seizures and had a hard time gaining back control. I learned my lesson, and so did he, the hard way. Don't give in when I whine about wanting carbs. —Heidi, adult with epilepsy on MAD

I bought raw almonds in bulk to use for grinding our own almond flour. I mixed some in a batch for microwave pancakes, tasted the batter, and realized it was incredibly bitter. Great, I thought, I bought bitter almonds by mistake! I added triple the amount of flavored Stevia to mask the taste, popped them in the oven, and when they were done I gave one to my son. As an afterthought I decided to check online to see if bitter almonds have the same carb count as regular almonds and was I in for a shock. Raw bitter almonds are not even sold in the U.S. (we live in China) because they contain cyanide, and in an uncooked state they are extremely poisonous! I panicked. I had micro-waved the pancake for several minutes, but was that enough to destroy the poison? We frantically called the hospital and several doctors, who honestly didn't know, said if he had any signs of nausea or pain within the next hour to bring him in immediately to have his stomach pumped. We didn't tell my son what was going on, but watched him like a hawk. I kept my cool for the next two hours while we waited, and when it was obvi-ous he was just fine, I went into the next room, quietly closed the door, and had an emotional meltdown. All my fear, panic, dread, and guilt seemed to erupt in one sobbing, quivering lava flow. It became a family legend. We try to laugh about it now, but I still can't think about bitter almonds without feeling kind of teary-eyed. —Jeanne Riether, mother of child on MAD

Mistakes happen. Sometimes you will feel discouraged and not want to do this anymore. The best thing to do when that happens is realize that the decision to quit diet therapy should not be made on a whim, and definitely not at midnight while sitting on the kitchen floor with tears streaming down your face because your efforts at batch cooking all just went up in smoke.

Sometimes just a good night's sleep can set things right. Rationally weigh the pros and cons of diet therapy. Has there been improvement in seizure control? Maybe you've lost one skirmish but are still winning the war. Have you given the diet enough time to work or are you frustrated by not seeing immediate dramatic results? Sometimes, it just takes time—weeks or months for some—until they see improvement. Are there things you can do to make all this easier on yourself? Do you need help from a friend or relative? More sleep? A night off? Do you need more varied meals, desserts, or some low-carb comfort food so that it isn't so hard to stick to the diet? Cut yourself some slack for being human, but try to find solutions that will work for you. And give yourself a big pat on the back for having made it this far. You're doing great.

Dealing with "Crazy Makers"

Sometimes in the war against seizures you may have to take cover from snipers. Thankfully, most people will be supportive of your effort to do a ketogenic diet, but when you encounter a sniper, be ready. Who are they? The relatives who invite you to Thanksgiving or Christmas dinner but insist on setting out platters of forbidden food and desserts on low tables within reach of your young child; the scoffing grandparent who dismisses a ketogenic diet as some sort of health fad; the clueless sister-in-law who brings your child a present of giftwrapped candy and then remembers "Oh that's right, you don't allow the poor thing to eat sweets. But maybe just this once wouldn't hurt?" Besides relatives, such "friendly fire" can also come from neighbors, teachers, friends, acquaintances, and everybody from the school janitor to the lady who runs the corner deli. Everybody seems to have an opinion about ketogenic diets, whether they know anything about it or not. Some may be quite pointed in their assault, expressing their concern that your child is "obviously not being put on proper medication." Others minimize your struggle with comments like, "I was on a diet once and lost 20 pounds. Dieting isn't so hard if you just have willpower."

Dana, mother of a child on MAD, describes this struggle:

I found the constant drain to be too much, trying to make people respect the diet, or educating people about the diet, or conversely having teachers and aides resent the diet and thus try to find ways to get back at us because of the extra work of the diet. Unfortunately, my son lost his older, hardworking teacher who did not mind the extra work and got a young fresh out-of-college teacher who really was not interested in doing anything beyond the bare essentials. The drain of educating people is real, and being the poster child all the time for the diet is like living inside the fish bowl. It's easy when you are not having any troubles, but very tough when you are working through a rough spell.

While you may occasionally get flack from people who don't understand Ketogenic diet therapy, it can also be all too easy to read judgment or disapproval into people's reactions that isn't really there. This is especially true when first starting out, when you are unsure of yourself and battling your own insecurities.

I wish I had picked up the phone or had more face-to-face conversations than relying on assumptions I made when I was feeling overwhelmed and vulnerable. I was so eager for validation and encouragement that I couldn't handle even neutral reactions. I adopted an "either you are behind me or you are not" mentality…it was too black and white. I know now that people need time to absorb information and collect their own data. —Heather P. Mother of a child on MAD

What can you do when you genuinely meet crazy makers who snipe at your efforts? Take a deep breath. Relax. Yes, it is frustrating, and yes, there will be times when the people around you…Just. Don't. Get. It. Remind yourself that it's usually ignorance, not cruelty. Choose your battles. If it's a well-meaning friend or relative uttering a thoughtless comment, it may be best to just let it pass. If someone is actually undermining your child's diet at school or home, be prepared to fight. Afterwards you can vent to your friends on your online ketogenic or MAD support group if needed. The people there will most likely have their own tales to tell. Educate when you can. If people choose to cling to their ignorance, shrug your shoulders and press the delete tab on the keyboard of your mind. Affirm your choices. Celebrate every little step forward. And remember, it's all going to be OK.

Siblings of Diet Warriors: In Pursuit of Justice

Kids constantly compare, and the attention you naturally invest in caring for a child with seizures who is on diet therapy can rankle with brothers and sisters at times. There is a certain stage in child development when "fairness" becomes something of a moral compass for kids. Granted, for young children "fair" is directly linked to their own self-interest, so many kids pursue justice like a prosecuting attorney if favoritism is suspected. To add to the drama, when kids find out they can use food as a dandy new device to aggravate their brother or sister, some Oscar-worthy performances may result. Your child may not even like being on the diet, but will suddenly rhapsodize over every bite of whipped cream when the others are looking. The non-dieter may retaliate by slyly pulling a bag of chips from under the table like a concealed weapon. No matter who started it, if the comparing war is escalating on your home turf, consider some of the following strategies:

- **Talk about it:** Don't explode when the drama starts. Instead, call a family counsel and remind everyone you're in this together. Talk about annoying behavior and try to negotiate a truce.

- **Love spelled T-I-M-E:** As the old saying goes, kids measure love by the amount of time you spend with them. As concerned as you may be for your child's medical condition and the time it takes you to invest in the diet, don't neglect giving your other children the personal attention they need and crave. Rotate "special time" so no one is left out.

- **Common pot:** When you're eating together as a family, it helps to center a meal around a dish everyone can eat, whether on the diet or not. Some easy-to-adapt meals can be chicken dishes, hamburgers, ribs, and steak, etc.

- **Reinforcement and rewards:** If you are using rewards and incentives for your child on the diet, try to arrange similar incentives for your other kids. Pick some behavior you'd like to encourage and reward them for their efforts. Kids usually respond well to this kind of motivation when you make it fun.

- **Super heroes:** As a sibling of a diet warrior, your child will undoubtedly make some personal sacrifices for the greater good. Let him know he is like a super hero who keeps seizures at bay by helping a brother or sister stick to their diet therapy. Enlist him in being a secret "guardian of the diet" who works behind the scenes, no longer eating high carb treats in his sibling's view. Acknowledge and reward his self-sacrifice, and encourage him in his secret role.

3
Calling All Comrades

Enlisting Help

Inherent challenges come with everything BIG and important in life. But keep this in mind as you continue reading about beginning diet therapy: both the authors of this book learned to make diet therapy work for our families, and our children found wonderful seizure control.

Beginning diet therapy, especially the Ketogenic diet, is similar to bringing another baby into the family, but without the joyous final moments of pregnancy. Before beginning diet therapy, you are likely at your wits' end, desperate, and possibly heartbroken that nothing has cured your child's seizures after myriad drug trials. Regardless of your situation before beginning diet therapy, the days after your return home from the hospital initiation—or after you've kicked out carbs and begun MAD—barely resemble the days before it all began.

In the hospital, while your child fasts and learns to eat new foods at a high-fat ratio for the first time, you learn how to navigate through the world of dietary therapy. You're taught to use a gram scale and calculate foods. You might hear from parents about how well their children did on the diet, and hopefully, you're full of that positive anxiety that comes with being excited and scared at the same time, because you know you're doing something BIG.

Just as when you carried your swaddled newborn into your home for the first time, everything you think you know seems to go right out the window. You will likely fumble with the scale and weigh two and three meals, though only one might survive from the kitchen to the dining table. Your son—who ate so well in the hospital that his doctor raved—suddenly decides he wants nothing to do with the Miracle Noodle macaroni and cheese meal you just spent your last hour's-worth of energy making. You steal away to the bathroom where you stare in the mirror, scream just loud enough that you—and only you—can hear, and then you fake a smile and say, "I can do this."

You somehow manage to convince your son that eating his macaroni and cheese would impress Buzz Lightyear, or the whole roster of Disney/Pixar characters for that matter, and with one meal under your belt, you are feeling better. I got this, you think. You check his ketones, help him brush his teeth with his low-carb toothpaste, and you are minutes away from the end of your first day. As dad puts the kids to bed, you calculate a couple of your son's new meals with the online meal program, KetoCalculator. What you thought would be a ten-minute deal ends up taking you an hour because you didn't know where to find peanuts (Are they a fat or protein? Are they under P or N for nut?), and you had a minor panic attack when you weren't sure whether your heavy whipping cream was 36% or 40%. Dad orders pizza because he's figured out that you're not cooking dinner. The pizza is cold before you get to it, but you're so hungry that you eat a cold slice as you stand and weigh out tomorrow's breakfast. You wash about ten small plastic bowls that you used to weigh all the ingredients, flashing back to nights that were bogged down cleaning baby bottles and rubber nipples.

With all of the next day's meals weighed and labeled, the kitchen clean, and your shirt soaking with stain remover because you spilled oil on it, you call it a day and fall into bed. You open one eye to see your husband laughing. You realize then that you forgot to undress. Three hours into your sleep, you wake not to the sound of a hungry newborn, but to a fear that forces you out of bed: did you weigh 10 or 12 grams of macadamia nuts in his banana muffins? And which was it supposed to be? You find your way into the kitchen and turn on the light above the stove. You read the recipe card twice. You try to imagine yourself at the scale. You look in the fridge at those tiny Tupperware containers. You decide that, of course, you weighed the right amount. An hour later, after thinking of every new recipe you can concoct in your mind, you finally fall asleep.

The previous scenario is fictional and not an indication of how everyone's first day home from a ketogenic diet initiation will go. (And you can probably laugh at some parts of it now if you're looking back on how you started.) What you can derive from the story, however, is that once the Ketogenic diet, and even MAD, enter your life, your days will change dramatically. This period of adjustment won't last forever, and thankfully after some time you will once again carve out familiar routines and a new sense of normal. Your sleep patterns will change, your free time might disappear for a while, and everything will be covered in oil, equaling more dish time and laundry time—just like bringing a new baby home.

While this section is not meant to overwhelm you and send you running from pursuing diet therapy, we want you to have a clear understanding of what's in store. Both the Ketogenic diet and MAD require thought, organization, time, patience, and a strong support system. In addition to finding the perfect Keto Team with which to partner on this journey, you should bring as many other people on board as possible. This includes your spouse and the rest of the immediate family, but in addition, consider grandparents, friends, even close neighbors. With a little creativity you can have your own Keto Team at your fingertips.

In the early days, when you are still finding your feet and you wonder how other parents possibly manage, cling to this thought: three months from now you'll be over the novice hump. Six months from now you'll have found a comfortable groove. Much of what is now a halting, nerve-wracking process will eventually become second nature. You'll figure out tricks and time-savers and establish patterns, just as new parents learn to care for a newborn. Life is going to go back to "normal," a new normal that may give your child a chance at seizure control.

In order to give you a better idea of how time consuming these diets can be, particularly when you are first learning the ropes, and to show you that you can become more proficient as time goes on, below are the daily schedules of three Keto moms. We asked moms at different points in the classic Ketogenic diet to provide us with a daily schedule of everything they do, diet related or not, in order to show how much of their day is taken up by the demands of diet therapy. As you read, note how each mom manages her time differently and how it's clear that over the course of time, they become more organized, systematic, and efficient.

Phase One: Just Starting Out—When Managing the Diet Seems to Take All Your Time, Thought, and Effort

The Novice. Lori's son Sam is four years old and has been on the Ketogenic diet for less than three months. In addition to Sam, Lori has a two-year-old boy, Finley, and is pregnant with her third child. She shares, quite candidly, what her days are like now that she's brought Keto into their lives.

7:00 a.m.: Wake up and make coffee for myself even though I am eight months pregnant, but need it! Eat a piece of toast as I empty the dishwasher, which currently gets run two times a day because the Keto diet is causing us to go through so many dishes.

7:30 a.m.: *Measure ingredients for son's favorite breakfast. Let chickens out and take a shower. Get Sam out of pjs, measure urine ketones, make his breakfast.*

8:30 a.m.: *As Sam eats I prep his morning meds. Sam finishes breakfast and then takes meds. I record meal, meds, and ketones on our kitchen chart. Husband wakes up with Finley and makes the rest of us breakfast.*

9:15 a.m.: *Clean up from breakfast and finish getting boys ready.*

9:30 a.m.: *Start prepping and measuring Sam's snack, which he is already starting to ask about because he is ALWAYS hungry. Try not to forget about making Finley something as well to take with us to the park... something kind of like what Sam is eating, something that Sam won't realize is totally different from what he is eating. Oh yes, and I need something for myself too.*

10:00 a.m.: *Load boys and snacks up into the car and drive to a park for some playtime. Can't distract Sam who wants his snack. Give him his three free olives.*

10:15 a.m.: *Play at the park.*

10:40 a.m.: *As soon as the timer on my phone goes off, feed the boys their snacks. Continue to play at the park. Drink lots of water.*

11:30 a.m.: *Sam is asking for lunch. Do what I can to distract him at the park. Wait until noon to leave.*

12:20 p.m.: *Arrive home from the park. Sam is begging for food. Make him a "snow cone" to calm him down until it is time for him to be able to eat again. Measure out Sam's lunch. Make Finley's lunch.*

12:45 p.m.: *Boys eat lunch. Clean up.*

1:00 p.m.: *Get boys ready for naps. Storytime. Boys nap. I lay down for 15 minutes to rest my pregnant body. Then I realize that since I am pregnant I need to feed myself something, otherwise this Keto diet would be a great way to lose some weight!*

2:00 p.m.: *Get on the computer. E-mail dietitian. Work on creating some recipes at our new ratio and calorie level. Search Charlie Foundation website. Go through ketogenic Yahoo! group e-mails for recipe ideas and for greater knowledge about the diet itself. Create a new recipe or two. E-mail these to dietitian. Catch up on other e-mail and household responsibilities. Talk to a friend. Cry.*

4:00 p.m.: *Sam wakes up. Prep his snack and feed him snack plus mid-day meds. Finley wakes up. Playtime inside or outside. Finley is grouchy...I guess I need to feed him a snack, but how do I do this without Sam wanting more food too? Give Finley a snack and tell Sam he already had his and remind him of the yummy mac "n" cheese he will get for dinner. Offer Sam some sparkling juice water for now. Play with the boys. Load up the dishwasher again. Throw in some laundry. A friend drops off a meal for John and I—dinner is set for us.*

6:00 p.m.: *Start making Sam his dinner. Try to also make something for Finley that is similar. Grateful for frozen mac "n" cheese from Trader Joe's for Finley.*

6:30 p.m.: *Boys eat dinner even though John doesn't get home until 7:00 p.m. That is when we used to eat as a family, but Sam can't wait any longer. Boys eat together.*

7:00 p.m.: *John gets home. John and I eat. We turn on* Thomas & Friends *even though we used to never put TV on for the boys. We just don't know what to do to distract Sam while we eat because he wants our food too.*

7:30 p.m.: *I am off child duty and John is on. But I still need to prep Sam's last snack of the day and get the meds ready. John plays with the boys while I clean up from dinner.*

8:15 p.m.: *John does bathtime, snack with Sam, meds, measures ketones, updates chart, storytime, and bedtime with the boys. I go to Trader Joe's and Whole Foods to get some cream and other things I need for Sam's diet.*

10:00 p.m.: *Try to measure out some things for the next day but I am so tired so I just go to sleep. John unloads the clean dishes and loads the dishwasher back up with the dirty dishes that are piled up again in the sink.*

Lori's schedule illustrates how not only does her day seem to be filled with either making or feeding her son Keto meals, but the emotional impact of having her son on the diet is constant. She must consider in every circumstance how to make this transition easy for Sam, while sticking strictly to the diet. Even when Lori isn't actively doing anything that involves Keto, such as playing at the park with her boys, she is thinking about the diet, anticipating her next move, and how she will navigate those challenges. This is normal and should be expected in the first couple months. For some, this period might even last longer, depending on any diet changes that the

Keto Team decides upon. Lori, however, is quite fortunate to have a husband who is so hands-on with the diet. Later in this chapter you will learn how to best utilize those who are willing to help you, just as Lori has done.

Next we'll show you two moms who have been doing this for a while. Though they're busy, they've developed time and stress-saving strategies that make the diet fit well for their families.

Phase Two: Hitting Your Stride—When You've Settled into a Busy but Familiar Routine

The Expert. Ashley is a single mom whose seven-year-old son, Aiden, has been on the diet for just over a year. Previous to beginning the Ketogenic diet, Aiden was on MAD for a year. Ashley has learned over the last couple years how to really manage her time. Though Ashley and Aiden live with Ashley's mom, who helps out considerably, Ashley is the sole Keto administrator. Below is the schedule of a typical weekday.

6:00 a.m.: Get up and put out Aidan's breakfast (already made the previous night), his meds, and his supplements. Finish the prep on his lunch for the day. Make sure he is dressed and ready for school.

7:00 a.m.: Leave and take my mother and Aidan to school and work.

8:00 a.m.–9:00 a.m.: Volunteer at the library at Aidan's school.

9:15 a.m.–12:00 p.m.: Batch cooking for things like chili or spaghetti sauce. Once these are done I put them in containers that have been labeled with all accompanying ingredients and freeze so that I always have these on hand, as chili, and spaghetti are very popular meals. Meanwhile I usually have laundry going during this time as well.

12:00 p.m.: Clean house, and other assorted chores that need to be taken care of.

1:00 p.m.: Lunch for me. Then I try to relax for a bit.

2:00 p.m.: Go to the grocery store and run any other errands that need to be done before picking up Aidan from school. (This is done after planning meals with Aiden over the weekend and making a shopping list of everything I don't already have.)

3:15 p.m.: Get home from picking up Aidan from school and give him his snack.

4:00 p.m.: Start dinner prep. Also work on Aidan's homework with him while doing dinner prep. This generally involves doing spelling words, listening to him read to me, etc.

5:30 p.m.: Serve Aidan his dinner and eat my dinner at around 6 p.m.

6:30 p.m.: Pick my mom up from work.

7:00 p.m.: Get Aidan in the shower.

7:15 p.m.: Give Aidan his meds and evening supplements.

7:30 p.m.: Aidan's bedtime. Read him a chapter from whatever book we happen to be reading (or listen to him read me the chapter).

8:00 p.m.: Breakfast and lunch prep for the next day. Also, this is my time to calculate and plan new meals.

10:00 p.m.: Catch up on whatever shows I happen to have sitting in my DVR.

11:00 p.m.: Bedtime for me.

Unlike Lori's days, Ashley's days are a little less defined by Aiden's diet. Over a period of time, Ashley learned that she could have easier days during the week if she batched foods on the weekends. "Batch" cooking is when you prepare multiple meals at the same time. This is particularly easy with all-in-one recipes that blend well, such at the flax bread from the Charlie Foundation. On a typical weekend, Ashley spends about eight hours creating meals and snacks for the week. She makes Keto lollipops (a great way to give fat), and other snacks or meals that freeze well. She uses a lot of berries for Aiden's meals so she weighs out his fruit in advance and freezes them in 2-ounce portion cups in the fridge. She also chops veggies and bags them. This cuts back prep time during the week when her time is more crunched. For more time saving tricks like Ashley has utilized, read Feeding an Army: Batching and Making Meals in Advance, in Chapter 4, "The Mess Hall."

The Professional. Abbie is a ten-year-old girl who started having seizures only a couple years ago. Like many other children, she did not respond well to drugs, so her mother, Heather, took her to Johns Hopkins for the Ketogenic diet. Abbie has now been on the diet for two years. Because Abbie has responded so well to diet therapy, her neurologist thinks she might be on diet therapy for life. Needless to say, Heather has become a professional at creating meals and measuring food, and will likely be more adept than anyone else in the years to come.

5:30 a.m.: I wake up, shower, get dressed, and put on makeup.

6:02 a.m.: In the sink are the oil-covered cups and containers from Abbie's meals the day before. I unload and load the dishwasher.

6:05 a.m.: *I start the meals for Abbie's day. Abbie has chosen a "milk-shake" for breakfast, ham rollups for lunch, and a "milkshake" snack. The KetoCalculator is bookmarked and ready for action. Luckily, I already know the milkshake recipe. It takes about five minutes to weigh the two containers for her milkshakes.*

6:15 a.m.: *Kirby is dressed and waiting as patiently as a seven-year-old boy can for his breakfast. Kirby chats with me as I look up Abbie's ham rollup recipe on the KetoCalculator. I weigh the ham, lettuce, cream, and oil. It all gets loaded along with the milkshakes into a mini cooler with two skinny ice packs. In about 10 to 15 minutes, I have created three fabulous meals for the day!*

6:20–6:45 a.m.: *During this time I might do the following: laundry, check e-mail/Facebook, decide about dinner and pull that out of the freezer, check my teacher bag and load the car for the day, and most importantly, I eat whatever I can grab.*

6:45 a.m.: *I wake up Abbie and get her dressed.*

7:00 a.m.: *I leave because I have to be to school by 7:30 a.m. Kirby rides with me to school. Daddy takes care of the rest of Abbie's morning routine.*

What happens with Daddy?

7:00 a.m.: *Breakfast. Abbie takes her required pills.*

7:07 a.m.: *Abbie brushes her teeth with baking soda.*

7:55 a.m.: *Daddy drops Abbie off at school.*

8:00 a.m.–3:00 p.m.: *I am in my classroom teaching. I know that Abbie will have a great day because we have a health plan in place to address all of it, including what to do if she has seizure activity of any sort, if she needs to use the bathroom, and how to make sure that her lunch is consumed and checked by the health room staff.* (For more about Abbie's health plan and IEP, read Chapter 7, "Warriors at School.")

11:00 a.m.: *Abbie eats lunch. After she has eaten her meal she is walked to the nurse's office/health room. In the health room her meal is checked and scraped with a spatula by a member of the health team to ensure that she consumes every last bit. It is recorded in her daily logbook that is sent home with her.*

2:40 p.m.: *School is dismissed. Her fourth grade teacher walks Abbie to the childcare center that is housed in our school.*

3:00 p.m.: *Abbie drinks her snack.*

4:15–4:30 p.m.: *I pick up Abbie and Kirby from daycare. They share stories about their day.*

4:30 p.m.: *I sign Abbie's daily logbook to indicate I have seen that her meals were finished and if she went to the nurse that day for anything beyond her usual activity.*

5:45 p.m.: *Start making our family dinner. Normally, Abbie will have a Keto version of what we are eating.*

6:00 p.m.–6:15 p.m.: *My husband is home from work. He makes Abbie's dinner. He has decided he wants to make Abbie's meals. YIPPEE! Let me tell you that it has taken over a year for me to give up control of measuring the food. After I allowed him to do it a few times I realized that he can actually make the meals, which takes a lot of the pressure off me.*

7:00 p.m.: *Dinner.*

7:45 p.m.: *Bathtime.*

8:15–8:30ish p.m.: *Bedtime! My husband or I read Abbie a book or she reads to us. We tuck her in, kiss her good night, and wish her sweet dreams. Dreaming is one of the things that she says she misses the most from having seizures. Then we move on to Kirby's room and do the same thing.*

9:30 p.m.: *Bed. I am lying in bed awake thinking about how much cream I have in the refrigerator and if I will need to stop at the store after school tomorrow. I, of course, get up to check. Old habits are hard to break.*

Beginning the Ketogenic diet or MAD is so time consuming in the beginning because it's not just a new way to think about food (i.e., fat is good, carbs are bad), but preparing food, from recipe creation to the prep work, is not a "normal" anyone has experience with. While beginning MAD is easier in some ways because protein is not restricted, calories aren't as closely monitored, and there is no gram scale, there is still a steep learning curve; just learning how to read a book on counting carbs, distinguishing between net carbs, and learning where to find hidden carbs is still a very daunting experience for many parents.

As you read in Chapter 2, "Boot Camp," the emotional commitment you make in the beginning of this diet is the fuel that will help you get through the early stages. Had Lori, our novice, not made the heartfelt and courageous decision to put her son on the Ketogenic diet, her final days of her third pregnancy might have had more free time, but she wouldn't go to bed each night with the satisfaction that she is doing everything possible to help her son. In a few months, as she adjusts to making meals and her son adjusts to a different kind of food, they will no doubt be able to go to the playground and run around without lunch looming before her. In the early days it truly feels like life revolves around food: what to make, how to make it, when to make it, when to feed it, how long your child takes to eat it, and cleaning up, with oil spills and degreaser a more integral part of your life than you could ever have imagined.

These early months are similar to those first days of feeding a newborn. From the moment the baby begins to feed, you are essentially counting down the two hours until the next feeding. By the time Baby has finished with his first feeding, perhaps because he fell asleep for 20 minutes in the process, you have only an hour before it's time to begin all over again. As days go on and weeks turn into months, the time between feedings is greater and Baby is a more accomplished eater, eating three times as much as he did in the beginning, but in half the time. The same holds true for ketogenic diets. Eventually you build a collection of recipes your child loves and you're not spending time creating recipes on the KetoCalculator every night. Or, you're not constantly jotting down carb amounts and measuring every bit of food that passes through your child's lips. Around the same time, you learn to recognize what a gram looks and feels like, so when you weigh your food it takes only moments. You figure out what foods to cook on the weekends, and with an hour or two here or there, you're saving countless minutes during the week. And best of all, your child has embraced his new diet and eats his meals quickly, or at least without a fight—most of the time.

The universal truth—no matter who you ask, no matter their history, their child's history, their love of cooking food—is that these diets are tough in the beginning. The miracles, big and small, make every gram of carbohydrate you count worth it. Just prepare yourself for the fight, including the long, hard days in the beginning, and know that in time the battle will become less daunting, and your time in the kitchen will dwindle as well.

The Importance of Seeking Help

When we first began writing this book we polled some of the online support groups to find out how parents were getting help from their families and friends. Surprisingly, most people who responded admitted that they had little help and that everything diet related fell under their jurisdiction of responsibility. Ideally, you are reading this book *before* starting on one of these dietary journeys, and we might have the chance to show you how significant it is to have a support team that you can rely on. In Chapter 2, "Boot Camp," we explained how your family's support is essential to your emotional resilience and, ultimately, to your child's success on this diet. But family and friends are not just there for emotional reassurance and stability; they can provide you with an incredible amount of help, from actually assisting you in preparing food to managing the house so that you can do at least one of the 300 things on your ever growing To Do list.

You might wonder why we're pressing the issue of enlisting people to help when we already told you that so many moms are doing the diet on their own. Quite frankly, just because that's how the majority of people seem to do it doesn't make it the best choice for you or your family. When managing these diets, especially if you're Mom—the one who seems to manage everything already—the weight of responsibility can be crushing. When, for instance, you have been up since 5:30 a.m. to prep your child's breakfast, followed by a long day at work, homework time with the kids, weighing out dinner, prepping meals for the next day, and doing everyone's laundry, the last thing that will be healthy for you on a physical or emotional level is to stay up until 11:00 p.m. weighing meals, creating meals on the KetoCalculator, or catching up on other chores while your significant other catches up on TV. This is not to say that it is always the mom who does the diet, because it isn't, and it certainly wouldn't be fair to assume that Dad gets an easy ride. However, as ever-present members of two online forums with hundreds of members, over time it has become abundantly clear that many, if not most, women are not only managing the diet nearly entirely on their own, but it is a struggle that weighs heavily on every relationship in their lives, and at the very least it exhausts them.

> *I did the diet by myself. Mike helped only if I was sick or when I had surgery and he had no choice. I can't really explain why he did this. He doesn't cook at all or bake so that probably played a part. In addition, because of that I don't think he really understood how the diet worked. He would mess recipes up and I would get so angry that I think it was just a silent acknowledgment that it was up to me. It has played a difficult part in our marriage. No doubt about that. Our families are in Chicago and were of no help either. I felt very alone and angry to have to save my son all by myself. —Amy*

Amy was also featured in Chapter 2 when we discussed how these diets affect significant relationships in your life, especially marriage. She is one of few moms who have been brutally honest about the challenges these diets have brought into their daily lives, yet she isn't alone in her feelings, as is evident in the questions posted on the various online support groups.

Aside from the physical exhaustion of preparing nearly 30 meals and snacks a week on your own for your warrior, you still make dinner for your other kids, and keep up with all the responsibilities you held before diet therapy entered your life. When things are going well for your child, going it alone doesn't seem impossible. When you've created some great meals, he's eating them, and seizures are improved, the Keto life can feel good. But when things are tough, going it alone is harder than you can imagine.

My son wanted ice cream for dessert tonight. I made the recipe, I made the ice cream...I got it all set. My other son spilled it all over my carpet (did I mention it was chocolate?). I got so mad at everyone. I'm mad at my eight-year-old who left his bowl on the floor to go to the bathroom. I'm mad at my ten-year-old for not watching where he is going. I'm mad at the world because it took forever to make and with one kick, it is all gone. My husband just says, "It's ok, he can have something else," but he just doesn't understand that means I have to make something else. I have to start over with another recipe and weigh everything else out. I'm so tired of my stupid scale. I'm so tired of having to weigh every single thing. I'm so tired of having to stop what I'm doing each time he wants a snack. I'm just so tired of the time all of this is taking. —Shannon

Shannon is in a classic stage of frustration. It began with something seemingly small (the spilt ice cream), but because the stakes are so high and she is clearly exhausted and overwhelmed by the stress of the diet, the ice cream spilling becomes a trigger for a bigger emotional explosion. This will happen to everyone at some point in time (unless you're perfect), so the fact that Shannon needed to vent is not an issue. The bigger issue is the fact that she feels her husband doesn't understand the weight of his suggestion. Replacing a spilled dessert or meal on diet therapy is not necessarily a quick and simple task. It takes time and thought. For a parent with a great deal on her plate already, a simple suggestion from a partner who isn't intimately involved in the process can feel clueless and insensitive, despite the potential good intentions of the spouse.

When both parents are involved with the diet, with each parent having an understanding of what is expected of them, the battles in the kitchen will be less overwhelming. Moments of sheer frustration and days of wishing the diet away will still happen, but the support system you've created inside your own house, both on a tangible and an emotional level, will decrease the duration of those jaw-clenching moments. Because we are not all accustomed to sharing such a great responsibility, the following section outlines several creative ways to get our spouses involved—and hopefully, some other family members or friends.

Creative Ideas for a Crowd

- **Cooking parties:** This is something you could do with a few of your closest friends or family members. The key here is to have people you trust. It's true that the Mama Bears in the epilepsy community have a hard time letting go of control, but quite frankly, weighing food is a pretty easy task that most people can do well if carefully instructed. If you don't trust anyone else to weigh but you, others can do the prep work. One can chop all the veggies or fruit, another can stir the batches of recipes, and one could even work on cleaning the gazillion little plastic containers so the kitchen doesn't swallow you whole. Serve some light snacks or even open a bottle of wine—if you dare.

- **Ice cream socials:** Have your spouse, or another close family member who understands the diet, take the kids out to an ice cream shop for sundaes. Make your warrior his sundae in advance and bring it along in a cooler. While the kids are distracted picking their ice cream flavors or choosing their seat, the adult can assemble the sundae in one of the shop's ice cream cups. While the kids are out of the house and you're left with some peace and quiet, you can catch up on weighing food or on other household chores.

- **Play dates:** Play dates have always been just as much for the moms as the kids. Moms need companionship, especially when you've been inundated with screaming kids and all your conversations begin with "no." If you have a close friend you trust and you've explained how your child's diet works, have a play date at your house, with the caveat that it will be a mom's working play date. While the kids are playing together (assuming they're of the age that they don't need constant supervision), both moms can do some prep work in the kitchen. You could batch a month's worth of chocolate chip cookies for your warrior, and as a reward, toss in some ready-to-bake chocolate chip cookie dough so the other kids can share in the fun. Or you could batch several pizza crusts and afterwards, have a pizza party for the kids. If your friend is extra gracious—and really, most are when they understand what you're taking on—your friend might offer to do this again!

■ **Romantic dinner dates:** This takes romance to a new level, and not a level that most of us parents ever really saw ourselves going. But why not order some take-out Chinese food or a local New York-style pizza, light a couple candles for ambiance, pop open a bottle of wine, and make some meals together? It will give you both a chance to have some quality time together, something that is often lost with these diets, and in the meantime, you can knock out at least a dozen meals in two hours' time. A note to the Mama Bears who have a hard time letting go: it will be tough, but once you've taught your husband the most efficient way to weigh, you have to let go and let him do his thing. This is a great recipe for success, but it's also a great way to squabble when Mom and Dad don't have the same approach to food preparation, so be prepared to be patient with each other.

■ **Get the kids involved:** This is one of those suggestions that won't save you on time, but it will give you a chance to educate your kids and turn what can be a tedious activity into a family-centered learning activity. Kids love to get involved in the kitchen, whether it's stirring a batter or measuring the ingredients. Obviously, the age of your children will affect the tasks you allow them to do, but consider letting them fill the measuring cups with chopped veggies or fruit (for MAD dieters), spreading peanut butter and butter into celery boats, or grating cheese. If your child is responsible enough, you can even have him weigh some foods on the gram scale. This activity will be a great confidence builder for your warrior, as it will give him a chance to contribute to his diet and it will help him to take ownership of it. It will give your other children a greater understanding of their sibling's diet while giving them quality time with their parent.

For those parents who believe in the "too many cooks in the kitchen" concept, there are other ways that your spouse or older children, even other family members, can help.

■ **Recipe brainstorming:** Check out a bunch of low-carb cookbooks from the library and have a family member peruse the book looking for recipes that could be converted into a Keto or MAD recipe. Provide a few basic parameters of what to look for, such as recipes that have a lot of butter, milk (to be replaced with cream), nuts, soft cheeses, eggs, or recipes that use low-carb veggies such as zucchini, spinach, asparagus, and spaghetti squash. Once they've tagged several recipes, you can convert them in the KetoCalculator or by hand if you're doing MAD.

■ **Redistributing other chores:** It's fair enough to say that you trust your spouse or other family members to do other chores around the house more than weighing food. After all, we each know our limitations. If you're managing the diet, then your spouse can do all the laundry or the grocery shopping. Our professional, Heather Ewing's husband makes breakfast every morning. That is something he thrives on and is proud of, and it certainly takes the weight off Heather so she can get her son off to school and be to work on time herself. Try to find something your spouse is good at or at least is acclimated to, and give him responsibility of that chore.

Teamwork At Its Best

Bethany explains how she and her husband manage the diet together for their son Oliver, who has been on the diet for a year and a half.

> *When we first entertained the idea of doing the Ketogenic diet, my husband and I felt overwhelmed, to say the least. Luckily, we're very similar in our approach to Oliver's care and we were in total agreement that if we were going to the do the diet, we'd both be as educated as possible about it. We both read up on the diet over a month before we were even admitted to the hospital to get started. When we were in the hospital for the diet initiation, we had family come to town to help with our older son, so that we could both be present for our "Keto lessons" with our diet team. In the past 16 months on the diet, I've done the majority of the cooking for Oliver, mainly because I'm a more experienced cook than my husband, but also because I like the consistency approach to the diet. I feel it's good to have one person make the meals the same way, every time to maintain consistency in what Oliver is eating. My husband is a huge help in that he will keep both of our kids happy and entertained*

while I spend the hours in the kitchen making meals. He will also help with all of the prep on a daily basis by weighing out Oliver's milk, cream, and formula for his breakfast bottle. He weighs the MiraLAX Oliver takes on a daily basis to stay regular, cuts up his pills and places them in a pill holder, shreds cheese for meals, and any other prep work I ask him to do. When I am having a rough week or am just so tired of being the Keto chef, I can hand him the printed recipes and he will happily take over and make the meals for Oliver so that I can get a break. —Bethany

Erin, one of the co-authors of this book, has had great success utilizing her family members in order to make the diet as seamless as possible. Here is her story of how she learned to give up some of the responsibility for everyone's benefit:

My son suffered a traumatic brain injury at four and a half months old. He awoke from his second medically induced coma on his five-month birthday. For the first three months after his injury he was seizure free on phenobarbital. Once we weaned the phenobarbital the head drops began. A year later when we started the Ketogenic diet, though he had improved dramatically on the Modified Atkins Diet, he was still having around ten head drops a day. Because of the devastating circumstances surrounding his injury, our family life personified the "it takes a village" approach to raising our children. When we began the diet in August, 2010, Noah was 20 months and our little guy, Avry, was six months old. Both the grandmothers joined us for our hospital stay in order to give Mike and I a break on occasion, and so that Avry could spend time with his brother in the hospital room. We wanted so much for our family to have as much normalcy as possible, even in the tiny hospital room at Johns Hopkins.

We moved forward with the Ketogenic diet using this same community approach. Though I did all the research and continue to hold the vast amount of dietary information within my own head, and I'm the one who continues to be the "boss" of the diet, from the beginning I chose to ask for help. At first, like most of us epilepsy moms, I had a tough time letting go of the reins, probably because we epilepsy moms live a life where seizures steal any control we have, so we fight extra hard to keep what little control we can get our hands on. In the beginning no one was allowed to weigh food but me. But while I was weighing out meal after meal, either my mom or my mother-in-law helped with the babies. My mother-in-law, who is tirelessly optimistic and endlessly patient, often fed Noah his meals, which depending on this mood, could take an hour. Every bite was a challenge. The "moms," as I call them, helped me clean the house, they grocery shopped, they followed my instructions about the diet to the T, giving me greater faith in them as time went on.

At some point, I realized that it was pretty hard to mess up weighing food. So I taught them to weigh.

Eventually, when I went to work and one of the moms was watching the boys, I could leave the recipe cards in the kitchen and trust that Noah's meals would be made correctly and he would be fed correctly. If they had a question, they called. The fear of making a mistake kept them diligent, just like it does for most of us. I bought a scale for both of the moms to keep at their homes so that when we traveled it was one less item we had to trudge along with us. My mom even started making my egg soufflé recipe for me at home. It was one of those recipes that we considered an "old faithful" because Noah loved it, but it was also ten ingredients and had to be baked. Even when batching, it was time consuming. In my mom's free time she would make two or three egg soufflés for me and bring them over each week when she helped watch the kids. This saved me hours of time and I couldn't have been more thankful.

One of my favorite things that we did in the months before we moved farther away from "the moms" is we had cooking nights every couple months or so, depending on everyone's busy schedule. Both moms would come to my house, we'd open a bottle of wine, and after the boys were tucked into bed, we'd make up to 20 meals in a couple hours' time. Using two scales, we'd chop, weigh, mix, bake, pack, label, and freeze meals. It was a great chance to chat, enjoy each other's company, and best of all, when we were done I felt so uplifted and free. Those couple extra cooks in the kitchen made it so that I could get my son back without losing myself.

Finding Additional Support Resources

As you move forward with dietary therapy, you will likely realize that most people have a hard time understanding your child's diet. First of all, the whole concept of a high-fat diet is foreign to people, as it likely was to you only a short time ago. It's difficult to explain to other moms that your child eats more fat in a day than their children will likely consume in a month, not to mention the fact that your new heart-stopping fear of Goldfish crackers and cookie crumbs will probably seem overly dramatic to a lot of people. The friends and acquaintances who want to understand your child's diet will likely ask questions with a quizzical expression, but take their desire to learn about your child's diet as a great opportunity to give them a little insight into the daily grind of your life. In time you'll perfect a short little speech that you'll come to rely on.

While your friends might grow to understand the basics of these diets, the real challenge will come when you are having a bad day, or maybe even a string of bad days, and you're looking for someone to vent to. Sadly, even our friends with the greatest heart and the most genuine desire to understand will simply not be able to grasp the gravity of the emotions you're feeling. Despite their best intentions to commiserate by sharing their own stories of picky eaters, or how tough a gluten-free diet can be, there is a vast difference. This diet is your child's medicine. Your child's well-being is literally in your hands as you weigh out his meals, as you hover over him forcing him to eat, and yes, even when nothing you do seems to work. We are not suggesting in any way that your closest friendships are no longer valid—quite the contrary, they are still essential. However, you will find the greatest understanding, comfort, and encouragement from other parents who are trudging up the same rocky terrain as you. For this reason, we cannot emphasize enough the importance of finding other parents out there with whom to share your experiences, from the unexpected miracles to the days when all you can think about is quitting.

I signed onto the Yahoo group before we started Keto to get more facts on the day-to-day aspects of the diet that only parents/ caregivers could provide. I am very fortunate that my dietitian and neuro are very knowledgeable and supportive, but they aren't in the "trenches" like we are every day. The encouragement of others doing the day-to-day battle against seizures like we are is a treasure to me, nobody else "gets it" like these families do. —Laura

Below is a list of online support forums, with a short description of what you can expect to find there.

- **Charlie Foundation**, www.charliefoundation.org: The Charlie Foundation will become one of your go-to sites. Not only do they publish the full list of Keto-approved, low-carb products, they have recipe ideas and an online forum where parents can join to seek advice and share experiences. The Charlie Foundation helps support over 100 diet therapy programs worldwide. They recently organized and sponsored the Third International Symposium: Diet Therapies For Epilepsy and Other Neurological Disorders held in Chicago in the fall of 2012. The event was attended by 450 scientists, clinicians, and dietitians from thirty countries. The family day was attended by two hundred and fifty families. It was the largest event of this sort to date.

- **Matthew's Friends**, www.matthewsfriends.org: Emma Williams, a mom with a son who has Dravet syndrome, started this England-based group. Matthew's Friends has excellent resources and tips for those starting out, as well as forums for parents.

- **Yahoo! groups:** There are groups for both the Ketogenic diet and MAD on Yahoo!. Each group has members from across the world and have proven invaluable to both writers of this book. In fact, Jeanne is the founder and moderator of one of the recent active MAD groups, the *Modified Atkins Epilepsy Support* Yahoo! group. Just do a search of Modified Atkins on Yahoo! groups and you'll find it. It's quite common for parents to write in with general questions, recipe ideas, questions on weaning drugs, and even the occasional e-mail just to vent or seek out someone else who can understand what the writer is going through. Some popular ketogenic groups where parents can find support on Yahoo! include the *Ketogenic Diet Support Group*, *Keto Kids*, and *Keto Café*. These groups might change over the years, so doing a search for Keto on the Yahoo! groups will likely give you the most updated list.

- **Facebook:** In the last year or so, parents have begun creating Facebook pages as an easy medium to provide support. Some are open to the public, but many are private. To find these groups, search "Keto" on Facebook, and you'll likely find numerous groups. After a while, you'll learn that many of the parents on Facebook groups are also in other online support groups. It's a testament to each parents' strong need for multi-dimensional support.

Sometimes there's nothing better than meeting a new friend face to face, someone who really shares in your experiences, especially when being part of the epilepsy community can make you feel isolated from the rest of the world. If you are willing, try to seek out parents within your community that might be on the diet. Here are a few ideas to get the ball rolling:

■ **Ask your child's doctor for references:** Most pediatricians know whether they have more than one child in their practice on the Ketogenic diet or MAD. Ask your doctor to put you in touch with another parent in a way that doesn't violate privacy laws. In Erin's case, her pediatrician asked another mom whose son was on the Ketogenic diet whether Erin could contact her. Two years later they are still friends and cheerleaders to each other's child's accomplishments. You might be surprised how willing parents are to meet other parents with whom they have something in common.

■ **Post notes at your local therapy locations:** Many children with epilepsy receive some sort of therapy service, and many locations have a bulletin board. Ask the center's permission to post a note about looking for other parents doing dietary therapy.

■ **Seek out volunteer opportunities at your local Keto Clinic:** Johns Hopkins has a program in which parents come in during the hospital initiation to meet and talk to families about the Ketogenic diet. This is a closed-door meeting with parents starting the diet and parents who are currently doing the diet. No doctors are welcome. Many other Keto Clinics are creating groups similar to this. If you participate, it's a great chance for you to impart your knowledge on new families and to make friends in the process.

■ **Talk to your child's school nurse:** Your child's school nurse is a wealth of information, especially because her role is significant to a child with epilepsy. Ask if she might be willing to help you find a local family whose child is also on diet therapy.

For the Boys

While it seems that moms have the majority when it comes to Keto and MAD initiators, there are fathers out there who have taken on this role with great success. We wanted to share a couple father's first-person stories so that you can see the world of dietary therapy through their eyes. We are so accustomed as a society to men who keep their emotions and their fears hidden behind a masculine façade. These fathers of children with epilepsy are not only open and candid about the myriad emotions they've felt on this journey, but they offer a valuable perspective often lost in a community full of women warriors. John, a father of a child on the Ketogenic diet, and Orlando, whose son is on MAD, give us a glimpse into their private battles in healing their children with diet therapy.

Later in this section is a Q&A with two fathers who aren't primarily responsible for the diet. We thought that getting into their state of mind might give others an idea of why they play a less significant role in the diet. The hope is that we can take these fathers' feedback and use it to encourage the men who are a little more hesitant about fulfilling a larger role in their child's diet therapy.

John's Story

Ayla is our only child and was adopted from China when she was 18 months old. She started having generalized tonic clonic seizures when she was one year old, but they were mostly controlled by Depakote. When she was a little over two years old she started having atonic (drop) seizures and then nighttime myoclonic seizures. The seizures became more and more frequent and severe over the next two years. There was no known cause for her seizures. We tried nine different anti-seizure meds and combinations with no success. In fact the medications seemed to be doing more harm than good. Ayla was almost four years old and she could no longer walk, talk, or even sit upright.

As a father I was devastated that my little girl was suffering these constant seizures and I could not help her. I knew that she was going to suffer permanent brain damage if we could not find an answer. I also knew that the medications were having a negative impact on her development and they were not helping with the seizures. Ayla's condition was also having an impact on our marriage. We could no longer function as a regular family. We couldn't do the things with our daughter that most families do, and our days were filled with stress, worry, and feelings of helplessness. I knew that I needed to find an alternative.

I called our neurologist in December of 2009. I told him that I wanted to find a way to get Ayla off medications, and I asked about alternative treatments. That was when we first heard about the Ketogenic diet. I started doing research about the diet.

I joined the Keto diet Yahoo group and the Charlie Foundation. We watched the Meryl Streep movie First Do No Harm *and we started to have some hope. We started Ayla on the diet the middle of January 2010.*

We knew that doing the diet would be time consuming. Both my wife and I work full time, and I was already the one who did most of the cooking and shopping so I took on the responsibility of doing the diet. My evenings were largely filled with cooking, measuring, packaging etc.—not just the Keto food but all of the supplements that went with it. We weaned Ayla off all meds in a very short time, and we saw an immediate improvement in her. Her seizures were down and her alertness improved. She started crawling and playing and mimicking words again. We continued to tweak the diet. On July 31st 2010, Ayla had her last seizure. She has been seizure free since her birthday, August 1st 2010.

The diet was difficult, especially the first several months, but we stayed with it because we could see Ayla making progress, and it gave us hope. I would much rather spend an hour working on the diet than giving Ayla another pill that was draining the life out of her. And during this process I believe that our marriage and our family grew stronger. We made it through some very difficult times, and although we are not out of the woods yet, we can definitely see sunlight again. As a father I feel like I was finally able to help my little girl get well again.

Orlando's Story

My son is 11 years old. He had viral encephalitis in October of 2007. Encephalitis is swelling of the brain. It happens when for some strange reason a virus passes the blood–brain barrier and infects the brain. He is the most wonderful boy in the world.

I found out about the Modified Atkins Diet and Keto three and a half years after my son's bout with encephalitis, when I was totally frustrated. Before learning about the diets, I was giving my son so many meds. My wife and I were really scared and had no idea how to start the diet. A few days before his birthday he started having clusters. The Depakote was causing some baldness, and I was going nuts. I decided to start MAD on his birthday because the night before he had had a few seizures. I just could not wait any longer.

We bought the Atkins for Seizures *e-book from Michael Koski,
and we bought a whole bunch of things from the Charlie
Foundation website. We started with only eggs and bacon as
we did not know what else to do. That was easy, since I can't
cook to save my life. Steak for lunch—it was a nightmare to get
him to eat—and dinner was salmon. After about two days he
lost about two pounds. I was frustrated again because he was
already skinny. That's when we discovered we could substitute
cream for milk. I would do half cream and half water and tell
him it was his "special milk." He liked it, and it was a blessing.*

*My wife does most of the cooking now and the diet is still very
basic for us. The good thing is that my son is a very picky eater
so it's not too hard to stay basic. Recently, he started eating a
little more variety like chicken and beef so we have been able to
go out and order him food instead of bringing it from home.*

*We have never had seizure freedom. My son seems to do well
with the diet and small amounts of natural sugars from fruits
only. We will keep tweaking away until we find seizure freedom or as close as we can get. Even if the diet never completely
works, I don't think we will ever eat the same again. Seeing
how the processed foods hurt my son has made me realize that
although we can tolerate this junk, our kids cannot. No matter
how we follow this diet, it will always be as pure as possible.*

For the Boys: Q&A

Because it does seem that the majority of the "food bosses" in the house
are moms, we ask three fathers who aren't active in their child's diet therapy to share some of their opinions on the role of either the Ketogenic diet
or Modified Atkins Diet in their family's life. We think it shows that even
when fathers aren't running the diet, they are deeply affected by it.

1. **Was it a mutual decision that your spouse would handle the diet?
   If not, how did your spouse become the administrator of the diet?**
   Dad 1: Overall, it was a mutual decision, based on a few factors: 1)
   My wife is a stay at home mom and prepares most of the food for the
   family. 2) My schedule sometimes limits me from participating in timely

dinner preparation. 3) My wife became a trusted cooking advisor for other Keto/MAD families and had done her homework on the complexities and nuances of the diets. 4) My cooking skills are dismal.

Dad 2: My wife believed this was the right path. I choose to follow my wife's lead. The diet is incredibly "exact timing and measurements." Work commitments are such that I was not going to be available day in and day out. On a funny note, I am pretty sloppy—2oz is a "small handful" to me.

2. **What do you think has been the biggest challenge this diet has brought into your marriage?**
Dad 1: The diet has been difficult at times and has limited our ability to travel on vacations, or go out to restaurants for meals. Additionally, the diets have required drop-everything scenarios in which one of us, or the entire family, has had to get ingredients at the drop of a hat.

Our son also is a picky eater, which has impacted enjoyment of meals for others at the table. If he doesn't get what he wants, he'll throw a tantrum that disrupts the flow of conversation and eliminates the "calm" that should accompany a family meal.

The feeling of guilt, at times, has also been overwhelming in the event that our son is required to eat something that no one else wants to eat. This has caused consternation and disruption at meal time, especially when a sibling wants dessert or something different to eat that the person on the diet cannot have.

At times, there is concern that nutritional needs are not being met through the diet due to reluctance of the patient to eat the variety of foods available. Additionally, perceived pressure by neighbors and friends to give kids snacks and non-Keto/MAD foods has made it difficult at times to maintain the diet.

Dad 2: It's a huge challenge for my wife. If she feels this is the right path, I believe her and put aside any doubts as best I can. I guess the challenge is my doubt. I will follow my wife's lead, no doubt. I believe in her resolve 100%.

3. **What fears or reservations do you have about the diet that keeps you from playing a larger role?**
Dad 1: Time commitment and complexity of recipe calculations are, at times, problematic. The possibility of screwing something up is a constant concern. Even with the best intentions, it's difficult to get it right 100% of the time. The stakes are high and not getting a recipe right could mean a trip to the hospital.

Dad 2: I don't think it's sustainable. My son wants to eat what he wants, and as he approaches his teenage years, I believe he will want to eat what his friends eat.

4. **What could your spouse do to encourage your participation more?**
Dad 1: Remaining positive about the diet has been a struggle and I think it's important to keep in mind the diet saves lives. Keeping it in that context is important, as is the teamwork required to make it successful. My spouse has been very positive and proactive throughout the process, which has helped me maintain momentum. Without that attitude, we wouldn't have been able to continue the diet for almost four years and still maintain our sanity, and marriage.

Dad 2: If I could understand the food science aspect. If we could get a better belief in the cost-benefit side of the diet, and cost obviously revolves around our son's inability to eat what he wants and when.

5. **What jobs would you be interested in having if your spouse were to ask for help with the diet?**
Dad 1: The peripheral tasks of shopping for supplies and cleaning up are preferable to me than preparing Keto/MAD meals.

Dad 2: Shopping for the ingredients. I actually like finding hard-to-find stuff! Getting involved in the menu, possibly. I am not sure I might have the skill sets, but would love to try. I actually like mixing stuff together in a pot. Does not sound very clinical does it?

6. **Has your spouse done anything throughout the course of this diet that you feel has discouraged your participation? If so, what?**
Dad 1: At times, emotions have run high, which has impacted our attitude towards the diet and each other. Maintaining the perspective of the diet having such a positive impact on our son has helped get us through the hard times.

Dad 2: My wife is fantastic. I don't understand how the diet chemistry works, and I feel so bad when my son wants to eat what his friends eat. I am slow to eat at family gatherings because of a guilt feeling. I would do anything to allow him a slice of pizza, a strand of spaghetti, or a coke. It's difficult for him and sad for both parents.

My wife is very precise when it comes to our son's diet. I have a math degree so it's possible that I could administer the diet. Maybe if my wife took a weekend off, she would be amazed that I can step up!

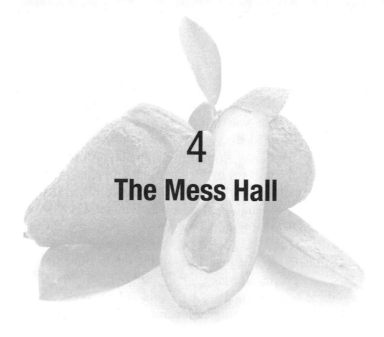

4

The Mess Hall

Re-Thinking Food

Look through your own pantry at home. Chances are you have boxes of brown rice, easy-cook macaroni and cheese, cans of chicken noodle soup, boxes of cereal, oatmeal, peanut butter, crackers, bread, and raisins. These are staple pantry items for a lot of families with children. With the exception of the peanut butter in very small amounts, these foods are on the *Off Limits* list that comes with ketogenic diets. Rice and wheat products are loaded with carbohydrates, while cereals and raisins—and many peanut butters—are full of sugar. When you think of taking these foods away from your child you may feel guilty or sad that your child won't be able to enjoy these foods. Just as we discussed in Chapters 1 and 2, the choice to pursue diet therapy is to give your child a chance at a healthy life, something he does not currently have, or you would not have considered this journey to begin with. Only after you've confronted all the emotional landmines that can come with kicking carbs to the curb, can you learn to salute the fats.

Once your child has been on one of these diets for more than a year, you will likely become a walking encyclopedia about fats: which have the highest fat content per gram or tablespoon, which are tough to enjoy no matter how you attempt to mask them, and which ones you or your child likes the best. You will become so familiar with the fats you use often that you'll be able to eyeball 10 grams of butter and 20 grams of oil (not that you would allow yourself to simply eyeball them if doing the

Ketogenic diet). All the foods you previously thought were too fatty, like sour cream and cheese, you realize all too quickly that not only are these foods not as high in fat as you'd like for the diet, they are also high in protein, making them less ideal in large quantities, except on the Modified Atkins Diet (MAD). Soon your love of finding high-fat foods might cause an embarrassing eruption of joy in the supermarket when you find a natural ranch dressing that has a whopping 16 grams of fat and only 1 carb! Let this chapter be the beginning of a new love affair with fats. After all, if you can't learn to love fat, you will never learn how to make appealing food to heal your child.

Fats come under several categories: saturated fats, trans fats, monounsaturated fats, and polyunsaturated fats. Saturated fats are the fats that come from animal byproducts as well as some plant foods. As a general rule of thumb, they are solid at room temperature. Butter and the fats found in hot dogs, sausages, and cheeses are saturated fats. Trans fats occur naturally in some foods, especially foods made from animals, but for the most part they are manufactured fats. Monounsaturated fats are found in a variety of foods and oils; these fats can improve cholesterol levels, so they're a great choice for Ketogenic diets, as the amount of fats in these diets often raises cholesterol numbers. Finally, polyunsaturated fats are found mostly in plant-based foods and oils. Omega-3 fatty acids, which are healthy for your heart and sometimes for the brain, are a type of polyunsaturated fat. Foods that are made up of monounsaturated and polyunsaturated fats are liquid at room temperature.

Coconut oil is an exception to the general rule about fats. While it is a saturated fat and is white and solid at room temperate, coconut oil is a great source of fat—and very healthy. Coconut oil is known for improving heart health, boosting the metabolism, and supporting the immune system. Coconut oil has nature's richest source of medium-chain triglycerides or medium chain triglyceride (MCT)s, a specific type of dietary fat. Because MCTs are smaller, they are more easily digested and are burned quicker by your body. In turn, because your body burns these MCTs quickly, it is able to produce larger ketones. Coconut oil is often suggested for children who have a difficult time staying in ketosis or when ketones need a boost. Coconut oil is easier to find sold as unrefined, and it smells like sweet coconuts and the beach. It's great mixed into fruity yogurts, baked into sweets, or sweetened and frozen as a candy. If the flavor of coconut isn't appealing to you or your child, you can purchase refined coconut oil. The consistency is the same, but there's virtually no smell or taste of coconut.

One of the best things about coconut oil is its ability to turn anything solid. Mix it into a runny yogurt and the cool yogurt will firm the coconut oil. Freeze coconut oil with cocoa and butter and you have the perfect "Keto chocolate." Many parents use these as a little desert served with each meal as a way to provide the fat in a more appealing way.

Another oil that you will encounter while on these diets is MCT oil. Unless you or your child is on the MCT diet, which we introduced in Chapter 1, MCT oil is used as a small portion of fat for children who either have high cholesterol or who need to stay in a higher level of ketosis. Like coconut oil, MCT oil is comprised of medium-chain triglycerides that are metabolized quickly. The oil can present unappealing side effects such as gastrointestinal issues if consumed in too high a quantity. For some children, however, MCT oil has greatly improved the results of their diets, and MCT oil is essential to the success of the MCT diet.

Just as you strived to create a balanced diet before a ketogenic diet entered your life, you can still maintain that approach when considering the types of fat you want to use in you or your child's diet. When you can, cook and bake with either monounsaturated fats or polyunsaturated fats, but any fat in moderation is fine. Here's an overview of your heavy-hitting fats:

Oils

Olive oil is great for cooking, but try not to use too much when preparing your child's food, as it has a tendency to turn the food green, and younger children find the taste too strong. Canola oil is a great oil to cook foods at high heats though the flavor can be unappealing to a lot of children.

TYPES OF FATS

Saturated Fat	Monounsaturated Fat	Polyunsaturated Fats	Omega-3
Cream	Olive oil	Safflower oil	Salmon
Cheese	Peanut oil	Corn oil	Mackerel
Beef	Canola oil	Soy oil	Herring
Pork	Avocados	Cottonseed oil	Ground
Sausage	Poultry	Peanut oil	Flaxseed
Hot dogs	Nuts	Poultry	Flax oil
Bacon	Seeds	Nuts	Walnuts
Lard		Seeds	Walnut oil
Butter		Mayonnaise	
Coconut, palm, and tropical oils		Sunflower oil	

Walnut oil is not only tasty in several recipes, it is also high in Omega-3. Try to get coconut oil in wherever you can, since it has great benefits all around. Safflower oil is another fantastic choice because it helps to lower cholesterol.

As you can see in the Types of Fats table, there are many different kinds of oils. Because fat is so essential to these diets, the variety in oils gives you freedom to play around with different flavors. When baking, making pancakes, and other sweets, consider switching from canola or another vegetable oil to a nut oil. Hazelnut, walnut, and macadamia nut oils all offer a slightly different flavor and complement sweet tastes. When sautéing, sesame oil gives any meal a strong, Asian taste, especially when paired with a touch of soy sauce and garlic.

Avocado

Avocados have to be the world's perfect food, and there is no doubt they are the perfect food for diet therapy. Not only are they the perfect 4:1 ratio, being high in monosaturated fat and low in carbs, they are a great source of vitamins B, E, and K, and they have more potassium than bananas. Avocadoes are also great for ketogenic diets because they are higher in fiber than prunes; this is important because constipation is often a common side affect of these diets, as you will learn in Chapter 5.

When looking for avocadoes in your grocery store, look for ones that are grown in either Mexico or South America, often called Haas. Avocados grown in Florida are lower in fat and therefore not the perfect 4:1 ratio. Avocados have an earthy, nutty flavor, and when perfectly ripe, are easily mashed with a fork. They can be sliced and eaten on sandwiches, cubed for finger snacks, or mashed into guacamole. Guacamole is one of the best ways to provide a healthy dose of fat to a meal. You can combine up to half the weight of avocado with oil (up to 15g of oil for every 30g of avocado) and the texture is still somewhat appealing, though, of course, the more avocado you can add to the guacamole, the tastier it is. Believe it or not, you can also use avocado in baking, in a frosting, or blended into a creamy drink.

Cream

Cream, for most children on the diet, becomes their "milk." When water is added it has a similar consistency as milk, though it lacks that slight sweetness, which can be added with a drop or two of sweetener. If your child will tolerate cream, it's a great way to get at least half of their fat for a meal. When looking for recipes and creating your own recipes, just swap the milk in the recipe for cream. In addition to being served as "milk" or for use in a recipe, cream is a perfect base for ice cream. Whether you whip it, freeze it alone with some sweetener, or add cocoa, yogurt, oil, or berries, Keto ice cream is a delicious and easy way to encourage your child to get the extra fat of his meal. You can also whip it with sweetener and serve it as a side of "whipped cream." What child wouldn't love that? Well…the truth is that several children refuse cream. Not to worry. There are plenty of other ways to sneak the fat in.

Mayonnaise

Mayonnaise is a wonder food. Don't let its reputation for being unhealthy—remember this is a new state of mind!—keep you from learning how to implement mayo into recipes. Added to muffins, soufflés, or egg dishes, mayonnaise can add extra fat while maintaining the shape and lightness of the meal. Toss together some meat, nuts, a little egg, and a hefty amount of mayo, form a patty and fry it, and you have instant "cakes" of any kind: crab, fish, chicken, you name it. For children who love to dunk their food, mayo is the perfect base for a variety of tasty dips.

Butter

Butter, whether the healthiest choice or not (ultimately it will be up to you), is quite possibly one of the kindest fats as far as flavor goes. Butter, mixed with almost anything, is pretty tasty. Mix two parts butter with one part peanut butter and you have a more Keto-friendly version of peanut butter. (Peanut butter on its own has too much protein.) Used in small amounts, butter adds great flavor to any cookie, muffin, or pancake. Butter is also a fantastic base for "syrups." Clearly the conventional syrup is off limits, but using melted butter as your base you can add liquid sweeteners such as Stevia, natural flavorings such as Bickford, or any of the low-carb products that are now available to make a sweet topping that will not only make your child's pancakes or waffles delicious and fun, but create a higher ratio as well.

Nuts

On a ketogenic diet, nuts are a new staple food. The big guns are macadamia nuts, which have the highest amount of fat, followed by pecans and almonds. These nuts are a fantastic way to cook healthy, high-fat foods (it isn't a misnomer!). For great ideas on how to incorporate nuts into cooking and baking, read Baking Without Flour later in this chapter. The next page has a table that shows which nuts are the highest in fat, as well as other nutritional benefits.

IN A NUTSHELL

Type of Nut	Amount of Fat per gram	Amount of Protein per gram	Additional Benefits
Macadamia	.76g	.079g	Good source of fiber, high in thiamin
Pecan	.72g	.092g	High in linoleic acid, an essential fatty acid, and copper
Brazil	.66g	.14g	High in thiamin, phosphorus, and magnesium
Almond	.49g	.21g	High in vitamin E
Peanut	.49g	.26g	High in niacin, folate, and linoleic acid, an essential fatty acid
Pistachio	.45g	.20g	High in vitamin B_6 and copper

Are All Carbs Created Equal?

The topic of carbohydrates is somewhat complex and varies depending on your Keto Clinic. The information provided here is to give you a general idea of how carbohydrates work and to give you some advice on how to get the most out of your carbohydrate allowance. Be certain to seek counsel with your diet center and any required reading they provide you with.

Carbohydrates, for people not on a ketogenic diet, are the basic component for making energy. In fact, your calorie intake probably comes from between fifty and sixty percent carbohydrates (that's the average). Our digestive system converts carbohydrates into glucose, which our body then burns. On a ketogenic diet, our body burns fat instead of glucose. Glucose that isn't burned is stored in our muscles and liver for future use. Simple carbohydrates include sugars found naturally in foods such as fruits, vegetables, milk, milk products, as well as any sugars added during food processing. Simple carbohydrates are found in these popular foods: white bread, white rice, potatoes, milk, and anything made with sugar. Complex carbohydrates are found in whole grains, starchy vegetables, and legumes. Foods high in complex carbohydrates include: brown rice, beans, whole wheat breads, and sweet potatoes. Complex carbohydrates don't spike the glucose levels in blood like simple carbohydrates do. In addition, complex carbohydrates are typically high in fiber.

When implementing these diets, your Keto Clinic might differentiate between total carbohydrates and net carbohydrates. To find the net carb number of any food, take the total carbohydrate number and subtract the amount of fiber. The fiber ultimately gives you a higher allowance for carbohydrates. The carb-counting books we reference later in this chapter will help you count carbs, and they can explain further how to take into consideration the total carb versus the net carb amount.

Now that it's clear not all carbohydrates are the same, how do you choose where your main carbohydrates come from? In theory it doesn't *really* matter where your carbs come from. If you wanted to give your child a candy bar and use his 10 daily grams of carbs that way, theoretically you could. That, of course, would create an unfair balance of cups of cream, tablespoons of oil, and a couple bites of a candy bar as your child's meal. When choosing the carbs to cook, bake, and eat in a day, the idea is to create appealing food so that you or your child can have some semblance of normal food. Normal, of course, is subjective; but tasteful is key.

When picking the staple carbohydrates of your diet, foods lowest in carbohydrates are going to give you the most out of your diet. Spinach, kale, and lettuce are fantastic choices because they are light in weight and low in carbs. Spinach can be added to foods and baked. It can be the base of a muffin. It's great sautéed plain, and it absorbs a lot of fat. Veggies labeled as *Group B* vegetables will become many of your main sources of carbohydrates. And, yes, there are also *Group A* vegetables. For people using the Ketogenic diet, consider the weight of foods before you select them. For example: carrots are relatively low in carbs, but they are heavy, so 10 carbs worth of carrot is going to be less than 10 carbs worth of spinach if you're weighing it on the gram scale. This is counterintuitive, and to anyone not on one of these diets, it probably sounds idiotic. After all, a gram is a gram. However, 20 grams of banana compared to 20 grams of spinach just *looks* different as far as a portion size. It might weigh the same, but weight here is not necessarily equal.

Later in this chapter is a table of some of the common foods used on these diets, and some foods that used to be an essential part of a healthy diet. If gives you an idea of how carbs can vary from food to food, even among vegetables. Low-carb bread is still too full in carbohydrates to be considered a part of a daily menu, unless you're considering the Low Glycemic Index Treatment (LGIT) diet, which has a higher daily carb allowance, or you are using very small amounts of it on MAD.

Group A Vegetables

Asparagus
Beet Greens
Cabbage
Celery
Chicory
Cucumbers
Eggplant
Endive
Green Pepper
Poke
Radish
Rhubarb
Sauerkraut
Summer Squash
Swiss Chard
Tomato, Raw
Tomato Juice
Turnips
Turnip Greens
Watercress

Group B Vegetables

Beets
Broccoli
Brussel Sprouts
Cabbage
Carrots
Cauliflower
Collards
Dandelion Greens
Green Beans
Kale
Kohlrabi
Mushroom
Mustard Greens
Okra
Onion
Rutabaga
Spinach
Tomato, Cooked
Winter Squash

A CLOSER LOOK AT CARBS

Carbohydrate Type	Carbohydrates per ¼ Cup	Additional Benefits
Broccoli	1.5g	High in vitamins C & K, high in fiber
Spinach	.027g	High in vitamins K & A
Zucchini	.96g	High in potassium
Yellow squash, sliced	1.23g	High in vitamins B_6 & C, riboflavin
Carrots, chopped	3.07g	High in vitamin A
Asparagus	1.30g	High in fiber and vitamin K
Tomatoes	1.75g	High in potassium and vitamin C
Onions	3.74g	High in vitamin B_6 & C
Apples	4.32g	High in fiber (pectin)
Strawberries	3.19g	High in fiber, folate, and vitamin C

Carbohydrate Type	Carbohydrates per ¼ Cup	Additional Benefits
Avocado	3.20g (cubed), 4.90g (pureed)	High in fiber, linoleic acid, copper, vitamin K
Orange	5.29g	High in fiber and vitamin C
Banana (1/2)	13.48g (medium size)	High in potassium and vitamin B_6
Blueberries	5.36g	High in fiber, copper, and vitamin K, antioxidant
Raspberries	3.67g	High in fiber and vitamin C, some niacin, antioxidant
Grapes (American)	3.94g	Antioxidant
Sweet potato, cubed	6.69g	High in fiber, copper, iron, niacin, vitamins A & B_6
Brown rice, medium grain, cooked	11.45g	Magnesium, typically enriched with niacin, thiamine, riboflavin, and iron
Sami's Bakery low-carb bread	2g net carbs, 10g total carbs	High in fiber, no cholesterol
Whole milk	2.93g	Calcium, phosphorus, vitamin B_{12}

Carbohydrate values are total carbohydrate and were calculated based on United Stated Department of Agriculture (USDA) food standards. All vegetables are raw and unprepared unless otherwise noted; if there is no indication of how a food is cut, either the food was left whole or there was no difference in carbohydrate value.

Carb Counting Tools

With the increasing popularity of low-carb diets, there are many carb-counting resources to choose from. In addition to books, there are online programs that will provide total calculations for you and even help you map out meal plans. There are even apps that you can download on your iPhone or iPad.

Books

The CalorieKing Calorie, Fat, & Carbohydrate Counter 2012, Allan Borushek
    Why We Like It: This is the book recommended in *Ketogenic Diets* (5th edition) by Dr. Eric Kossoff, et al., which gives us peace of mind.

Complete Guide to Carb Counting: How to Take the Mystery Out of Carb Counting and Improve Your Blood Glucose Control, Hope S. Warshaw and Karmeen Kulkarni

Why We Like It: This book provides a background on what carb counting is, how to do it, and tools to help guide you. It also includes advice
on eating out and reading labels.

*Dana Carpender's NEW Carb and Calorie Counter-Expanded, Revised,
and Updated 4th Edition: Your Complete Guide to Total Carbs, Net Carbs,
Calories, and More*, Dana Carpender
Why We Like It: This book contains information about carbs, fiber, fat,
and protein for each entry. It also provides specifics on fast food chains
and common brand name foods.

*The Ultimate Guide to Accurate Carb Counting: Featuring the Tools and
Techniques Used by the Experts*, Gary Scheiner, M.S.
Why We Like It: Written by a certified diabetes educator, this book provides many specifics on the glycemic index, as well as carb counting
in the real world.

Online Resources

Fat Secret: http://fatsecret.com/
Why We Like It: This free online source is a way to keep track of your
diet online.

Calorie King: www.calorieking.com/
Why We Like It: This online source provides a place to set goals, record
daily food intake and exercise, and receive guidelines about improving
your health. It does unfortunately have an annual fee.

Different Camps of Thought about Food

This is a topic that continues to spark controversy. What it comes down
to, we believe, is how each parent is fundamentally different, with diverse
ideas on what is right for their child. We support variances in thought and
approach when trudging through the muck of figuring out these diets, and
most importantly, we respect your desire to heal your child—or yourself—
according to your own values and heartfelt decisions.

There are two main camps of thought that parents tend to follow when
pursuing diet therapy. One is natural, using only whole foods and nothing
artificial. For the sake of clarity in this book we will call this way of thinking Natural, though it can also be referred to as clean or pure. The other
camp of thought we'll call Typical, meaning that nothing is necessarily off
limits within moderation, much like the average American's diet.

Proponents of the Natural approach to these diets generally don't use packaged foods, processed foods (such as hot dogs, sausages, and deli cheeses such as Kraft American cheese), or anything containing artificial sweeteners, colors, or added preservatives. Michael Pollen, the world-famous food writer, would likely fall under this camp. Their perspective is something like this: if it has a bar code, you should think twice before feeding it to your child with seizures—or at least read the ingredient list very carefully. Parents arrive at this camp for various reasons. Some have been raised on the idea of simple, clean food. Others, and this is most often the case, believe that the fewer components that need to be accounted for in your child's diet the better. This is a beneficial way of thinking in the beginning of the diet because it takes a lot of guesswork out of what could be potential seizure triggers. It also makes tracking foods in your journal far easier than writing down a dozen or more ingredients for one serving of packaged food, whether it's low-carb or not.

Most Keto Clinics don't seem to subscribe to this Natural way of thinking, but that's not to say they won't support your choice to pursue the diet this way—if that's the approach you want to take. For many Keto Clinics, Jell-O pudding mix and sucralose-sweetened low-calorie sports drinks are free foods (meaning their consumption isn't limited), but for a family who doesn't use artificial sweeteners, these products are off limits. KetoCal, a product that has been shown to improve the results of MAD if consumed in the first month on the diet and is a product many people swear by, has aspartame in the 4:1 vanilla formula. The 3:1 formula does not have aspartame. While KetoCal is a product that has improved the palatability of food for families across the world, for some it just doesn't jive with their personal view on food.

Those in the Typical camp have a more no-holds-barred approach to feeding their children. Packaged and processed foods are not out of the equation, especially if they can provide comfort to a child who ate those foods before the diet. Fast food, though not a norm by any means, is fine on a rare occasion and if it can be worked into a meal. Think how glorious a McDonald's French fry or chicken nugget might taste to a child who feels as though she's lost all the fun from her food. While one parent might think that treat isn't worth the potential negative side affects, another parent might revel in the simple smile of her warrior enjoying those measly grams of fast food. Fast food is an extreme example of what the Traditional camp will try for their children, but it clearly shows that this group believes more in taking away as many restrictions as possible in order to help their child remain compliant long term. In short, artificial sweeteners, flavorings, colorings, and additional additives are fine, depending on each child's sensitivities and seizure control.

Finding a Compromise

There is a great benefit to beginning these diets the Natural way. When seizures are out of control, the best tactical move is to take away as many potential triggers as possible. There are several parents who have learned along the way that their child has food sensitivities and allergies that they might never have otherwise realized, simply because they had never been forced to confront each food on an individual basis. If your child has always eaten packaged foods with dozens of ingredients, how will you ever know that one of those ingredients might be the cause of some of your child's seizures? Whether you are a Naturalist by heart or not, we believe that it can't hurt to eliminate all factors that you don't have any control over.

By starting the diet using whole foods, you can use fresh produce, unprocessed meats such as chicken and steak; dairy products; eggs; nuts; natural, low-carb sweeteners such as Stevia; and a variety of oils. Mayonnaise is debatable to some, but if you can find an organic version, there are far fewer ingredients. Cheese, while technically processed, is still a whole food. Avoid processed meats full of nitrates and additives such as caramel coloring or monosodium glutamate (MSG). Packaged foods, even those approved as low-carb foods, are best skipped in the beginning since they are loaded with a variety of artificial ingredients. Even foods containing "natural flavorings" can be seizure triggers for some children. This might sound challenging, but it's actually pretty easy. You're limited to shopping on the outskirts of the grocery store and your cost of food—aside from the expensive nuts and oils—might be lower than if you were using a lot of packaged foods.

After the first month, if you see seizure improvement that is consistent, you can slowly begin to add foods back into your child's diet. Think about the early days when you were feeding your infant solids for the first time. You gave one food at a time for several days to see if there was a reaction. This is a great approach to these diets. Using your food log (which we will discuss at length later), write down every new food and any changes in your child's seizure activity. Introduce new foods every few days.

If you've seen consistent seizure improvement, or if after doing the diet using whole foods for quite some time and you're convinced that your child was never affected by the foods you have eliminated, you can decide what other food products you'd like to add back into the mix. Some parents might opt to keep this natural approach the entire length of their child's diet. Other parents might find their child needs more foods that resemble the pre-ketogenic diet life.

The children on this diet have already had so much taken from them, and these diets take away a lot of the "normal" foods kids love, foods that in some ways define childhood (think pizza and hot dogs). Few of us have a summer memory that doesn't involve a hot dog. So, when you're ready and your dietitian is on board, we advocate that you add whatever foods back in that you think will ultimately make the diet easier for you and your child. If every meal is a struggle, throwing a hot dog into the meal plan, or some pepperoni on a Keto pizza, could be the difference between a smile and a tantrum and an evening without fights versus an emotional breakdown on your behalf.

Ultimately the choice is yours and yours alone. Most dietitians don't advocate one way or the other, and there is no evidence that suggests a natural diet will produce greater seizure control. Every child is different. Every seizure trigger is different. And all of us are very different parents, with varied tastes and experiences that flavor our physical and emotional responses to food.

Just a Reminder: Epilepsy is the Enemy

There have been several situations when we have either witnessed or been in the middle of the sometimes silent, sometimes deafening battle between these two camps of thought. Having epilepsy or a child with epilepsy makes us accustomed to fighting. We argue with doctors about drug weaning and treatment. We fight our way in to see new doctors, and we fight with the nursing staff when our child is not getting the treatment he deserves while staying in the hospital for a 24-hour EEG. And of course, we battle this beast that threatens to steal our lives. It's natural for some of that energy to be unleashed on the wrong people, but what we find disheartening is when parents mock or judge other parents because their parenting choices are different than our own. We would never stop another mother in a grocery store to tell her she's buying the wrong food for her children. We would never tell a parent he's hurting his child when he stops by McDonald's for a special treat, whether or not we advocate feeding our own child fast food. Social rules keep us in check. When encountering parents in the numerous support systems out there for these Ketogenic diets, think carefully when providing advice and read over your e-mail carefully before sending it on to dozens of readers. Every parent is desperate for advice, but the goal is for those parents to read their e-mail feeling empowered and creative, to feel heard and understood, never to feel judged because their core values—even if we're only talking about using diet soda or ketchup—are different from yours.

Crossing Enemy Lines: The Ketogenic Diet and MAD

One of the reasons we are writing about both the Ketogenic diet and Modified Atkins Diet in this book is because they are inherently similar, and it makes sense to group them together. In fact, aside from *Ketogenic Diets* (5th edition) by Dr. Eric Kossoff, et al., there are no other books out there that attempt to tackle the similarities and differences of these two diets. We believe these diets complement each other; they don't compete with each other. In Chapter 1 we provided potential reasons that you might want to pick one diet over the other. These are based on medical circumstances as well as personal circumstances.

It has become more popular in recent years to use these diets together. Dr. Kossoff mentions in *Ketogenic Diets* (5th edition), "...These diets are more alike than different, and the Ketogenic diet is probably just a 'higher dose' of dietary therapy than the MAD." Because MAD is similar to a 1:1 ratio, it makes a nice introduction to the Ketogenic diet, as well as a great option for parents stepping down from the Ketogenic diet. By using MAD for a couple months when you have already decided to try the Ketogenic diet, you give your child a chance to get used to his new foods and you become a pro at cooking and baking with fats. You will learn what foods your child likes and what foods she wouldn't touch even if Justin Bieber pleaded with her. The Ketogenic diet, after this introduction via MAD, will be much easier for you and your whole family. Who knows, as an added bonus, your child might find the seizure freedom he needed on MAD.

As you will learn in Chapter 10, the idea of stepping down from the Ketogenic diet after years of weighing food on a gram scale is overwhelming. Parents are filled with fear on every level. Will the seizures come back? Will I be able to adapt to giving my child normal foods? It's a transition that wreaks emotional havoc. For parents too fearful to let go of dietary therapy all together, MAD is a great way to step down. It makes sense that as you wean the diet you go from 4:1 down the scale until you get to 1:1. Staying at 1:1, or MAD, for a while gives everyone in the equation a chance to get used to the idea of eating more protein, having less restricted calories, and having some freedom again.

There is great value in learning the way both of these diets work. One simple way to do this, if you have the time, is to become a member of both the Ketogenic and MAD online forums. It's amazing what reading e-mail chains of other parents will teach you. Because these diets are similar and we're all buying out our local grocery store's selection of oils, mayonnaise, and eggs, why not let our knowledge cross over the line? You can learn a great deal from a mom who is doing MAD, just as a MAD mom can learn so much from a mom using the Ketogenic diet.

Mess Hall Duty

Baking Without Flour

A truly confounding thought when you've grown accustomed to muffins and pancakes baked with flour is "How can I do it *without* flour?" The bottom line is that low-carb baking is never going to be the same as a baked good made with flour. It's like trying to compare a turkey made of tofu with the typical turkey we're served at a Thanksgiving meal. When there is no similarity in the ingredients, everything about the final product is going to be different: texture, density, sweetness, crunchiness, etc. This is not in any way meant to discourage you from baking without flour. The point is to make you aware that there are great possibilities and delicious foods that are baked without flour. Just don't set the bar too high—i.e. trying to make a moist, fluffy, chocolate cake just like grandma's on the Ketogenic diet—you'll undoubtedly fail. (Although, we have to admit, our chocolate hazelnut cupcake recipe is pretty darn fantastic for a 4:1 cupcake!) However, you can find success and extreme satisfaction in baking a desert that your child will love.

When it comes to baking or creating a recipe like pancakes, waffles, or muffins, you have several great choices of ingredients. What you choose to use will depend on the ratio (i.e., how much fat you need) and what flavor you're trying to achieve.

- **Macadamia nuts** have a salty, nutty flavor and a dense, moist consistency when ground in a processor until just before they turn into butter. Because they have so much fat, macadamia nuts are the first choice when you're on a high ratio of the Ketogenic diet. Because they have a neutral flavor, they are suited for both sweet and savory recipes. If your child likes dense, moist cupcakes and muffins, macadamia nuts are a great choice. When cooking with macadamia nuts, try to bake your recipe at a lower heat so the macadamia nuts have enough time to soften. They tend to stay slightly crunchy when used in pancakes that don't cook long on the range. To soften them, you can also try soaking them in water after you've weighed them.

- **Pecans** are not only super high in fat, they grind up well to create a great muffin or pancake base. Because they are often seen in recipes loaded with fruits and sugars, they lend themselves particularly well to sweets. Ground up pecans can be mixed with a little egg and sweetener for a crust of a cheesecake or fruity desert such as a cobbler. Mixed with apples in a waffle or combined in a cookie recipe and you have a meal that virtually no one would refuse—even someone not on one of these diets!

- **Almond flour** is truly versatile, though because it's higher in protein than macadamia nuts or pecans, it is best used in smaller amounts unless on a lower ratio or on MAD. Almond flour is finely ground so that when combined in a recipe it creates a nice batter. It's great for sweets and for savory recipes alike, though if used in higher quantities, without sufficient wet ingredients, it can have a tendency to make foods a little dry.

- **Coconut flour.** While coconuts are not actually nuts, coconut flour is another low-carb baking staple. Coconut flour has a consistency very similar to white flour. Because the flour is so light, it only takes a few grams to equal a lot of flour, which is another plus because it does contain a small amount of carbs, limiting excessive use in a 4:1 ratio. Coconut flour can dry out a recipe, making it almost "sandy." Make sure to compensate with liquids. Coconut flour also doesn't seem to bind as well as the other nuts. To improve the consistency and texture of your finished product, try adding extra egg, mayonnaise, or xantham gum to help bind your food.

- **Flaxseed meal.** Ground flaxseed meal is both high in fiber and high in fat, including Omega-3, making it an ideal food to cook with on a ketogenic diet. A little goes a long way. It makes a nice, nutty bread, and in smaller amounts can be added to muffins and pancakes. It can even be used to make a warm cereal, though it does have a tendency to become solid if you don't add enough liquid.

Later in this book are recipes that incorporate many of these nut flours, including hazelnut flour, into the mix. There are sweet choices, savory choices, and even recipes in which the nut owns the flavor of the whole meal.

Arming Your Kitchen

Before you initiate any of these diets, it is essential to prepare your kitchen with the tools that will make life with diet therapy more organized and efficient. In this section we highlight several solutions to organize your kitchen, as well as a wide array of supplies that will make everyday meal prep as simple as possible.

- **Create a Keto Corner:** No matter the size of your kitchen, you should quarantine at least a corner of the kitchen for supplies and meal preparation. For those of you who will do the Ketogenic diet, this is where you will store your gram scale, recipes, and the items you will use most often on the diet, such as a squirt bottle of oil, rubber spatulas, and small bowls, containers, and labels. If doing MAD, you can store your recipes, carb-counting books, and measuring cups. If you have a bigger kitchen, consider reorganizing your cabinets so that one cabinet can be dedicated to the diet. There you can store a variety of oils, ground nuts and nut flours, supplements, liquid sweeteners and flavorings, an assortment of prep materials such as small bowls, a food processor, silicone baking cups, plastic storage containers, food labels, and markers.

The idea behind this is to have everything at your fingertips when it's time to prepare a meal. If you've ever been behind the line at a restaurant and have observed how the chefs prepare food quickly, the key is that all food ingredients are neatly prepared, organized, and within an arm's reach. No time is wasted rifling through cabinets and pantries. If you put foods in the same place in your cabinet every time, you could prepare a meal even in the most chaotic of situations because you have eliminated the obstacles that can bog you down.

- **Reserve a spot in the fridge:** This concept is the same as creating a Keto Corner. Rearrange the fridge so that a shelf or a drawer is dedicated to the diet. There you can store high-fat yogurts, butters, mayonnaise, pre-blended eggs in a squirt bottle, any high-fat meats, and anything else for the diet. What is great about having a diet station in your fridge is that you can make it off limits to other family members. Because so many of the ingredients used in these diets can be expensive, and because only certain items are in the KetoCalculator, the last thing you want is for one of the children to finish off the cheese that you had saved to make your warrior dinner.

- **Containers:** You will marvel at how many tiny dishes you will use in a day's time, not to mention all the plastic storage containers used to freeze, store, and cart food from one location to the next. Unless you want to spend your free time—what little you have left—cleaning every tiny dish you own, purchase a dozen or so. Small plastic bowls can be found in the baby section and often in the seasonal dishware section of stores.

Why all the silly plastic containers? Especially for the Ketogenic diet, in the early days it's a smart idea to weigh out each food item separately. This way, if you add too much of one ingredient you don't have to toss out the other foods that you'd already weighed in the same bowl. This will seem incredibly tedious in the beginning, but it will help you to become more efficient at weighing and will help to train you to judge how much a gram—or 10 grams—is of any given ingredient. Learning to judge a gram versus several grams by eyeballing it will save you time in the end. You will be able to know that 10 grams of butter is about a half-inch slice of a butter stick. By judging these ingredients individually you become faster and more confident, and at that point you can weigh every ingredient into one bowl.

Plastic containers with lids, of every shape and size, will become monumentally important during your years doing diet therapy. Look for containers that close tightly so that no oil will spill out. The Rubbermaid Easy Find Lids containers are great because they come in several small sizes and they hold oil without any leaks. Take & Toss by The First Years are fun and colorful and last throughout several dishwashing cycles. These containers are especially friendly for the younger crowd.

When preparing food in advance, either for your own convenience or for a family member or school, many parents love to use the tiny clear plastic condiments containers. They hold about two ounces and are great for storing the ingredients of meals to be assembled later, or for dips, butters, an so on. These can be purchased online or at a restaurant supply store.

■ **Labeling supplies.** Living the Keto life will require you to be almost unnaturally organized. Even if you are the only one doing the diet and no other family member touches or gives your child food (which we sincerely hope will not be the case), labeling food will help keep you organized, especially in the days when you are so frustrated and over this diet that you can't think straight. (Yes, they will come.) Here are items to consider labeling:

■ Foods you have prepared in advance to freeze.

■ Pre-prepped meals for school or other outings.

■ Food items you have prepared, such as homemade peanut butter, macadamia nut butter, ground pecans, etc.

■ Individual ingredients you have weighed in advance and are storing in the fridge, such as chopped veggies or pre-cooked meat.

There are a lot of great options out there for labels. Browse the office supply aisle at your local grocery or super store, and hit the office supply stores to see what you think will work best for you. Labeling comes down to personality and personal style. For those of you who like to write, Post-it has some great supplies. Their Label Roll comes in different colors and is basically a Post-it note on a tape dispenser. Roll out as little or as much as you need at a time. Post-it also has Super Sticky pads that come in different sizes and bright colors. Unlike regular Post-it notes they are sticky on the entire backside. Both of these kinds of labels remove easily by hand or they also eventually dissolve in water. All-Purpose white labels also come in small packs, as well as larger sheets. You can cut these to size and use them on anything. They virtually dissolve in water so removing them is simple, though they do sometimes leave a slight sticky residue.

In the beginning, and certainly when other people are involved in the diet, even if they are your child's teachers of daycare providers, labeling can take the guesswork out of the diet for everyone. It will help you stay organized and keep track of what you have stored in your fridge and freezer, and it will help others to learn how to successfully provide a meal. When it comes down to medical necessity, it is absolutely better to be safe than sorry; in other words, you can never be organized enough.

■ **Kitchen tools:** You'll be making the majority of your child's food by hand. In the ever-important effort to save time, here are five kitchen items that we have felt indispensible in our daily meal preparation.

■ **The food processor:** Walk into your local Bed Bath & Beyond and a walk down the appliance aisle might make your head spin. There are so many food processors of every shape and size conceivable. Here's what to look for: 1) Multiple sharp blades. You will be chopping nuts into nut flour, which requires a mean blade. Likewise, if you are chopping raw chicken, you need something to power through the meat. 2) A container without many nooks and crannies. If you have weighed all your ingredients and are blending them, the last thing you want to do is spend ten minutes trying to scrape food out of the cavities of the lid. 3) Something relatively small. The small portions you will often work with will be lost in a giant container. Brands we like are the Ninja, Magic Bullet, and for softer blendables, the Cuisinart Mini Prep.

■ **Stick blender:** This is an item that gets more action in our kitchen than anything—except maybe the coffee machine. This detachable, hand-held stick blender is strong, blends beautifully, and is easy to clean by popping it in the dishwasher. If you bake a lot of muffins, make pancakes galore, or just use mixed raw egg often, this tool will become your best friend. Blend eight to ten eggs at a time and store them in a tall quirt bottle for easy measuring. We like the Cuisinart Smart Stick Hand Blender, but there are several versions out there, some with interchangeable parts.

- **The condiment squirt bottle:** This little friend goes right along with the stick blender. If you have ever tried to weigh eggs without blending them, you will soon realize that you can go from 3 grams to 30 grams instantly, because the heavy egg whites are impossible to control. Once they've been blended, pour them into a tall condiment squirt bottle. It gives you great control when weighing eggs. In addition to storing eggs in these containers, you can store oils, flavorings, or pre-made cheesecake mixes. For thicker fluids, cut the top down a little bit.

- **Individual silicone baking cups:** These come in regular muffin size and mini muffin size, and are most often available at higher-end cooking stores, but as they continue to grow in popularity, they are sometimes found elsewhere. There are several reasons why these are fantastic. First, having the ability to put one or two of these on a baking tray instead of a whole muffin tin saves cleanup time and it's easier to pop out the muffin. These are not just for muffins; use them to bake your Keto cookies, to make perfectly-shaped crackers, such as the Cheese Crackers in *The Keto Cookbook*; use them for making frozen candies; or you can put dipping sauces in them for a fun way to present food.

- **Silicone spoon spatulas:** You can go ahead and toss out the thick plastic scrapers that aren't shaped like a spoon. They are hard to manipulate and they aren't thin enough to slide underneath the tiny amounts of food you'll be scraping up. We recommend you have at least half a dozen of these. When batching and using several ingredients, have a container of them right in your Keto Corner. Use one spatula for each ingredient. Toss a colorful spatula in with your kid's lunch for school, and keep one in your bag or car just in case. When it comes to maintaining the perfect ratio, these are your wingman. And for some reason, they make a super fun toy for the little ones— especially the oral ones—so be prepared for a couple to be lost in that toy chest or under the couch.

Feeding an Army: Batching and Making Meals in Advance

When you have all your ingredients out for one meal, why not take the extra five to ten minutes and make additional meals for later? This is the basic idea behind batching. Batching can be done in a variety of ways, for both the Ketogenic diet and MAD. While batching can be time consuming, it can reduce stress during those hurry-up-and-go mornings, and, among myriad other reasons, having batched meals packaged and stored for easy grabbing can make a night with a picky eater easier. After all, who has time to cook three meals for a child who proclaims she likes nothing? No one. By having something in the fridge or freezer that you can pull out and heat up, you might have averted potential disaster.

The concept of batching can be applied to anything: cooking meats such as sausage and bacon in advance, blending a cartoon of eggs for easy weighing each day, making muffins to freeze for easy on-the-go meals, or chopping veggies to weigh out and add to meals throughout the week.

Here are several suggestions of foods that you can batch and either store in your fridge or freeze in labeled containers for future use. If you're super organized, you can create a list on your freezer or in your notebook that outlines the foods you have available and cross the items off as you use them. (Don't worry, not many people are this organized, so if you were thinking, "yeah right," you're not the only one.)

- **Chop vegetables:** Spend some time one day a week and chop veggies you use often in your child's meals. Most *Group B* vegetables can be frozen, while many *Group A* veggies such as zucchini and spaghetti squash don't freeze as well due to their high water content. You can either weigh or measure out the appropriate portions and you can store them in a baggie or container to weigh later when you're making meals.

- **Make nut flours or butters:** If you do a lot of baking, chances are you will use a lot of nut flour. In a matter of minutes you could chop a bag of pecans and macadamia nuts for use in future recipes. If you prefer nut butters, it takes only moments to puree nuts into butter. Add some carb-free sweetener and a little salt and you have a fantastic homemade butter. Store them in an airtight container in your pantry or fridge.

- **Blend eggs:** As we mentioned earlier in this chapter, eggs are much easier to weigh when they are blended to a liquid consistency. The average condiment squirt bottle can hold about eight blended eggs.

- **Pre-cook meat:** Bake chicken or turkey breasts, cook hamburger, or fry bacon and sausage over a weekend and store it in the freezer. You can weigh out the meats according to each meal and label them, or just divide them into smaller portions for later. This way it's easy to pull out a couple sausages for a breakfast, grab some chicken to thaw and toss into chicken salad, or add hamburger to a last-minute meal.

- **Make Keto chocolates:** Keto chocolate recipes vary, but they usually consist of coconut oil, cocoa, sweetener, and sometimes butter. Make a huge batch and freeze them in ice trays or candy molds. Once they are frozen you can pop them into single serving containers or baggies.

■ **Make multiple snacks:** Crackers, mini muffins, and cookies are all great items to batch. For snacks that include a fresh fruit and a fat, you can weigh out the fat ahead of time, label it, and freeze it. To make it easier on you later, write how much fruit you need to serve with the fat. Snacks such as yogurt and applesauce can also be made in advance. Instead of making one or two recipes at a time, if it's a food your child eats often, make ten recipes. Write the weight of a single serving on the container for snacks so you know how much to weigh out later.

■ **Bake muffins:** Whether your child likes breakfast muffins, savory meal muffins, or egg soufflés baked in a ramekin, these are easy to batch. Most muffins and egg soufflés also freeze well. The 100 Ways Egg Soufflé and the Spanakopita Bites in our recipe section always freeze well.

■ **Compile entire meals:** While this can be more time consuming, you can also weigh entire meals and freeze them. Keep in mind that not all veggies freeze well. You can either cook these meals or have all the ingredients weighed or measured and then cook the meals after they defrost. This is a great option if you're leaving town or you have someone who cares for your child while you're at work.

■ **Measure and freeze small portions:** For those who serve small amounts of butter, coconut oil, or any small food portion, you can weigh ingredients in small plastic containers, such as the 2-ounce condiment containers with lids, and label and freeze them.

■ **Whip up ice cream:** Ice cream obviously freezes like a dream, and it's easy to make additional batches in one bowl and then freeze individual portions.

To save additional time batching on the Ketogenic diet, here is the quickest way for all-in-one meals such as muffins, pancakes, cheesecakes, candies, and so on. Try batching the Summer Muffins, Baby Puree, Baby Puffs, and the Chocolate Hazelnut Cupcake this way.

1. Multiply each ingredient by how many servings you want to make. If you want to make ten servings of yogurt, multiply the cream weight, the yogurt weight, and the oil weight all by ten.
2. Measure each ingredient into a bowl large enough to hold whatever quantity you're working with.
3. After weighing, mix everything well, making sure there are no chunks that might weigh unevenly in the next step.

4. To determine each individual serving size, add up the total grams of the original recipe. If one serving of the recipe calls for 44 grams of yogurt, 5 grams of oil, and 15 grams of cream, your total weight of the meal is 64 grams. Each serving size is also 64 grams.

5. For the next step you can either weigh out each serving size and prepare accordingly (i.e., baking if necessary), or you can keep the entire recipe in one container with a label for the weight of each serving size, and weigh out an individual serving whenever you want.

Keep in mind that this method will only work with meals that are relatively smooth in consistency. If you are working with a meal that has significant chunks of food, you can batch foods using the assembly line method. To do this, take out several containers for each meal you want to prepare. Weigh the first ingredient into each container. Then you can put that ingredient away. Follow this step for every ingredient until you have completed the meal. With practice, you can prepare several assembly-line meals in a short period of time. The 100 Ways Egg Soufflé and the Toasted Coconut Trail Mix are two recipes that will work best with the assembly line method.

Recipe Creation

One of your biggest challenges in this great battle against seizures is creating and maintaining a collection of delicious, exciting meals for your warrior—or you. We all fall into habits, especially it seems, in the kitchen. We make what we're accustomed to, what our kids and spouses like, and new recipes often take a back seat to the comfort meal you know the whole family will eat without a fight. It's easy on these diets to fall into a rut and to end up panicking when mealtime is approaching, with the question that lurks in the shadows of everyday life, "What am I going to feed my warrior today?" How do you hold onto the creativity and the motivation to continue making meals your child will want to eat—even when playing around with a recipe is the last thing you have the time or energy for?

Our goal in this section is to not only teach you how to seek out recipes to adapt them to a high-fat version for one of these diets, we want to show you how you can continue to be creative in the kitchen. We're not all chefs by nature. Some of us would rather clean a toilet than bake. But our children depend on the food we're preparing, and the pressure is on. Our hope is that after reading this chapter, you'll be armed with a few tricks and tips to keep your creative juices flowing, without making you feel like you're the one in the pressure cooker.

How to Search for Recipe Ideas

- **Cookbooks:** Cookbooks are a fantastic resource for inspiration. Of course, you won't be able to use all the ingredients in recipes so you'll be swapping a lot of ingredients out with Keto-friendly versions. However, cookbooks are great to see what ingredients pair well together, how to create a recipe that might be new to you, and really, they're just great at getting you in the mood to cook. When looking for cookbooks, consider specialty cookbooks that you can check out at your local library. There are cookbooks on using Stevia, baking with almond flour, and using coconut oil; you can try raw cookbooks for ideas on using nuts in baking (though of course raw diets don't cook their nuts, but you can!); gluten-free cookbooks offer a lot of nut-based baking ideas; and of course, low-carb books, which are abundant, have hundreds of potential recipes you can tweak and tailor for your needs.

- **Online forums and Facebook:** One of the greatest assets of the online forums and Facebook groups is the opportunity to share recipes with other parents who are doing these diets for their children. When parents come up with a good recipe, they are often so excited that they want someone to share it with. Just remember that when another parent shares her recipe, you have to play around with the recipe to get the right calorie amount, as well as the fat, protein, and carbohydrate count for your child. Never just take a recipe and sprint into your kitchen with it!

- **Online resources:** As we mentioned in Chapter 1, you are coming into diet therapy at an exciting time. Resources are popping up all over the place as more and more creative moms take diet therapy into their own kitchens. Dawn Martenz's Ketocook.com is the first online resource to really give Keto parents what they've been looking for: recipes, sage advice, and a place where parents can be inspired. In addition to Dawn's website, other parents are blogging about their children's experiences on the diet, and those blogs revolve around food. Ask around in your online forums to find parents who blog about their experiences. In the next section, Dawn Martenz, KetoCook.com's creator and co-author of *The Keto Cookbook*, shares her secrets of how she keeps her kitchen life exciting. Pinterest.com, Tastespotting.com, and good old Google are also great places to search and browse.

■ **The food network:** Foodies from all over rely on the Food Network to keep abreast of new recipes and trends in the kitchen. You can catch a cooking show, or even better (and less time consuming) you can go to foodnetwork.com and search for recipes. Search for recipes that include ingredients that are Keto friendly, such as: avocados, macadamia nuts, mayonnaise, spaghetti squash, coconut and coconut oil, pecans, almond flour, eggs, and cream. Most recipes you'll find with these ingredients can be tailored. You just need to know which ingredients to swap, which we'll address later in our Use This Not That chart.

■ **Your local kitchen supply or super store:** With a wide array of kitchen gadgets on the market, you can find simple inspiration just by buying a new gadget, whether it's small or big. Many Keto moms have raved about the mini doughnut makers, pizzelle makers, and popsicle makers. Even a new ice tray or candy tray can prove to change things up just a bit.

Finding Your Inner Keto Cook—Dawn Martenz, Co-Author of *The Keto Cookbook*

Dawn is spearheading the Keto recipe revolution, dedicating countless gram-weighing hours in her kitchen towards creating fun and exciting recipes for kids across all age groups. Her daughter, Charlotte, has Dravet's Syndrome and has been on the diet for more than two years. Here's what Dawn had to say when we asked her to give us a little advice on staying organized and inspired:

First of all, I would not consider myself a "naturally creative" person. I work very hard at trying to come up with new idea and recipes. For me, creativity is more of a result from habits and routines that I stick to in other areas of my life...

The biggest thing that has helped with learning how to create Keto recipes is learning the substitutions for ingredients that are non-Keto friendly, like flour, sugar, bread, etc. Once I figured out how to replace these ingredients with Keto-friendly ones, adapting recipes became a lot easier.

Here is how I stay organized and creative:

    •   **Plan meals ahead of time.** *A huge part of devoting time to my Keto cooking experiments is being organized in the* *other areas of my life that I can control (unlike epilepsy). Meal planning and grocery shopping for the family and Keto cooking is HUGE for me. I have found that if I plan meals and ideas for Keto food ahead of time (I usually do this on Sundays), I have time later in the week to work on a recipe that I have not tried yet.*

• **Rely on meals your warrior likes.** *I rely on meals that I know Charlotte will eat. For example, she will eat yogurt and her cheese stick meal everyday for breakfast and lunch. That leaves only one meal a day that I have to "figure out." When I find that she does like something, I'll try to make several at a time and freeze them or prep them if I can.*

• **Keep a list of meals you want to try.** *I keep a list of meal ideas that I want to try, and I'll aim to try only one or two new recipes a week. This way I don't feel like I'm stressing myself out creating a new meal everyday.*

• **Always be on the lookout for new meal ideas.** *I constantly keep an eye out for new meal ideas by just looking around at the grocery store (especially pre-packaged kids food), and looking on the Internet. Sometimes I ask Charlotte what she wants to eat; I never know what she'll say, but I can usually figure something out after researching a low-carb version online. Sometimes I just pick a new ingredient and search for recipes. I'll pick one that jumps out at me!*

• **Don't try to replicate food that just won't work.** *I drew the line at trying to replicate things like bread, rolls, pasta. It was too complicated and too much work. The results just never measured up either. That eliminated a lot of stress.*

The Mission: Swapping Out Ingredients

When you are taking the time to become inspired and you're on the hunt for a new recipe, just as Dawn mentions above, you need to have a basic understanding of what items can be substituted with Keto-friendly items in order to make the meal appropriate for a high-fat diet. This chart provides you with alternatives to the ingredients that are found in most recipes that can be adapted towards a ketogenic diet. Also use this table if you're looking for an alternative due to allergies. Just keep in mind that we have not separated out ingredients according to allergies so you need to double check with your dietitian if you have a question about using any of these ingredients.

USE THIS NOT THAT

Standard Recipe Ingredient	Keto-Friendly or Allergy Substitute
Milk	Heavy cream, almond milk, coconut milk, hazelnut milk
Sugar	Stevia (liquid or powder), Truvia®, Splenda®
Flour	Almond flour, coconut flour, ground macadamia nuts, ground pecans, hazelnut flour, flaxmeal, whey protein, Ketocal 4:1 or 3:1, KetoCuisine 5:1, unsweetened coconut
Eggs	*For binding in baking*: Flaxmeal and water or oil; unflavored gelatin and hot water; applesauce or other pureed fruit; Xantham gum *Binding and thickening in non-baked recipes*: Chia seeds *Leavening*: Oil, water, and baking powder *Eating or cooking:* Tofu
High GI fruits	Low GI fruits
Peanut butter	Macadamia nut butter, almond butter, cashew butter, pumpkin seed butter, sunflower seed butter
Butter	Dairy free Earth Balance, Spectrum Organics' palm oil shortening, ghee (clarified butter)
Pasta	Shoestring sliced zucchini, spaghetti squash, Miracle Noodles
Breadcrumbs	Almond flour, ground macadamia nuts, ground low-carb tortilla
Tree nuts	Pumpkin seeds, sunflower seeds
Mayonnaise	For a soy free version, make your own; for an egg-free version, find a vegan mayonnaise

Now that we've introduced you to basics of how to come up with a meal idea, those of you using the Ketogenic diet will need to learn how to take an idea and bring it to the dinner table using the KetoCalculator.

Camp KetoCalculator

If you've read any of the books on the Ketogenic diet and seen the math involved in calculating the diet, you should be over the moon that your dietitian has allowed you access to the KetoCalculator, the online program that calculates the perfect ratio for you. Many of us have been so spoiled in fact that we could not calculate the diet without the KetoCalculator. (If you are one of those people who always prepares for an emergency, perhaps you will decide to learn calculating the diet by hand; if so, you are more awesome than most of us!) For the rest of us who choose to use those rare moments of our spare time in other ways, the KetoCalculator will be your greatest ally in this great food fight.

Most Keto Clinics provide you with a short tutorial where the dietitian—who is so accomplished and fast that you are afraid to blink—walks you through the basic steps of creating and altering a meal. Most of us learn a little slower and certainly require a lot more hands-on time. Our advice is that as soon as you are given your user name and password, you start practicing right away. Learn the major food categories and determine ahead of time where most of the ingredients you cook with are located. If there are ingredients that you depend on, make sure they are in the KetoCalculator. If they aren't, your dietitian can manually add them for you. The more familiar you are with the KetoCalculator, the less time it will take you to create your child's meals.

KetoCalculator Q&A with Beth Zupec-Kania: Answers to Questions You Might Not Have Thought to Ask

Beth Zupec-Kania, a registered dietitian, created the KetoCalculator and continues to mentor families on the Ketogenic diet through her work at the Charlie Foundation. While Chapter 9 of the *Ketogenic Diets* (5th edition) by Dr. Eric Kossoff, et al., provides a visual tutorial on how to work the KetoCalculator, we thought our readers could benefit from a Q&A-style conversation that would provide answers to questions that arise often in forums and online groups.

Q: Is the KetoCalculator designed only for people administering the MCT, LGIT, Keto, or MAD diets? If not, who else uses the KetoCalculator?

A: Those are the most common diets that KetoCalculator is used for. It is used for many different conditions other than epilepsy including autism, Alzheimer's and Parkinson's diseases, cancer, severe allergies, and also for weight control. The KetoCalculator is also used by over 40 countries outside of the United States.

Q: Should any of the foods on the KetoCalculator be considered "off limits" for those on any of these diets? If so, which ones?

A: Foods that are "off limits" are restrictions for the condition that the diet is treating. The nutritionist who is managing the diet should provide those instructions. For example, I don't allow my patients with epilepsy to eat foods that contain sugar-alcohols, but I allow them for people who are using the diet for weight control. The Charlie Foundation publishes a booklet for the Ketogenic diet that explains hidden carbohydrates such as sugar-alcohols.

Q: Why do some of the foods have a note to ask your dietitian?

A: The master database of foods does not have a note of this nature. Each dietitian has the ability to add foods and notations like these to their KetoCalculator account, which only their clients or patients have access to.

Q: How are foods chosen that are listed in the database?

A: The database was designed initially for the classic Ketogenic diet, with whole foods as the primary content. Commercial foods have been introduced to add variety and convenience to the diet. Again, each dietitian has the ability to add foods into her account, which in turn her clients will have access to.

Q: How often are foods added and what is the process?

A: The master database is reviewed annually and edited if there is a change in the food composition. Some foods that are commonly used on the diet like processed cheese, hot dogs, and yogurt are checked twice a year because they have a history of being reformulated. I recommend that if you are using commercial foods that you check the label each time you purchase the product to check to see it is the same. It is often users who notice the change in a food label and then notify us. There is a Frequently Asked Question (FAQ) link in the program for assistance. You can e-mail us your request directly through that link.

Q: If a parent has a food they'd like added to the KetoCalculator that they think multiple people would benefit from, how can they go about that?

A: Obviously if they ask their dietitian, only their KetoCalculator would have the product. If it is a food that is appealing to many people and is available nationally, then I am happy to add it. You may make that request through an e-mail in the FAQ link within KetoCalculator.

Q: What advice would you offer a parent who is using the KetoCalculator for the first time?

A: There is a step-by-step instruction guide in the Handout link in KetoCalculator. There is also a FAQ link that addresses each feature of the program.

Q: Can you offer any time-saving tricks when using the Keto-Calculator?

A: The "Standard Meals" and "Standard Snacks" are meant to save time. I start most of my families out with the Standard Meals that include food groups. These meals are timesaving from the standpoint of creating a variety of meals from one recipe. You can also create a Standard Meal and then completely re-design it. The Standard Meal provides you with a template to guide you in creating a meal. For example, "Meat/Vegetable" can be used to create a turkey salad or pork with broccoli. Once people are comfortable with these and understand the type and amount of food in a meal, modifying the meal becomes much easier and quicker.

The biggest challenge with a meal is usually figuring out how to incorporate fat. The Standard Meals were designed using the mathematical formula for the classic Ketogenic diet, where heavy cream provides half of the fat in each meal. Not all people like cream and some can't have it at all, therefore the meal needs to be modified. The Standard Meals can be used for any ratio but were designed for the 4:1 and 3:1 ratios. Lower ratios such as 1:1 and 2:1 allow much more carbohydrates and/or proteins and need more editing for palatability. The majority of users select the Standard Meals then modify them. This is much faster than using the "Create Meal from Scratch" option, which requires knowledge of food composition in order to design meals.

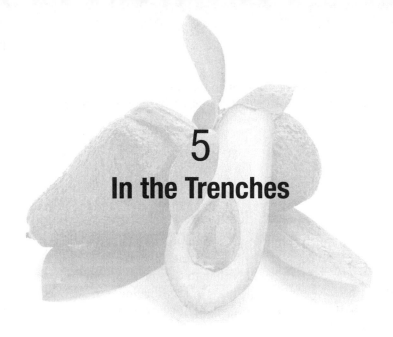

5
In the Trenches

Marching Forward

Remember when you started your first job and someone told you to give yourself about three months before you feel comfortable and confident in your new role? The same holds true for starting a ketogenic diet. Whether you are beginning the Modified Atkins Diet (MAD) or a 4:1 ratio on the Ketogenic diet, the first few months are going to be a challenge. Because you are new to the ritual of counting fat and carbs, food will feel as though it has taken over your life. You will think about it, dream about it, make it, feed it, and clean it up. Try to be patient with yourself. Know you will make mistakes. Know that your child might struggle with the foods you make, and that you might have to try dozens of meals before you find a meal he will eat without complaining. Allow yourself this learning curve.

In this section of the book, we try to address some of the common challenges you will encounter in these early months and moving forward. Because every child is different, and every child will react to these diets differently, please know that we could not tackle every side effect that might happen, nor are we medical experts. Your child's dietitian and neurologist should always be your primary source of counsel when making decisions and when facilitating your child's care, but the content within the pages of this book is meant to supplement your expectations with the experience of many parents who have been in your boots. As we will say often in one way or another in this book, the more information you are armed with, the more weapons you have in your arsenal to fight the enemy: epilepsy.

The Emotional Trajectory

Each person's journey is unique due to the variety of emotional baggage we bring to this adventure. In the beginning, we can't tell you exactly how you're going to feel, but you will likely be overwhelmed, perhaps a little confused, and the pressure to get it right might challenge you further. This is the time to fall back on the lessons and the perspective we introduced in Chapter 2, and it is absolutely time to lean on your support system. Just know that however difficult it feels in the beginning, it will get easier. It simply takes time. Below, parents describe how their first days and weeks on the diet affected them emotionally.

When we first started the diet, I really didn't let it get me too overwhelmed. I had lots of friends that have/had kids on the diet and I saw that they could do it, so I figured we could do it too. It was a little time consuming and scary at first, but once we got a system going in preparing the formula and meals, it got much easier. I think we were just so focused on trying to find something to help with seizure control that we would have done just about anything! —Krista

We were so excited and apprehensive to start the diet, hoping for seizure relief since medications were only making her seizures worse, but also thinking, "why should this work when nothing else has?" As we got the diet underway I felt overwhelmed and stressed at trying to keep a two-year-old with low muscle tone in the mouth from losing a drop of food while she ate. As we gained experience and knowledge, our confidence increased, we settled into a routine, and could find and fix most glitches that came our way. Seeing an 80% drop in seizures and getting rid of medication side effects made all the struggles worthwhile. —Machell

I was overwhelmed. I was scared of making a mistake. I didn't think we'd make it through breakfast let alone the entire day.

But we just kept on going. We learned to take things literally one bite at a time. —Laurie

After a rough Keto induction that involved lots of vomiting, very little eating, and no change in seizure activity, it was another three days before I was able to set a meal in front of Riley that earned a big thumbs up from him. I was so happy and relieved and hopeful again that I cried tears of joy. Within another week, we realized Riley had had half his typical number of seizures, and that alone made the struggles with planning and weighing his food, making it palatable, and making him eat it worth it all! —Wendy

Question from the Trenches: Will There Be Any Side Effects?

As concerned parents this is one of the first questions most of us ask. This is a medical therapy and as with most therapies there can be side effects, which is one of the main reasons you need to be under a doctor's supervision. The good news is that the side effects of the diets can be less severe than the side effects of most anticonvulsants.

Below are the most common side effects of these diets. They can rear their ugly head early on, or they can appear later on down the road. For more in depth information on any of these, contact your Keto Clinic or reference *Ketogenic Diets* (5th edition) by Dr. Eric Kossoff et al., which outlines these issues from a medical perspective. And by all means, if your gut tells you something is wrong, act on that impulse.

- **Kidney stones.** Kidney stones are not as common on MAD as they are on the Ketogenic diet. Signs your child might be developing kidney stones are rusty crystals in the urine or on a diaper or blood in your child's urine. Most clinics now offer a supplement called Polycitra-K, which helps to prevent kidney stones; other Keto Clinics will have you give your child baking soda. If you see signs of kidney stones, or if your child is complaining of severe pain in his abdominal area, seek medical counsel immediately. The stories of having a child's kidney stones removed are enough to terrify any parent.

- **Constipation.** The lack of fiber and excess fat in these diets result in constipation issues for many children. Start by increasing fiber in your child's diet by increasing the amount of high-fiber vegetables, and depending on the ratio, fruits. Avocados are wonderfully high in fiber, as is broccoli, turnip greens, spinach, raspberries, and apples. Medium chain triglyceride (MCT) oil, or its natural alternative, coconut oil, is another great choice. For chronic constipation, Miralax is Keto-safe and recommended by most Keto Clinics. Above all, make sure your child is well hydrated.

- **Hair loss/thinning.** With proper supplementation, this should not be a big issue, but for some children who have trouble taking their supplements, hair loss and hair thinning is a problem. Be sure your child has a good supplement, one that is high in selenium and zinc. For additional selenium, which helps promote healthy hair, add Brazil nuts to a few recipes, as Brazil nuts are very high in selenium. *The Keto Cookbook* has a very tasty recipe for Brazil nut cookies.

- **Calories/hunger issues.** This is a complex topic that truly varies from child to child, and it certainly varies whether your child is on the Ketogenic diet or on MAD. Hunger is most often caused by insufficient calories. If your child complains of hunger, contact your Keto Clinic and ask what they recommend. They might provide you with another snack during the day or very slightly adjust the calories of each meal. If your child is on MAD and experiencing hunger, try increasing the fats since they are going to fill your child up. You can also add in an extra couple snacks during the day.

- **Dehydration.** This can happen relatively quickly on a high ratio of the Ketogenic diet if your child is not drinking enough. Watch for symptoms such as lethargy, dry diapers or urinating less frequently, sunken eyes, or drier skin. As long as you really push the fluids, however, this should not be an issue. If your child is refusing to drink, try ice cubes sweetened with a zero-carb sweetener, or sweetened water frozen into popsicles. In the Toddler section of Chapter 9 are several suggestions on how to get your child to drink sufficient fluids.

- **Reflux.** Any child who had an issue with reflux before the diet will undoubtedly have reflux issues while on the diet. The high fat content seems to affect a lot of children, even if they didn't suffer from reflux before. Signs your child might have reflux can include burping, vomiting, refusing to eat, or in some extreme cases, extreme physical reactions such as throwing the arms out or arching the back. Your child's doctor will likely suggest an over-the-counter medication to alleviate the symptoms.

■ **Vomiting.** Vomiting is worrisome and miserable for your child, and all us parents have a tendency to panic. While it can be a sign of acidosis, which is very serious, a child's body adjusting to the diet and to ketosis can cause vomiting in the beginning. If your child had reflux before the diet, vomiting might be a side effect of his reflux. Or, vomiting could just be a sign of another illness not at all diet related. Work with your child's doctor and dietitian to determine what might be the cause in order to create a solution.

■ **Acidosis.** Acidosis basically means the body has become too ketotic and symptoms such as lethargy, sleepiness, or vomiting can occur. Your warrior's ketone reading on the Ketostix might be so dark that it is near black. This can be scary, and if not treated, can become serious. Push fluids so that your child doesn't also become dehydrated. Once you've talked with your neurologist, you might try giving a very small amount (usually 30 ml) of orange juice to lower your child's level of ketosis. Watch your child carefully. If she worsens, take her to the emergency room. Just be sure you are prepared with information on the diet and a number that the emergency room doctor can reach your neurologist.

■ **Hunger strikes.** There can be medical reasons that your child might refuse to eat or these reasons could be emotional. If your child refuses to eat, it could be that he is too ketotic, has reflux, or is perhaps painfully constipated. Other reasons usually have to do with your child trying to exert some control over his life again. If your child is a toddler, you might just be dealing with a developmentally appropriate picky-eater stage. We will discuss more on encouraging your child to eat and dealing with power struggles in Chapter 9, but initially, stick to all-in-one meals and make sure your child stays hydrated. Ketogenic diets mimic fasting, so the biggest issue you have to contend with is your child being overly ketotic.

■ **Cholesterol.** Your child's cholesterol will increase; it's nearly impossible for it not to. In many cases cholesterol levels seem to level out after your child has been on the diet for several months. Because these levels are checked before every ketogenic checkup (this is the reason for fasting before the bloodwork), try not to spend too much time worrying about it. If your child's cholesterol level reaches a level that concerns her doctor, then you can add more MCT or coconut oil to help lower it, as well as high-fiber vegetables such as broccoli or macadamia nuts, which are also a cholesterol-reducer. Replace butters, when possible, with an oil such as safflower oil, which is known to lower cholesterol, and moderate higher cholesterol foods such as processed meats and egg yolks. Often cholesterol levels come down over time for children on diets without any intervention, too.

Testing Ketones

Some clinics test ketones using a blood test, though most families are instructed to test ketones at home using Bayer Ketostix. They are usually found near the pharmacy by the diabetic equipment. These Ketostix measure the size of ketones in the urine on a scale of 5 mg/dL to 160 mg/dL. Five is considered to be a trace amount, while 80 to 160 are large. Generally, the goal is for ketones to be at least 80 on these diets. Some people do better with lower ketones than others. It just varies from one person to the next.

For MAD, you likely need to only check ketones once a week. Pick the same time every week for consistency. When beginning the diet, or if you're in a stage of tweaking or of increased seizures, you can increase the times you check urinary ketones and chart the results in your journal. On the Ketogenic diet, you will likely check the ketones twice a day in the beginning, once in the morning and once at night, then less frequently over time. For consistency, try to pick the same time each day and chart the results in your journal. Most children seem to be within the 160 range in the evening and around 80 in the morning.

For infants and children in diapers, put a cotton ball in the diaper and either squeeze out the urine onto the Ketostix or press the strip into the saturated cotton ball.

Charting the Journey

As the parent of a child with epilepsy, or perhaps as a person with epilepsy yourself, you know the value of tracking seizures. If you can find patterns you can seek out triggers. If you can eliminate potential triggers and positively impact the seizure pattern, it's a small victory in this war against epilepsy. Just as you would chart whether a new anticonvulsant was successful at managing seizures, you should chart the ketogenic journey. Consider the Ketogenic diet a new form of medication; however, because you are dealing with many variables—including all the ingredients used in a day—the process can be a little more complex. The end game is the same: see what is helping seizures, and determine what could be making seizures worse.

Not all Keto Clinics or neurologists believe in seizure triggers, but most parents do. In the ketogenic online forums, triggers are a common topic, especially where foods are concerned.

In many ways, the beauty of doing a ketogenic diet is that it gives you power in this fight that you never had before. You are relying less on the time-release of an anticonvulsant in your child's bloodstream and more on the foods you choose and the meals your prepare. This can be exciting and it can be frustrating. It is exciting because you have control over everything your child puts in his mouth; it is tough because sometimes, just like the drugs, the combination might not work for some reason and your child might have a seizure. Instead of blaming yourself for doing something wrong and taking on a weight you won't be able to shake, write down everything. This will give you insight as you move forward to determine trends, food sensitivities, difficulties managing ketones, and of course, to have a visible confirmation of seizure improvement.

Like creating labels, you can create a custom tracking sheet using Microsoft Word or Excel. Print out several weeks' worth of copies, hole punch them, and place them in a binder in your Keto Corner.

Here are suggestions of items to include on your custom tracking sheet:

■ Date and day of the week

■ Meal name, ingredients, calories, and time served

■ Snack name, ingredients, calories, and time served

■ Ketone readings, both am and pm, or at a particular time you are observing seizure increases.

■ Blood sugar/glucose readings if you test them

■ Fluid consumption

■ Enter any new foods

■ Potential triggers, such as falls, headaches, sleepiness, and activities such as swimming, anything that might be relevant to you or your child

■ Seizure count, including type of seizure and time

■ Medications and supplements and time given

Battle Tip: My Epilepsy Diary

The Epilepsy Therapy Project offers a very useful tool, *My Epilepsy Diary*, which you can find on their website at www.epilepsy.com/seizurediary. It is also available for iPhone and iPad, so if you carry either of these with you, you can instantly record any seizure activity. When you or your child experiences a seizure, side effect, or mood change, or you want to enter dietary notes or other personal events related to epilepsy, use this app. Before your next doctor's appointment, simply print out a report, which provides an organized, easy-to-read record of you or your child's epilepsy history. This is very helpful in tracking the effectiveness of diet therapy treatment over the long term and helps you see whether any changes are in order.

Allergies, Sensitivities, and Intolerances

You might wonder what the difference is between an allergy, sensitivity, and intolerance, and to be honest, so did we when we began writing this. In the parental world these terms are often used loosely and interchangeably, but medically there is a difference. An **allergy** is characterized by an immune system reaction to a substance that can result in all sorts of symptoms ranging from mild to deadly. Most people have heard about some of the life-threatening ones, like peanut allergies, that have sent some kids into anaphylactic shock. But allergies can also include milder reactions, like hives, swelling, respiratory problems, or a runny nose. Usually, even just a tiny amount of the offending substance can cause an immediate reaction. If you have a food allergy you need to avoid the offending food entirely.

A **sensitivity** involves no system immune response, but the symptoms can still be nasty, ranging from digestive complaints to neurological issues. To make it more frustrating, sensitivities can present a variety of abstract symptoms like nasal mucous, generally feeling unwell, or fatigue, so identifying and tracking down sensitivities can be difficult. Common sensitivities include reactions to food additives found in processed foods. As with allergies, sensitivities can range from mild to extreme, and some can even be life threatening, particularly if exposure to the offending substance is repeated.

An **intolerance** means your body lacks the ability to process a certain type of food; most people are familiar with lactose intolerance, for example, which is caused when the body lacks an enzyme needed to process foods containing lactose, such as milk. Gluten intolerance to the protein in wheat is another common problem many people suffer. Food intolerance symptoms usually come on gradually and in some cases you may be able to eat small amounts of the offending substance without a problem.

After first learning about allergies, sensitivities, and intolerances, it's easy to become paranoid and suspicious of every bite you eat. That is not our goal, and to be honest, we have seen some parents nearly paralyzed with fear once they learn that their child (like all kids) might react to certain foods. We'll use straight talk here: food is not the enemy. You've got enough to worry about without panicking that your daughter's runny nose is possibly being caused by a food sensitivity doing its evil job. Chances are, she just caught a sniffle and everything will be fine. But sometimes, some kids have issues, and if your child does, it's good to be informed.

When things aren't working with the diet, before throwing up your hands and quitting, it can be a smart idea to rule out the possibility that seizure control may be compromised by reactions to offending foods. If you suspect your child has an allergy, sensitivity, or intolerance that may be affecting seizure control, talk to your doctor. Be forewarned, however, that you might get some raised eyebrows. Reactions to foods do not commonly cause seizures in children, and yes, it is definitely not the first thing you look for when treating epilepsy. However, if you are already at this stage of the game and you still don't have good seizure control on the diet, you are already searching for that elusive needle in the haystack that is causing trouble. Eliminating the possibility that some foods are causing unusual problems for your child is a simple step, so it makes sense to look into it. If it is not the culprit, then no harm's done. If it is the problem, then the key to improved seizure control might be as simple as just not giving a particular food.

We want to make it clear that we do not want to give parents on these diets more work. We know you are already busy, busy, busy. Finding out if a reaction to a certain food is causing problems should not become a difficult and convoluted process, the elusive search for the holy grail of seizure control. Most likely foods aren't the culprit. However, we suggest if you suspect reactions to foods might be a problem, take these simple steps to find out.

Allergy Panel Test: Allergies can usually be determined by ordering an allergy panel test at a lab. If your child has an immune related reaction to foods or other substances it usually (though not always) will show up. Bear in mind that allergies can change or develop over time, so sometimes it has to be done every few years. Meridianvalleylab.com is an online resource that will do a full allergy panel for a cost. Marilyn, a mom to a daughter on MAD with multiple allergy and gut issues that she has been dealing with for 26 years, comments, *"You do not have to have a doctor's prescription, but some insurance companies will cover it if you do."*

Finding out that your child is dealing with allergies on top of being on a ketogenic diet can be a tough call. On the other hand, knowing about them is going to help you fine-tune things so you can give your child the best care possible, as Lynette found out:

> *It was really hard when we first found out about Zach's milk allergy. I felt like someone punched me in the stomach, but again, another flicker of hope that maybe THIS would help the seizures. In some ways, it felt like I was starting Keto all over again. On a positive side, his meals became very clean...basic meat for protein, a fruit/vegetable, and then typically we created "crunchy candy"—a mixture of coconut oil, butter, ground mac nuts, and pecans melted together with two drops of English toffee Stevia and frozen. He really missed cheese in the beginning. The kid LOVED Colby jack cheese. In fact, pre-diet, it was a joke in our house that it was Colby Zach cheese because he ate so much of it. I found a couple dairy free cheeses (that smell awful) that melt nice in meals and he likes them. It isn't anything I would slice and allow him to eat alone, but on a pizza or for mac n cheese, they are fine.*

Sleuthing Problems: The Process of Elimination

Many parents lament that they did not receive a user's manual describing their child's own unique set of operating instructions at birth. Finding what works for your child can be a fine art, but this is why parents can make the world's greatest diet detectives. Nobody knows your child like you do, so you can watch and observe subtle changes and influences in ways no one else really can. There might be times when you feel like a cartoon version of Sherlock Holmes, outfitted with a cap and hat and a magnifying glass, looking into every corner of your child's life trying to figure out how to get rid of those remaining seizures.

While an allergy panel test can help you track down immune-related problems, sensitivities, and intolerances won't show up on these tests, so the best way to find out if they are the culprits is by the simple process of elimination and observation. We touched on this topic in Chapter 4 when we talked about the two different camps of thought, Natural and Traditional. Scale back your menu for a while to include only a small selection of basic whole foods, such as vegetables, several types of protein, and fats. Don't add commercial packaged products with multiple ingredients while you're on a sleuthing "mission"; it just makes it harder to find out what is causing the trouble. During this time your food and seizure records are your new best friends. Refer back to them each day to see if there is a link between increased seizure activity and certain foods. You will usually be able to note a reaction within a day and often within hours. If you do find something causes trouble, all you have to do is stop using that food. You can gradually add in new foods, one at a time, and keep notes looking out for any unusual problems. Every child is different and most have no trouble with foods, but if you suspect your child is one of the few who do, it's good to find out. If you find no correlation between food and seizures in your child, then at least you know what the problem isn't, and there can be real peace in that.

If you are still in the clueless stage as to what could be causing problems, if possible, ask your child's teacher to also write down what happens at school: art supplies used, scheduled activities—anything. The more information in front of you, the better chance you have of finding patterns in seizure behavior. For example, if you note that every Sunday your child has a seizure, you can look into what happens consistently on Saturdays. Is he consistently handling play dough or painting at the activity center that day each week, or is he scheduled for a swim class? Or is that the day you serve his favorite dessert containing (fill in the blank)? Or perhaps the seizures seem to consistently occur in the bathroom or the bedroom immediately after a shower. One parent discovered the chlorine fumes in the closed bath stall were doing their dirty work. Incredibly, a filter installed on their shower faucet solved the problem. This process takes time and patience, but many parents have found success over time.

We would like to insert a word to the wise, however, along with a little warning about approaching sleuthing in the right spirit, otherwise it may drive you into an obsessive-compulsive guilt-riddled frenzy. Go back and review Chapter 2 of this book about handling the emotional minefield of epilepsy if you find yourself heading in that toxic direction. You cannot control every unknown factor in your child's life and it is not healthy for you (and definitely not for your child) should you try to do so. Sleuthing is a wonderful servant but a terrible master, so don't let it begin to rule your life. Most seizures just seem to happen without our ever knowing why. Sometimes hearing anecdotal evidence from other parents can be confusing or even disheartening. What works well for one child might send another into a cluster of seizures, so where do you begin? Our advice: keep it simple. Try not to let this search define your life and stress you out or you'll start seeing seizure triggers behind every blade of grass and drive yourself crazy in the process.

On an encouraging note, some parents have found that after their child is weaned from the diet, certain foods or ingredients that once triggered seizures might eventually be well tolerated. Don't ask us why; we don't think anyone really knows. Perhaps in much the same way an injured ankle needs rest following a sprain, some kids need to give their bodies a break from certain foods for a time, but later can consume them without incident. Though sometimes it's hard to find any rhyme or reason to it, the important thing is to find out what works for you.

Here are a few diverse examples that we gleaned from parents who managed to track down their own personal 'public enemy number one' that was causing their child's problems. The list shows a wide variety of tolerances and intolerances and certainly proves the adage, "what's one man's meat is another man's poison."

Sleuthing: Sweeteners

There are many low-carb sweeteners on the market. Some are natural, like Stevia, which is extracted from plants. The liquid version, without alcohol or fillers (such as Sweet Leaf brand), comes in various flavors and is very popular among parents. Because it is a plant, sometimes people who have ragweed allergies don't tolerate it so well. Other sweeteners are artificial, such as saccharin, Splenda, and aspartame and are more commonly used in commercially sweetened drinks, syrups, and low-carb products. As you can see below, different parents report different results when using them.

Throughout her life, something Kimberly would eat would set off seizures, sometimes immediately, but often the next day. We initially saw improvement [on MAD] but then saw her backslide, and I realized it was the Sweet and Low we were using to sweeten her drinks. We switched to plain powdered Stevia by KAL and her seizures settled down again. We even stay away from the flavored liquid Stevias because our daughter is so sensitive. —Marilyn

Stevia was a real problem with my son in the beginning. Splenda too. The only thing that did not cause seizures was saccharin, so we sweeten everything with it. —Holly

It took some sleuthing but I figured out the Splenda in my daughter's Fruit20 water was the culprit for her seizures. When I removed artificial sweeteners, dyes, and flavorings we got back on track quickly. —Heather

Sleuthing: Additives and Preservatives

Some parents have reported trouble with additives, commonly found in processed foods; eliminating the additives from their diets was their personal key to seizure control.

It was not until I eliminated nitrates from my son's diet that he became seizure free. Nitrates are found in many processed foods, such as hot dogs and deli meats. I also eliminated yellow dye #5, red dye #40, and sodium benzoate. After two years on the diet, my son remained completely seizure free and anti-epileptic medication free. He was then weaned off the diet and remained seizure free. —Michael

We've had to eliminate the KoolAids, Crystal Lite, DaVinci syrups or anything else that has either red dye #40 or yellow dyes #5 and #6 because Sean will have seizures from those dyes. —Mom to child on MAD

We found that our daughter quickly lost the very good and very quick seizure control she found with MAD when we introduced whipping cream. We had a strong suspicion carageenan in her heavy whipping cream was the culprit. Once we were able to find a brand without carageenan she regained control within about a week. —Joanna

Sleuthing: Various Foods and Drinks

Keeping your seizure and food record updated daily is a great way to determine if something just isn't working. Here are some examples parents found in commonly consumed foods and beverages.

My helpful hint that I believe was a big factor in getting seizure control was the elimination of low carb products such as tortillas. Once I omitted those we saw a HUGE change in his behavior, better concentration, bigger vocab, and seizure control. —Holly

In our case, my son cannot eat wheat in any form or he'll have a seizure...so no bread of any kind other than the ones made from almond flour or other nut flours. —Mom of child on MAD

*By rotating oils I have learned which ones she can tolerate
and just stick to those, rotating them every fourth day. For
her, the safe ones are canola oil, sunflower oil, ghee (clarified
butter), and avocado oil. I need to stay away from coconut oil.*
—Marilyn

Sleuthing: Spices, Herbs, and Essential Oils

Many people use essential oils for massage; however, oils are absorbed
through the skin, and some people have trouble with them. Common herbs
and spices used in cooking can sometimes cause reactions for certain people, so don't forget to add them in your food record.

*I react to lavender and rosemary. However some of the chemi-
cals that most people react to, like aspartame, I don't react
to. Our bodies are unique and intricate and wonderful, yet
strangely made.* —Heidi

Sometimes it is not a particular food or additive per se that seems to
cause trouble, but other factors that cause trouble. Tracking some of the
more common ones can sometimes reveal problems.

Sleuthing: Vitamin Deficiencies

*For no reason apparently, my son's seizures would go away in the
summer and come back around Thanksgiving, become a real problem by March, and then start to go away again, year after year.
I started having his doctor monitor vitamin D levels and giving
him a vitamin D supplement. This has helped a lot.* —Dana

Sleuthing: Chlorine Reactions

*My son has been on the diet for about eight years. He is gener-
ally seizure free, but I noted a sharp increase in his seizures
about two years ago when he was introduced to swimming
at school. He started having one per day. We took him off the
swimming and his seizures stopped. Sadly, most public swimming pools are chlorinated, but you could look into making
your pool a saltwater pool if it is your own.* —Dana

*When my son was on MAD and we had gained about 60%
improvement in seizure control, we took him swimming in a
public baby pool. He swallowed a gulp of water and the next
day he had 32 seizures, more than he had ever had, and almost
four times as many as he was averaging after starting MAD.
Since that day, he has not put a toe in a chlorinated pool, and
for a while, we even cut out public water because of the small
amounts of chlorine in it.* —Erin Whitmer

Sleuthing: Sleep Trouble

Getting sufficient rest plays a large part in seizure control. Making sure
your nighttime routine is a calm and relaxing one, and sometimes offering
a high-fat snack before bed, can often help. Some parents discuss the use
of supplements with their doctor such as melatonin and L-tryptophan, or
the popular magnesium drink, Natural Calm, if their children develop sleep
issues while on the diet.

*As the summer approaches and there is light longer, many
children have bouts of insomnia, but for our kiddos, sleep is so
important. Without it, they are left more vulnerable to seizures.
We have used melatonin for years with no issues. Doses vary
from child to child. Some children on my caseload (and I work
with preschoolers) require 9 mg per night for ideal sleep. There
has been research to show that not all children make appropriate
amounts of melatonin and without supplementation have severe
sleep disturbances. Dev always has sleep issues, but they are usually the worst during med changes...the diet is like a med change
if you think about it. Make sure there are no hidden ingredients
in the form of melatonin you are using. The liquids and chewa-
bles likely have sweeteners. Other OTC remedies are L-tryptophan
(chemical found in turkey that makes us sleepy), Natural Calm
Magnesium Drink (powder that you dissolve in water), or
lavendar essential oil massaged into temples after warm bath.
Camomile tea can also be relaxing for those who can tolerate it. I
have Devyn's Pandora app on her iPad loaded up with classical/
calming music to play while she is falling asleep.* —Heather P.

As you can see from the examples above, and as we repeat endlessly
in this book, every child (and adult) is different. What works for one does

not work for another. Sleuthing to find what works for you can be a tedious process, but when you do find valuable clues, like Sherlock Holmes, you will be able to proudly declare, "Mystery solved!"

Sleuthing: Detergents

A few weeks ago, we had a cluster of TC seizures, five of them in the period between 1:00 a.m. and 5:00 a.m. one night…and this was after not having had a TC seizure in nearly two years. In trying to figure out what might have caused them I realized someone who was helping me changed my son's bedding and dug in the linen closet for a particular sheet that had not been used in months. It was washed in some detergent that I had discontinued due to suspecting Sean was reacting to it. Sure enough, as soon as we changed the sheets to those washed with the detergent that is safe for him, the TC's stopped and he hasn't had another. —Carol

Sleuthing: Behavioral Changes

Our son never reacted to a food/spice/supplement by having an actual seizure around the time of consuming whatever it was that he turned out to be sensitive to. Rather, his seizure threshold would be lowered. It was as if he would have increased sub-clinical activity, which probably would have shown up on an EEG but didn't necessarily manifest itself in an actual seizure. He would get really confused and disoriented or laugh uncontrollably or act more "child-like" (he's eight now but would regress for a time to a two to three year old). It was as if a seizure was getting ready to hit, but it didn't always happen. Following the diet in a way that's appropriate for him would keep the seizures/activity at bay, but when he was consuming something that didn't agree with him, his seizure threshold would drop and a seizure would eventually push through. —Karolina

Sleuthing: Blood Sugar Spikes

For us, it's important to BOTH keep the carbs low and to keep Sean's blood sugar from spiking. He will have seizures from too many carbs at once and also from going too long without eating. So, we try to portion out the carbs fairly equally among breakfast, snack, lunch, snack, dinner, and sometimes another snack before bed. —Carol

Off Limits! Tackling Dietary Restrictions

Many children are already on special diets because of food allergies, and often parents are puzzled about how to work around those issues when starting the Ketogenic diet or MAD. Thankfully, high-fat low-carb diets can be adapted to almost every specific dietary need. *Ketogenic Diets* (5th edition) by Dr. Eric Kossoff, et al., has an excellent chapter that covers this. "The Diet for All Cultures, Religions, Food Preferences and Allergies," Chapter 6, explains how to make substitutions when certain foods must be avoided. To quote their work, *"The trick to allergies is to look at what the child is currently eating and pair it with a fat they can tolerate."* Here are a few examples from different parents on Keto and MAD showing how you can work around your own child's food restrictions, no matter what type of diet they are following.

> *My daughter has multiple food allergies especially to wheat, gluten, milk, eggs, white potatoes, and sugars. We had already put her on the Specific Carbohydrate diet (SCD) a couple of years ago because of her many allergies and gut pain issues, along with eliminating the foods we knew she was allergic to. We started the MAD diet in December, mainly just adding lots of fat to what she was already eating. However, after seeing a nutritionist he recommended the Low Glycemic Index Treatment diet. So we are doing the SCD diet, using low glycemic index vegetables, and following the MAD protocol for high fat, moderate protein, and low carbs (20 grams for her). And it is working! Soon after, Kim was able to lower one of her meds (Lyrica) by one pill, and her seizure control continues to improve, plus she feels so much better on less meds.*
> —Marilyn

If your child can't tolerate certain fats, finding ones that work well can take some experimentation. If your child tends to tolerate certain types of oil for a time but then begins to have trouble when it is constantly used, rotating different oils each day can sometimes solve the problem. There may also be fat sources you haven't thought of trying before that could work for your child. A dietitian can point you in the right direction in your search for food substitutes.

> *Finding fats my daughter can tolerate has been the hardest issue. Olive oil seems to be safe. We tried coconut oil because*

of the high MCT in it, but she developed a rash. She also didn't tolerate palm oil, flax, or safflower oil. Butter is high in MCT, but since Kim is allergic to milk, I was concerned that she would not be able to tolerate butter. The nutritionist suggested ghee (clarified butter), and, sure enough, she handles it fine.
—Marilyn

Gluten Free/Casein Free

Many children with autism or behavioral issues follow gluten free/casein free (GFCF) diets. When breaking out of a familiar dietary routine, it might help you to do it in small steps instead of jumping in with both feet. Heather shares below how she worked with her daughter who has autism and was on a GFCF diet when she transitioned to MAD.

I gradually weaned my daughter from some of her favorite things, first her rice milk, which was a staple for her. Then I invented a "brownie bite" to replace her love of GFCF chocolate bars. Little by little we replaced things and when she had her last big cluster of seizures at the beginning of December, we knew it was time to go all the way. . My advice is to figure out four or five meals/snacks that your child is really going to enjoy before you go full force into the diet. It takes some of the stress out of it. —Heather P.

Working with a dietitian is the best way for you to work around dietary restrictions, as they can offer valuable direction and advice. Otherwise, if you are already dealing with a restricted diet and attempt to move ahead by adding a ketogenic diet into the mix without any support, you're going to wind up feeling like a marginalized "minority within a minority."

I do not think that I can express clearly enough how extremely lonely, frightened, and overwhelmed I felt when beginning MAD. To add to my feelings was the fact that many people on MAD are not gluten/casein free so much of the advice for foods included items my son could not eat such as whipping cream, cheese, and butter. Knowing he was already sensitive to some foods, I decided to take this opportunity to keep my son's diet as simple as possible and as pure as possible. I chose to eliminate all artificial sweeteners, preservatives, dyes, sugar/

sugar alcohols, soy, and any known seizure triggers such as rosemary, sage, and fennel. We now have a newly stocked pantry and refrigerator, filled with pork rinds, coconut oil, light olive oil, eggs, chopped low carb veggies, homemade mayonnaise, Stevia, and a freezer filled with fatty meats and fish and frozen low-carb vegetables. —Pam

Problems with Nuts or Soy

Often on the Ketogenic diet or MAD, products using nuts and soy are included as they are a good source of protein. They are not essential, however, and alternatives are available. For those with problems with soy, avoid low-carb products with ingredients such as "flavorings" or "natural flavorings," "vegetable gum" and "vegetable starch," as they often contain soy.

Molly experienced seizure freedom after six weeks on the Ketogenic diet. Just as I began to breathe, after she had been seizure free for a month, I noticed small red hives around Molly's mouth, neck, and belly after she ate peanut butter for approximately the 30th time. We took her to a pediatric allergist, who tested her skin and blood for a variety of common allergies. In both the skin and blood tests, she showed that she had allergies to peanut and soy. We decided to play it safe and avoid all peanuts, tree nuts, and soy products until we were able to see an expert pediatric allergist at Johns Hopkins.

During the months waiting for the appointment, I spent hours searching through grocery and natural foods stores, reading articles and recipes online, and seeking out advice from people on restricted diets. Luckily, Molly was two and didn't mind repetition of the same foods each day. She ate a lot of eggs mixed with butter and cream. We would mix up the fruits and vegetables to keep it interesting and healthy. Also, we found Earth's Balance Soy-Free Spread, a canola mayonnaise, and a ranch dressing made with canola oil. We created grilled cheese sandwiches and buttery pizzas using Oopsie Rolls. I baked muffins in Christmas tins using canola oil, egg beaters, baby food bananas, and Fiber One flour. She didn't particularly miss the peanuts or soy, but I hoped that she wouldn't grow tired of her meals because I felt limited. —Lynn

It's great to know that no matter what your child's needs, these diets can accommodate a wide range of preferences and restrictions. With some creativity and a little research, you'll be preparing suitable meals in no time.

Supplements

Your dietitian should provide you with a list of supplements that are already Keto approved, and you can always check out the low-carb list of products on the Charlie Foundation site, but the question about supplements is always brought up in the ketogenic communities. We have provided a list of potential online sites for you to find vitamins and supplements that are 100% natural and free of various allergens. When searching for a supplement, look at the ingredients and the carb count. Avoid vitamins with alcohol sweeteners, starch, sugar, gluten, and other potentially high-carb ingredients. When you find a supplement you think might work, always check with your dietitian before using it to make sure it is Keto friendly and to ensure correct dosing for you or your child. In general, tablets are better than liquids, and certainly better than chewable tablets or gummies.

- Country life. www.country-life.com. Vegetarian, hypoallergenic supplements for children and adults.

- Freeda vitamins. www.freedavitamins.com. Vegetarian supplements that are all free of yeast, gluten, lactose, sugar, and salt.

- Kirkman. www.kirkmanlabs.com. Specially formulated hypoallergenic supplements, many of which are free of soy and starch.

- NuLife. www.nulifevitamins.com. Wide range of formulations for different age groups. Most are hypoallergenic and vegetarian.

- Nutricology. www.nutricology.com. Adult and children's multiple vitamins, specially formulated for individuals with food sensitivities.

The Question of Carnitine

At some point in your ketogenic journey, you or your child might be prescribed carnitine as a supplement. Carnitine is an amino acid that is found in nearly all cells of the body, and it plays a critical role in energy production. It transports long-chain fatty acids into the mitochondria of the cell so they can be burned to produce energy. (We bet you're wishing you paid better attention in biology right about now!) In healthy adults and children, our liver and kidneys produce enough amino acids to meet daily needs. However, there have been several studies that state that while on the Ketogenic diet, serum carnitine levels decrease. Signs of a potential carnitine deficiency can include fatigue, low ketosis, and lack of energy.

Most Keto Clinics test for carnitine levels at each ketogenic check-up. If your child has any of the above symptoms and you have already ruled out other potential causes with your dietitian, ask that your child's free and total carnitine levels be checked. This is done through a blood test. If levels are low, most neurologists will supplement carnitine at that point.

There is an ongoing debate over how much carnitine equals the most benefit. Many children on the diet don't require supplementation, while other clinics and dietitians prescribe it more readily. Further research is needed to determine what its overall benefits—or lack of benefits—are to children and adults on a ketogenic diet. However, there are some people who believe that carnitine supplementation was the missing link in the chain to seizure control.

Carnitine, as a supplement, is not appealing for most children, as it tastes pretty terrible. If introduced at higher doses too quickly, it can cause unappealing side effects, sometimes including an increase in seizures. You can also try to increase carnitine levels naturally by increasing foods such as meat, fish, and poultry. Generally speaking, the redder the meat, the higher the carnitine content. 4 ounces of beef steak, for example, has between 56 and 162 milligrams of carnitine.

Drug Weaning and Adding Medications

One of the absolute trickiest topics to tackle with epilepsy in general, and certainly within the specific boundaries of a ketogenic diet, is when to wean drugs. We want to be very clear that we are not medical profession-als, just a pair of moms who felt compelled to share our stories and to share other people's stories about how best to survive the life-changing choice of pursuing a ketogenic diet. We are only two stories of hundreds, and of those hundreds of stories, not one child is the same. As parents of children with epilepsy we all seek to compare our children. Sometimes we do it in the hopes our story might be as uplifting; at other times we make the comparison to feel better that our child is not as bad off as another. When it comes to the topic of weaning drugs, the same tendency to adopt other people's experiences as our own tends to motivate us, whether for the better or for the worse.

In this section, because talking about weaning meds specifically is impossible, we hope to enable you to be your child's best advocate: educated, with the ability to balance all the advice you are given, and most of all, to be brave in your responsibility and to trust yourself.

Educate yourself: Every medication has a long list of side effects, and certain drugs have reputations for creating adverse reactions when coupled with a ketogenic diet. Get all the information you can from your neurologist and also do some online digging. Be forewarned, however, not all content out there is true. Try to stick with reputable sites when doing your research, such as hospitals or epilepsy foundations.

Learn about other experiences: No single person's experience is indicative of what will happen to your child, nor do two people's similar stories equal a general conclusion about a drug. However, by learning of other people's experiences with a drug you open up yourself to seeing things differently, and maybe that similarity will prove to be a clue in what your next steps should be. Tread carefully when mentioning other children's experience with a drug to your doctor; it doesn't seem to be a popular topic.

Use your journal: The decision to wean drugs is another testament to the importance of keeping a journal. If you can pin down seizure activity to timeframes that a drug is taken, or if seizures increase or decrease with the change of a drug, you have very significant data that you can present to your child's neurologist to argue your case.

Watch your child: No one knows your child better than you. Watch for changes of behaviors that might correlate to the medications he is on. If he has a tendency to be more tired at some point in the day, and you've already tweaked the diet to add a snack to power him through, perhaps it's that morning dose of his medication that is slowing him down. The potential for side effects and the unique ways they can manifest themselves will only go noticed by someone who knows your child as well as you do.

Stand your ground: As your child's advocate, as the one who knows him best, you might feel that you are not being heard by your child's doctor. While there are no doubt medical reasons that, in your doctor's mind, outweigh your parental instincts, you can still present your case and fight for what you believe in. We are not suggesting you defy doctor's orders—there is great potential for hazard in that—but we believe that an educated parent who knows her child has just as much to say in the argument concerning medication as your child's doctor. Just be certain you can present and support a solid argument; that's where education and knowing your child weigh heavily.

There is a misconception out there that the goal of a ketogenic diet is to be drug free. While that might be one of the expectations you discussed with your doctor and a personal goal, it is not a fair expectation for everyone. Try shifting your expectations so that seizure control is the goal. This way there is less stress accompanying the idea of either weaning or adding medications. Ultimately, you want your child to stop seizing. You want his brain to heal. Sometimes the best combination is the diet and a medication, or maybe two. For other children they find better seizure freedom once the drugs are out of the picture. You will never know how your child will react to the diet until you are deep in the trenches. At that point you can discuss weaning or adding a medication. Many neurologists see the diet and drugs as a partnership. As long as you remain diligent in educating yourself—and you learn to trust yourself—the question on how to handle drugs will feel somewhat less convoluted.

The following are several first-person accounts of parents' experiences weaning medications.

Owen, who is six years old now, started MAD at two and a half and started Keto at three years. He was on the diet for three and a half years. He had been on the diet and the Depakote for so long that I felt something had to give since his seizures were still not 100% controlled. Owen also has liver tumors and we felt that the Depakote might be interfering with his liver so that was another reason for the wean. We took the Depakote wean extremely slow, 1/4 of a capsule every month or so. One book that helped me through all this was Ben Carson's, Take the Risk. *This book helped me tremendously to evaluate a situation and know when to take a risk. —Amy*

We started the diet with the same hopes as so many other parents, seizure freedom—but ultimately I wanted him off the Depakote if nothing else. He'd had lots of side effects and we were just hoping to get our little guy back from the constant yoyo between lethargy and impulsiveness. Levi had five glorious days of seizure freedom at the beginning of the diet. His seizures then started coming back and we made lots of tweaks. I asked the doctor if we could try weaning Depakote when seizures got worse than they were before the diet. She agreed, though very hesitantly. He weaned off the Depakote over a six-month period. Today, Levi's much more alert, has his sense of humor back and has also been able to wean off of the two meds he was taking for ADHD behaviors. He continues to have seizures daily but there has been some slight improvement off the meds. —Rebecca

We started the diet a year and a half ago and Max was on Keppra, clonazepam, Trileptal, and Zonegran. We weaned Trileptal after three months on the diet. I took about a month to do this. He had a bit of a little breakthrough seizures, but this stopped as quickly as it started. We then tried to wean his clanazepam 12 months into the diet. He was having more breakthrough then I wanted (I believe this was due to the speed at which the Neuro had me wean), so I put him back to the prewean dose and waited two months to try again. I took about six weeks to wean it, with a bit of breakthrough, but just for a few weeks. Very livable! Next month we will start to wean his Zonegran! —Shannon

Our story is a bit unique in that most families start weaning meds after achieving seizure freedom with the diet. We started weaning Oliver within two months of the Ketogenic diet initiation, even though he wasn't seizure free. Since the medications he was taking were both advised for short term use we figured we'd have to wean them eventually anyway. Why not begin as soon as possible and give the diet a chance to work on its own? When we started the diet, Oliver was on Sabril (vigabatrin) and clonazepam on a daily basis. We started weaning the clonazepam first. The wean went smoothly, with maybe one major seizure a few days after each dosage drop. As we got closer to getting off the medication, the wean became harder, and we had to slow down our timing. Oliver experienced withdrawal symptoms (very cranky and irritable) but leveled off once he was off the medication for several weeks. We followed a very similar, very slow wean with the Sabril and experienced much of the same behavior from Oliver (fine in the beginning and irritable and cranky toward the end of the wean). Once we had him off of all of his medications we noticed he became much more alert and able to stay awake during the day. Having his awareness back was worth the wean, even though we still haven't achieved seizure freedom over one and a half years into the diet. —Bethany

My son is autistic also (along with other disabilities) and the first thing we saw with starting MAD was almost complete cessation of stimming and other autistic behaviors, as well as very noticeable cognitive gains and a huge change in mood to a much lighter and more fun guy. The MAD journey for my son has been that every time we had a period of time with no seizures, then they started again, it meant he needed a decrease in meds. The neurologist we were seeing at that time said it was "counterintuitive" to drop meds when seizures increased and recommended we go back up in meds. We did that the first couple of times he recommended that and our result was that the seizures became more violent. We changed our neurologist. We dropped his Topamax 1/4 tab and immediately saw a huge decrease in seizures. We left him at that dose until seizures started increasing again and then dropped another 1/4 tab, which resulted in another decrease in seizures. We have weaned off Topamax, Zonegran, Depakote, and Lamictal this way. He is still on a low dose of Lamictal and is holding steady at about one mild absence-type seizure every two weeks or so. —Pam

Doctor's Visits and ER Trips

Don't be fooled: when it comes to ketogenic diets, there are few medical professionals who know what these diets entail and the limitations the diet presents as far as treating your child. It is a constant complaint among many parents that an ER trip turns into an argument between the educated parent and the medical professional who hasn't learned the nuances and restrictions of a ketogenic diet. We are not faulting the medical community; after all, there is a reason there are specialists: there is simply too much information out there for one person to absorb. The responsibility of ensuring your child is appropriately cared for, then, is yours.

Take it upon yourself to be as educated as possible about your child's diet. By participating in online forums you have the advantage of learning through other parents' experiences. Though your child might never have had kidney stones, you will certainly benefit from learning how they are treated and the challenges parents have had when dealing with this common side effect. This is true for just about any medical issue that will come your way.

Have your child's Keto Clinic provide you with the following forms, if possible: 1) Keto-approved medications, and 2) an explanation of the restrictions of the diet and general DO's and DON'Ts. For example, if your child is dehydrated, many ERs will give your child glucose in the saline. Glucose will knock your child out of ketosis. Instead, your child should have only a saline drip. Whenever possible, travel to doctor's appointments with medical records or ensure that medical record copies have been faxed to your child's doctor. When at the pediatrician, instead of finding yourself in a bind over how to treat your child's ear infection, these forms will provide the information essential to ensuring your child's diet is maintained, while also dealing with external medical issues. You should also have your neurologist's phone number and e-mail for emergencies. There will be situations when it is appropriate for the attending at the ER or your pediatrician to talk to your neurologist about treatment for your child.

Trust us, it is terribly frustrating to have your child's doctor tell you that a medication is fine, even though in your gut you know it is not. Unfortunately, parents aren't paid to have gut feelings, and we're not medical professionals; therefore, our word will likely be taken with a grain of salt. Having resources at your fingertips to assist you in being your child's advocate will save you a lot of anxiety.

Lab Work

Before each checkup with the Keto Clinic, your child will have an extensive panel of blood work and urinalysis done. Typical lab tests include: a complete blood count with platelets; electrolytes, including serum bicarbonate, total protein, calcium, zinc, selenium, magnesium, and phosphate; serum liver and kidney tests, including creatinine; fasting lipid profile; serum acylcarnitine profile; urinalysis; urine calcium and creatinine; and anticonvulsant drug levels. Clearly, this is a long list and several vials of blood will be drawn from your child, which can translate into an unpleasant experience for your child.

Here are several tips to make the process a little easier.

■ **Find a lab that specializes in children.** You are limited to some extent due to your insurance, but if possible, call around and ensure that there is a skilled technician who can make your child's blood work as painless as possible. Because children's, and especially infants,' veins are so tiny and because they can be tough to hold still, it takes an artful hand to draw blood without distressing your child.

■ **Make your child's appointment as early in the morning as possible.** Because fasting is required for the lipid panel, your child will be hungry and cranky if you wait to schedule an appointment in the afternoon. Make the appointment super early, get it over with, and have a snack for your child to eat after his appointment is finished.

■ **If your child doesn't urinate on command, of if dehydration has been at all a factor during your diet experience, consider getting a couple urine cups and urine bags in advance of your child's lab appointment.** If you have a young baby, you can attach the urine bag and cut a hole in the diaper to accommodate the bag. Do this first thing in the morning and you are guaranteed to have a urine sample by appointment time. Store it in the fridge and bring it to the appointment; just be clear with the lab technician that this was indeed done after fasting. After your child has several vials of blood drawn, you will not want to wait around in a lab waiting room for your child to urinate.

■ **Bring toys or items that will calm your child.** Considering you have a child with epilepsy, you are likely no stranger to getting through long doctor visits and grueling ER trips. Music works wonders for many children to soothe them, so consider bringing your cell phone or iPod with music. A new book or small toy can also take the sting out of the experience.

6
On the Move

Once you've gotten in the groove of preparing ketogenic or Modified Atkins Diet (MAD) meals at home, the time will soon come when you'll want to "mobilize your troops" and travel to visit friends and family, or take off for a well-deserved vacation. You'll also want to open your doors and host diet-friendly birthday parties and celebrations, or send your child to attend parties at the homes of friends. You certainly don't want to let diet therapy put a damper on all the fun of living, so let's learn about Keto-on-the-go!

Making Parties Fun Again

Birthday parties have long revolved around food. Until now, the food side of things might have been one of your child's favorite qualities about the parties he's attended. However, once the traditional cupcakes and chocolate cake covered with colorful, sugary frosting is placed off limits, birthday parties can quickly transform from lively social occasions to anxiety-inducing events everyone in the family dreads. So, how can you save the day and ensure parties remain all-time-favorite activities? Whether you're throwing the party or you're attending someone else's, sugar might be off the table, but fun needn't be.

How to Throw a Keto-Friendly Party

The key to a successful party, without tears on anyone's behalf, is to shift the focus away from food. It might seem unfair to you at first, especially given society's emphasis on food at social events, but younger children are easily distracted if the environment is exciting. It will take the pressure off you and your child if you highlight other types of fun at the parties you organize.

- **First, consider throwing the party at a location other than your house.** Children's museums, public parks, indoor recreation centers, bounce houses, national parks, and public pools are all locations that shift the focus from food to activities. The children will be so immersed in the action around them that they won't have time to think, "Where are the cupcakes?"

- **Time the party so that it isn't centered on mealtime.** Morning parties or midafternoon parties are great because people will have eaten before they arrive, or they will choose to eat afterwards. Throw a party at 12:30 p.m. and you'll have hungry kids with an expectation of food.

- **Decide whether you'll provide food, and choose your menu carefully.** If you plan on serving food, consider serving low-carb snacks to all the kids. Cold cuts without bread, sliced apples and peanut butter, a tray of assorted cheeses and olives, or a veggie platter served with dressing and dip are all great options. The last thing you want to serve your guests are off-limit goodies like peanut butter and jelly sandwiches (torture for your child watching the others feast on his big day), crackers and cookies that could drop crumbs that your child might pick up (instant panic attack), or a giant cake that everyone but your child can eat (just plain mean).

- **If you do have food, keep it away from the party activities.** In your home, pick a room or a table in back, where it isn't a focal point. Kids will want to eat quickly so they can head back to the "center ring" where all the action is happening!

- **If this will be a food-free party, specify this on the invitation.** Be up front on the invitations regarding your choice that no food will be served at the party. When people RSVP, take the extra time to explain about your child's diet so they know what to expect when they arrive, and they can prepare their child for a party that might be a little unconventional.

- **Consider posting signs around the party reminding people not to feed your child.** If your child is still young, you might want to consider putting up a few strategically posted reminders as a precaution. You can't watch everyone, and because you might worry that someone will somehow give your child food that he can't have, signs can provide you with a sense of control and help settle your fears that your child may get into food that will knock him out of ketosis. If your child and his friends are older and can read, however, it is likely best to skip the signs and focus your attention on educating the parents and chaperones.

■ **It's hard to have a birthday without candles to blow and wishes to make, so instead of the conventional frosted cake, consider making cupcakes.** You can make standard cupcakes for the children attending the party and make your diet warrior a special cupcake frosted to look like the others. Decorating each cupcake with a small toy not only makes the cupcakes fun and identical, but provides a party favor each child can take home. We have a great cupcake recipe in this book that can be altered according to ratio, and the frosting can be colored with natural food coloring to make it festive and fun.

■ **When it comes to a party, anything goes!** You just need to think outside of the box to come up with an idea that your child will love. As you will see often in this book, creativity is the key to survival. For example, if your child loves pancakes, have a pancake party. Macadamia and almond-based pancakes are delicious and perfect for the diet; they are also fun because you can use pancake molds, food coloring—anything really—to make them unique for your child's birthday celebration.

Tips for Attending a Party

When your child is invited to someone else's birthday party, you will have little control over how the party plays out. Will there be carbohydrate-loaded food around every corner? Is the party centered on pizza and soda? Is it guaranteed to be an event that will leave your child in tears and you feeling guilty for the role this diet plays in your life? Worrying about it all in advance can be quite nerve wracking.

I can still remember the panic I felt when we went to our first birthday party. What if Devyn cried and wanted foods she wasn't allowed to have? What if the people there thought I was being mean by limiting her diet? There had been people who thought her GFCF restrictions were "just plain silly" and I worried that something that was even more restrictive would be viewed with even greater scrutiny. I was ready to spout off the research and made sure we literally stuffed Devyn with her favorite MAD foods before we left so she wouldn't be hungry.

We were armed with her favorite toys and her iPad. She didn't notice the forbidden foods and instead of people judging me, they praised me for following my gut! They all noticed big changes in her overall disposition and without me having to justify it, they embraced it. That experience made all the ones to follow easier. —Heather P.

There are things you can do to minimize the chance of tears at the parties your child attends when forbidden foods will definitely be served and enjoyed by the other kids. You know your child best, so follow your gut and do what you have to do. Following these simple tips can help ensure greater success when you are the guest.

■ **When you call to RSVP to the party—or even before you consider RSVP-ing—call the party's host to learn more.** First explain your child's dietary restrictions and then find out what food will be served, including what kind of cake or cupcake will be offered to the children. If it's a pizza party and your child will be content with his Keto pizza, that's great. If the menu is something that you could recreate in a high-fat version, then prepare his food and bring it to the party. Ask if the parent would mind saving you any special non-food type of decorations she'll be placing on the cupcakes or dessert, so you can add one to the dessert you bring from home for your child. This will help your child feel included.

■ **If the food isn't conducive to the diet, find out what activities will be done at the party** to help you determine if there will be enough going on to keep your child distracted from the food. If not, plan to bring fun things to do from home.

■ **Consider bringing a special treat or small toy to occupy your child when the birthday cake is served.** You can take your child into another room to play with his toy or eat his own special treat. This is not an effort to spoil your child; it's an effort to give your child something to remind him of the importance of his diet, despite the challenges, and of course, it's a chance to make him feel special.

■ **Remind your child that even the birthday kid doesn't get to eat cake all the time,** but on his special diet, he can eat ice cream every day for dinner if he wants. Take this opportunity to empower and encourage him.

■ **Talk about it before you go.** This is especially true for older kids who
are past the distract-them-with-a-toy stage of life. Even adults on the diet
can feel uncomfortable at social occasions when they realize they can't
eat anything served, so discuss how to handle such dilemmas. While
you don't want your child walking into the party totally unprepared
for cake and candy, you also don't want to be guilty of trying to over-
protect him from every possible disappointment life may hand him.
Remind your child that there will still most likely be plenty of fun things
to enjoy and that friendship is a lot more important than food. Work
out a plan together to deal with temptation, and praise him for being
a warrior.

Holidays and Festive Occasions

Now that diet therapy is part of your life, you have a wonderful opportunity
to steer holidays away from food, and create new enjoyable family traditions chock full of meaningful memories. You can address holidays in much
the same way you approach birthday parties, shifting the focus onto something other than food such as a fun activity, game, or outing. Christmas
stockings and Easter baskets can be filled with games and puzzles instead
of candy, and the pre-holiday excitement can center on decorating the
house or reading stories together about the meaning of the festival.

> *Holidays are less about candy and more about books, toys, or
> giving back to a charity. At Easter we adapted our Easter egg
> hunt to have clues written in each egg that leads you to another
> egg until you finally reach a basket of fun things that includes
> books, clothes, games, etc. No candy!* —Chris

Halloween can still be filled with costumes and pumpkin carving,
but it often poses a dilemma to kids who are used to going out trick-or-
treating and collecting bags of sugar-laden loot. Most parents get around
it by bartering with their child to turn in candy in exchange for cash or a
trip to the toy store (if he can be trusted not to snitch any), or by going
ahead to the neighbors on the route their child will follow and distribut-
ing small prizes to hand over in lieu of candy when their child rings the
bell. Some parents skip the door-to-door part of Halloween altogether
and host a costume party for kids instead, followed by a movie or other
fun activity.

One of the most important things you can do for your own self during the holiday season is to educate your family and friends about diet therapy and all it entails. Whether it's Christmas, Hanukah, Eid al-Fitr, Thanksgiving, Chinese New Year, or any other festival, encourage them to help you in any way they can (consider it part of their present to you and your child). When you take action and educate others, you create a support system and make them aware of how they can help you during the holidays. This can include taking the incentive to restructure an event so that your child won't be left out, helping you to prepare foods for your child that are similar to what everyone else is eating, or even just spreading the word to other family members and guests. Teach them how to provide you with the kind of emotional strength you need to deal with challenging situations—such as holidays—that will no doubt arise in the two or more years that a ketogenic diet will be part of your life. It may turn out to be a blessing in disguise and bring you all closer together than ever.

And remember, diet therapy isn't only about biting the proverbial bullet and sacrificing. Food can still be fun. You may even be surprised to learn how others view all the interesting things your child gets to eat. You might start to take the heaped mounds of whipping cream and daily ice-cream bonanzas for granted, but it could well be an object of envy to siblings and classmates. Even older teens can fall prey to lusting after their younger brother's or sister's low-carb, high-fat delicacies.

When my older son Chris had his 18th birthday and we were discussing inviting a couple of his friends over for a fancy dinner party, I asked him what he wanted me to make for this special meal. Without hesitation, he told me, "Jordan's food!" He thought his 14-year-old brother on MAD got to eat way better than he did, especially since Chris has recently been subjected to the monotony of college canteen meals. Whenever Chris comes home from university he's always caught sneaking some of Jordan's leftovers, and you can't blame him when his younger brother gets to feast on almond pancakes, coconut flour cake, bacon burgers, and cheesy casseroles. For our birthday bash we served a cheese and olive platter, homemade cream of mushroom soup, roasted lemon chicken with dill, egg and cauliflower fried "rice," tossed green salad with dressing, and a cheesecake topped with frozen raspberries. Jordan could eat every bite along with his older brother and friends. —Jeanne Riether

Cookies, Cakes, and Goodies Galore

When it comes to holiday cookies and treats, which are hopelessly abundant during the holidays (hence everyone's expanding waistline), you are fortunate that there are great options for your diet warrior. In the recipe section of this book, we have included several treats that will lend themselves nicely to holiday festivities. In addition to the always-popular cheesecake, consider making fudge, a peanut butter pie with whipped cream, frozen chocolate candies, coconut cookies, and pastries with macadamia or pecan crusts. Look through holiday cookbooks and spend some time brainstorming meal ideas, to see how you can adapt things to Keto-friendly fare.

Don't forget about the great appeal of creative packaging. Use holiday cookie cutters, muffin tins, and silicone cups, play around with food colorings, invest in some bright, festive plates and cups—anything to give an ordinary meal that holiday twist.

Visiting Relatives and Friends

If you're heading "over the river and through the woods to grandmother's house" for dinner, here are a few tips to remember to help things run smoothly when you are the guest.

- Feed your child something before you arrive so he doesn't hit the door ravenously hungry and surrounded by all sorts of delicious forbidden food.

- If you are bringing your own food, try to bring already prepared dishes that only need warming up, as the stove may be busy.

- Offer to bring diet-friendly contributions to the meal that everyone can enjoy.

- If your child is very young, try to arrange for temptation to be kept out of reach of little fingers. Call in advance to explain the situation and enlist support. Arrange for trays of snacks, candy, and desserts to be kept off of low coffee tables if at all possible. While it would be unreasonable to expect others to keep forbidden food entirely out of sight, keeping the delicacies up on higher tables or counters, and not right at preschooler eye level, can temper the blow.

- What do you do if the tears start? Distraction time! Head for the next room with a favorite toy or book, or an interesting DVD. The storm will soon pass and life will go on.

■ Consider hosting the event yourself. It's a lot of work, but if you invite everyone over to your place you can call the shots about how the meal is displayed and what is served. Give them all a taste of turkey stuffed with crushed pork rinds and diced almonds, a creamy cauliflower casserole, and blueberry cheesecake. And if they don't like it? Send them to the next room with an interesting DVD. (Payback time! Snicker, snicker.)

Restaurant Adventures

Most people enjoy eating out, and you won't have to forego that pleasure while on the diet. MAD is particularly restaurant friendly, but even children on the Ketogenic diet can find ways to incorporate a fun restaurant adventure while sticking to their eating plan. Thankfully, for young children much of the fun of the restaurant experience revolves around the change of scenery and being served at a table. Even if you opt for bringing most of the meal along with you from home, your child will still enjoy participating with your family in a new environment. Particularly if your family has always enjoyed going out to dinner, it's important that you try and continue that tradition and include your warrior in the process.

■ **If on Keto, you can bring along a small portable scale and weigh portions of diet friendly foods at the table**. The success of doing this is in part dependent on the ratio and wholly dependent on your creativity and advance preparation. We would never recommend a family with a child on a 4:1 ratio go to a restaurant without already having an idea of what's available on the menu, and preferably, you should go prepared with a recipe you've created in the KetoCalculator, using the menu as your guide. It is tough to make foods on a 4:1 that are savory and delicious without planning and a little innovation. Should you come to a restaurant with your child without any prep work, your child might be stuck eating about a tablespoon's worth of grilled chicken, a couple small broccoli florets, and a tremendous amount of butter packs or oil. That would surely sour any restaurant trip. When taking your warrior to a restaurant on the Ketogenic diet, try bringing some fats with you that you can calculate into the meal. For example, coconut oil candies or a very high-fat chocolate yogurt. Choose foods on the menu like sliced avocado, soft cheeses that are higher in fat, and maybe grilled chicken that can be dipped in mayo.

■ **If on MAD, take a measuring cup or get used to eye-balling the size of a half-cup serving of various vegetables.** (If you're new at this though, stick to measuring until you are confident about amounts). Keep a list of the common carb counts of foods in your purse, and look for low-carb options on the menu. You can always politely ask your server to substitute fries or chips or other forbidden foods for a salad or steamed vegetables. Most restaurants will be happy to accommodate you and provide foods that will work on the diet, so don't be afraid to ask.

■ **Or you can choose to bring food from home in containers and ask the restaurant to furnish a plate** and heat it up for you. When children on either Keto or MAD have numerous food sensitivities, or when a child is on a higher ratio that is difficult to manage "on the fly," parents often prefer this option so they'll be certain of exactly what their child is eating. Be forewarned, however, that not all restaurants will reheat your child's food, as it is sometimes against company policy. To avoid possible disaster when a restaurant won't accommodate you, bring along a meal that doesn't need reheating, and simply ask them for an extra plate for your child.

■ **A phone call and a letter.** It is wise to phone the restaurant in advance to explain the situation and ask if there will be a problem with reheating, as some establishments are concerned that they may be held responsible when serving food not prepared on site if a customer becomes ill from food poisoning. Bring along a signed letter confirming that, for medical reasons, you have furnished the food and asked them to reheat it, absolving them of responsibility. (You can keep some copies in your purse or car, and fill in the restaurant name and date when needed). Keep in mind that restaurants have policies for a reason, and unfortunately, some employees aren't aware of these policies. We've heard of situations when an establishment heated food up one day, only to refuse to do it another day, leading to a very frustrating experience for everyone, especially the warrior.

■ **Fun ways to participate.** Even if the food options are limited, let your child participate by ordering his own glass of water and a side order of melted butter, or take him to make a trip to the salad bar for leafy greens. Sometimes just a few little touches can make a young child feel like part of the action even if he can't eat most of the food on the menu.

Getting Menu Savvy

Older kids can quickly learn to scout out acceptable choices on menus. Non-breaded meat, poultry, or fish that is roasted, grilled, poached or steamed make good selections. You'll often find that the secret is in the sauce—the secret hidden carbs that is! Ask them to hold the condiments and dressings that often contain hidden sugars. Carb counts vary considerably with brand, so when in doubt, look it up. Some salad dressing options that are usually in the lower carb range are blue cheese, ranch, or Caesar salad dressing. If you aren't sure if it's a good choice, just ask for plain olive oil and vinegar. Or better yet, bring your own salad dressing from home. Carry a bottle with you and you'll know exactly how many carbs are in it.

Fast Food Restaurants: Ronald McDonald on Diet Therapy?

We usually think, "Do you want fries with that?" when we talk about fast food, and though the diet-friendly pickings may be slim, there are still acceptable options for warriors on MAD at many fast food restaurants. Fast food isn't generally Keto friendly under any circumstance, though parents who desperately want to give their child a taste of normal will sometimes weigh out a small portion of a McDonald's hamburger or chicken nuggets. The amount of chicken nuggets allowed on a 4:1 ratio is pretty sad so for warriors on the Ketogenic diet, consider getting a Happy Meal box, a toy, or something else fun and non-edible to give them that fast food experience again.

For those on MAD, consider taking a good look at the menu before you arrive. Most of the big chains have online meal calculators that will evaluate the carb content and other nutritional information of listed menu items. We asked some MAD users for a short list of fast food items they've found that worked well on the diet and these are the top choices:

Wendy's: Double Burger without a bun, and a Caesar salad

KFC: Kentucky Grilled Chicken pieces

Subway: Turkey Breast Salad with cheese, veggies, and oil dressing

Burger King: Tendergrill Chicken Sandwich without the bun

McDonald's: Angus Mushroom Swiss Burger without bun, or the Boneless Chicken Breast with a small lettuce salad

El Pollo Loco: Flame Grilled Chicken Breast

Chik-Fil-A: Chargrilled Chicken Sandwich without the bun, and a side salad

In-N-Out: They offer a "secret menu" that is not advertised with two low-carb choices: the "Flying Dutchman" (two meat patties with two cheese slices), or the "Protein Style" meat patty wrapped in lettuce leaves with tomato and onion. Ask at the counter.

Parent-Approved Restaurant Guides

A very handy book to bring along when you are out and about is *The CalorieKing Calorie, Fat, and Carbohydrate Counter.*

And if you are looking for a quick online review of low-carb options in various chain restaurants, check out the ***"Low Carb Guide to Chain Restaurants"*** at **About.com** found at: http://lowcarbdiets.about.com/od/chainrestaurantsad/LowCarb_Guide_to_Chain_Restaurants_AD.htm.

Theme Park Restaurants: Mickey Mouse Definitely Does Keto!

If you are planning to spend time at a theme park or resort, call ahead to ask customer services if they offer any services at their restaurants for visitors with special dietary needs; you might just uncover a gold mine of assistance. Disney is a great example that many parents rave about, but other parks, resorts, and cruises may offer similar services. At Disney, you can request Keto or MAD meals to be prepared at most restaurants within their parks with advance notice (72 hours is the minimum, but we'd suggest allowing more time than that. The more specific your needs, the more advance notice you should give them). When you make advance reservations at the restaurant of your choice, they will make note of your special dietary needs and you will be put into contact with the executive chef to arrange the menu and ingredients used. When you arrive, the chef-on-duty will come to your table and review your requested special menu before the meal service starts. When provided with recipes, they will gladly prepare Keto quiche, turnip fries, chicken nuggets with almond flour, sugar free chocolate mousse, or whatever foods you order, right down to using keto-friendly products such as specific brands of salad dressing or mayonnaise. Additionally, most Disney theme parks have vendors that sell assorted items a la carte that work well with Keto and MAD, such as smoked turkey legs, barbecued chicken, and ribs. This delightful service gives parents of kids on diet therapy a wonderful break from cooking while on vacation, and we hope more parks and resort centers copy their excellent example. For more information see: http://disneyworld.disney.go.com/guest-services/special-dietary-requests/.

Battle Tip: Disney Guest Assistance Card

Children that do not have a visible disability, like many children with epilepsy, can benefit from a Guest Assistance Card that can be issued from Guest Relations at Disney. If your child has issues with heat (as many children on seizure medications do) or you need to use your stroller like a wheelchair in places where strollers usually are not allowed, having a GAC can ensure you get quick assistance from staff, including moving through special lines when needed.

Planes, Trains, and Automobiles

Travelling farther afield on road trips or flights while on the diet isn't as complicated as you might think. Taking your show on the road just takes thoughtful planning and wise packing. The key to success is making sure you have the basics on hand to put together simple, balanced meals at a moment's notice even if there are flight delays, traffic mishaps, or other travel glitches. Being prepared will help you rest easy and enjoy the trip instead of constantly worrying you'll be caught short without an important ingredient. What you want to avoid, as one parent blogging their cross-country Keto experience described, is to find yourself in a strange city rushing to the store with a hungry, frustrated toddler in tow, fumbling an explanation to the traffic cop who pulls you over that you need a jar of mayonnaise and it's (sort of) a medical emergency. (*And no, Officer, I have not been drinking.*)

Plan out your trip day-by-day, bring the essentials, and figure out where you can buy what you need along the route. If a particular brand of a product is important and substitutes really won't work, take that into account in your packing. Just because you can buy a particular brand of cream at a national supermarket chain in your hometown doesn't always mean they'll carry the same brand elsewhere. If a substitute won't work, carry an emergency backup with you and only open it if you can't find what you need in shops. Also take into account that occasionally regional varieties of the same product can have changes of ingredients, so if your child has sensitivities, read labels.

Basic Traveling Equipment for Extended Trips

If you plan on eating solely at restaurants during your journey—and we don't advise this for those on Keto—your supply list will be shorter; however, most people find being able to prepare meals and snacks for their child and supplementing with restaurant food to be a much more practical option in the long run. Having a portable version of the equipment you use at home to prepare and measure food makes travel simple. The list below may seem lengthy at first glance, but look again: most of the items are small and can fit well inside a collapsible bag with pockets, and, apart from the scales and cooler, are inexpensive. Keep a travel bag packed with these basics and you will be ready whenever it's time to jump in the car and go.

- Several copies of easy meal plans (laminated if possible).

- Good lightweight travel scales for Keto (emphasis on "good," so don't just get the cheapest—see our recommendation below).

- Small plastic measuring cups and spoons.

- Lock-top food containers that won't spill.

- Rubber spatula.

- Microwaveable bowl and lid.

- Condiment containers with tight fitting lids for oils, mayo, and other items. These are good for day trips; you can keep larger bottles and containers in your cooler or hotel fridge, and fill up small ones for your day out. Disposables can be easily found at stores like Walmart).

- Small ziplock food bags.

- Plastic bags to wrap around bottles that might leak such as oil, etc.

- Disposable plates, bowls, cups, and cutlery (makes cleanup on the road easier).

- At least one non-disposable plastic cup with snap-top cover.

- Small wide-neck thermos for soups.

- Several metal spoons for stirring and mixing (plastic ones tend to snap easily).

- One knife for slicing vegetables and a vegetable peeler (pack these in your check-in luggage on flights).

- Sponge, dish soap, drying towel, and paper towels for clean up (store inside plastic food bag when wet and dry out at night in hotel room).

- Napkins and wet wipes.

- Flashlight and batteries. (You don't want to be caught with the lights out in an emergency trying to weigh food.)

- A small insulated shoulder bag (your school lunch bag works great for this, so you don't need to buy another). You can leave your bigger food cooler in the car trunk or your hotel room, and just take what you need in your smaller bag.

- A durable bag (canvas works well) to carry the above equipment. Side pockets and flaps are good for stuffing in this and that.

- An insulated food cooler with reusable cooling packs (smaller cooler sizes fit more easily on planes, bigger ones go well in the trunk of a car) or a collapsible, insulated cooler bag. If you are flying and then renting a car, you could consider buying an inexpensive larger cooler when you arrive that fits in the trunk.

- Salt (OK, its food, not equipment, but you KNOW you're going to forget it if we don't mention it here).

Parent-Approved Travel Scales

The American Weigh Black Blade Digital Pocket Scale
Why We Like It: This scale, which measures in 0.1 gram *increments*, is powered by two AAA batteries and comes with a ten-year warranty. The platform is only 2.7 × 2.7 inches and is lightweight. The scale comes with two expansion trays, a retractable backlit display, and is pre-calibrated. On Amazon, this scale costs around $9.00.

The American Weigh SC-2KG Digital Pocket Scale
Why We Like It: This scale measures in 0.1 gram increments, with a platform of 4 × 4 inches. It has an LCD, backlit screen, 10-year warranty, and is powered by two AAA batteries. On Amazon, this scale costs around $19.00.

Food for the Trip

If you have a cooler equipped with freezable cooling packs you can easily carry almost any prepared meal, take along assorted cooked foods to weigh or assemble into meals, or take along raw food to cook. Easy no-fuss choices are luncheon meats, cooked chicken breasts, or other prepared meats, cheese, steamed vegetables or raw vegetable sticks, and salad fixings. Of course you don't want to forget your all-important fat sources such as oils, mayonnaise, cream, butter, and nuts. Double check that the foods you are bringing include everything you need for your meal plans, so you have what you need.

On the Go

One of the easiest ways to prepare for a trip is to plan your meals out in advance. Look through your recipes and figure out what meals you want to make, and pack the ingredients essential to prepping those meals. If you'll be making a berries and Greek yogurt, for example, you'll want to make sure you have the yogurt, cream, berries, oil, and your sweetener. Using the small plastic containers we suggested in Chapter 4, "The Mess Hall," you can either pre-weigh your ingredients before packing them, or you can pack ample supplies of each ingredient if you think you'll make the meal more than once. For places you visit often, such as a grandparent's house, we suggest stocking their house with the staples such as coconut oil, mayonnaise, and nut flours you always use for Keto pancakes. The less you have to pack and think about, the better!

Suggested Foods and Snacks that Travel Well without a Cooler

Sometimes bringing along a cooler just isn't convenient. If you are looking for foods and snacks that travel well to supplement restaurant meals, here are a few ideas. For those on Keto, just remember that if these foods aren't already in a recipe, you'll have to create a recipe to accommodate any food you decide to bring.

■ Almonds, macadamia nuts, pecans, and walnuts

■ Boiled eggs (eat as soon as possible the first day out)

■ Hard cheeses like cheddar, as well as string cheese

■ Home-made cheese crackers (microwaved sections of sliced cheese on parchment paper to form crackers, that can be stored in food bags)

■ Pepperoni or other dry or semi-dry sausage that does not require refrigeration

■ Pork rinds

■ Just-the-Cheese snacks

■ Low-carb muffins (see recipe section)

■ Peanut butter

■ Cherry tomatoes

- Cucumbers (if you wash well and eat with the peel, they keep for a few days)

- Cans of tuna packed in oil

- A small jar of olives

- A small jar of pickles

- A container of mayo to slather on restaurant meals for extra fat

- A container of oil with a tight lid, wrapped in extra plastic

- Packets of Stevia or other sweeteners

- Herbal tea packets

Where to Stay on the Way

Hotels: If you're staying in hotels along the way, call ahead to explain your situation and ask to have a refrigerator placed in your room to store food from the cooler. If the room doesn't have a microwave (most don't, but some do) ask if your child's special medically necessary foods can be reheated at the hotel restaurant or coffee shop. Another great option to consider is a hotel or vacation cabin that offers self-catering facilities. Having your own kitchenette or hot plate available to prepare meals relieves a lot of pressure, and keeps down vacation costs as well.

Camping: Do camping trips work on the diet? Of course! Many Keto and MAD moms and dads testify that they've weathered all types of camping scenarios. The trip will take diligent planning, simple menus, and well-packed supplies, as well as good communication with camp organizers, but whether your child belongs to a scout troop, you're RVing with your family, or you're setting off on a hike in the hills with a tent on your back, your child doesn't have to miss out on the fun. And who knows where you'll end up! One of us had a marvelous camping experience at a once-in-a-lifetime destination.

Camping in Inner Mongolia on MAD

*Before Jordan was diagnosed with epilepsy, my two boys and
I had planned an adventure trip to Inner Mongolia. Epilepsy
delayed our plans but when Jordan was 13 and had been on
MAD for a year, we decided to go for it and experience life with
people who still herd animals for a living. He loved the fatty
roasted lamb (you couldn't have found a better fat source as
they skewered and roasted whole chunks of fat with the meat!)*

as well as the wild greens picked fresh each day. I didn't let him
eat the grassland flowers the herdsmen cooked and ate though,
as I had no idea of the carb count. We lived in a yurt and my
son learned to ride horses and herd sheep on the rolling plains.
It was an amazing experience and probably one of the crazier
things we've done, but we didn't want to be afraid to attempt the
things we dreamed of before his diagnosis. And I learned that
if you can pull it off in the grasslands in a yurt, you can make
this diet work just about anywhere. —Jeanne Riether

If you don't have the benefit of a Mongolian herdsman cooking for you, don't despair. You can heat any MAD or Keto meals you've brought along using a mess kit over a campfire or on a simple propane camp-stove such as a Pocket Rocket. If your child is attending an organized camping event, such as Scouts, and you won't be accompanying him you should:

■ **Communicate:** Check with the camp counselors in advance about exactly what services they can provide for a child with special dietary needs. Many structured camps require that all meals are prepared in advance and sent along with your child. Be aware that some camps do not offer facilities to freeze pre-prepared meals. Work out clear instructions (laminated sheets work well) about what is to be eaten at each meal, along with heating directions, to give to the counselor assigned to oversee and assist your child.

■ **Pack wisely:** You can pack clearly labeled, easy-to-heat meals in Tupperware-style containers, or in small resealable bags stacked in layers inside a large ziplock bag, and placed in a foam cooler with dry ice, frozen water bottles, or cooling packs. Soft coolers that can clip on to backpacks are great for one day trips or day hikes.

■ **Meals on Wheels:** For local programs, rather than packing food for an extended stay, some parents find it easier to arrange to bring out meals to the campgrounds every few days. Keep your meals simple and chances are, even if your child is eating nearly the same thing nearly every day, she will be having too much fun to notice.

Airports, Flights, and All Things Keto

"Know before you go" is the slogan to remember, starting with a call to the airline to explain your needs and inquire about current regulations regarding bringing food onboard in carry-on luggage. At the time of this writing, passengers traveling within the United States do not need a doctor's letter to bring medically necessary food with them on flights as long as it is declared at Transit Security Administration (TSA) inspection. However, procedures and regulations are subject to change, so a confirming phone call to the TSA overseer at the airline is always a smart move. This may take more than one call, but it is worth the trouble.

Plan to arrive at the airport early (and in some cases, *very* early) and declare your situation when you get in line. If you have any trouble, ask to speak to the TSA manager on duty. Non-sealed food containers will most likely be thoroughly checked by security so allow enough time for these procedures. If you are traveling with a small or active child, one nerve-saving tactic is to have one parent accompany the child through TSA screening while the other accompanies the food cooler and any needed equipment. This way your little one doesn't have to endure the extra pat-downs, questions, and waiting while they examine the foods you are carrying.

Liquids brought on the plane must be declared to be part of a medically necessary diet and put in a separate security bin from other items to be tested. In general, Jell-Os, puddings, and gel-like substances will receive greater scrutiny. You can speed things up by choosing to carry solid food items (i.e., meals of meat and vegetables) if your child can eat them, and avoiding gel-like foods for the flight. Bring along sufficient food to allow for missed or delayed flights, since we all know it happens. Taking too much food isn't usually a problem, but taking too little could spell trouble.

Dawn, an intrepid parent with a child on the Ketogenic diet and who has a nose for reporting, offered to help us out by researching further details regarding TSA requirements on food and meds. Here's the scoop:

- **Letters are NOT required** to get medications, medical equipment that is non-powered (i.e., AMBU bag), food, or beverages through security checkpoints. However, a letter is highly recommended to make the process go smoothly.

- **You need to declare that you have some of these items, or any liquids greater than 3.4 ounces that are not in a clear resealable quart size bag,** to the **first** TSA agent in the security line. They will then move you to go through a more intensive screening.

- **Have all prescription medications labeled** with the name of med and to whom it is prescribed.

- **Plastic ice packs are preferable** to use in a cooler. If ice is used, you will have to remove the melted water from the bottom of the cooler.

- **Coolers containing medically needed food do not count as a carry on.** Coolers should be 9"H × 14"W × 22"L, or no larger than this. Sometimes they will let you put these in the overhead compartment; however, they are supposed to go under the seats.

- **There is no limit to the amount of medication you can bring with you.** If you are traveling with a large quantity of medication, put it in a separate bag and keep it all together. This includes dosing devices such as needles, syringes, glucometers, and such. This will not count as a carry on either.

- **You do not need any formal paperwork to bring medical devices.** Only portable oxygen concentrators (POC's) need prior approval and paperwork submitted.

Additional Travel Tips for Smooth Flights

- Carry a list of emergency phone numbers with you (in case you lose your phone it's good to bring along a written list as well) including your neurologist, pediatrician, and a family contact familiar with your child's medical history and diet.

- Carry a printed menu of your child's food plan.

- Bring enough cooling packs in your insulated bag to keep your food safe.

- Phone the airlines well in advance and try and arrange for seats near the bulkhead so that you will have room to handle the cooler bags at meal times.

- If you have a vagus nerve stimulator (VNS), have your registration card handy when passing through airport security.

- Make sure you are carrying sufficient amounts of anti-seizure medication to last the entire length of your time away from home.

- If you are traveling out of the country, bring a signed doctor's letter explaining the medical necessity of the special food you are carrying, as well as a description of your child's epilepsy and prescription for anti-seizure medication, as security regulations may vary abroad.

Home Alone: When Someone Else Stays with Your Child

Family emergencies, work obligations, hospital stays—if you are your child's main cook and caregiver and you're suddenly called away, you'll need a clear plan for whoever stays behind. It's always a wise idea to keep a good supply of frozen, clearly labeled ready-to-eat meals on hand, and rotate them as needed.

When the freezer's near empty, however, you'll have to rely on clearly written instructions to carry the home team through. It's worth the time to write up meal plans in advance, before you're unexpectedly called away, so they'll have a plan in hand in case of emergency. You can keep this on your computer desktop, as well as in a clear plastic folder in the kitchen. If you have an older child or teenager who can be responsible for handling his own food while you are out of the picture, teaching him to cook is a smart move and also a fun family activity that doubles as emergency prep.

If you aren't working with a KetoCalculator (and though most parents on MAD don't use it, Keto parents kiss the ground beneath she-who-invented-it), then print a list of the net-carb equivalents of commonly used foods and attach it to the fridge. If you're doing MAD it will be a real time saver, especially when your stand-in newbie chef gets nervous or has to change the menu. And if a food isn't on your list or a substitute is needed, we suggest MAD cooks check out a handy little site called fatsecret.com to quickly find the net carb value of most foods.

Besides a meal plan and preparation instructions, if there are any other special instructions you'd like them to follow, make sure you have it written out and posted as well. Does your child need an extra high fat snack before bed to help ward off nighttime seizures? Does your teen do better when he wakes up with a cream drink first thing in the morning? Does your toddler need you to make airplane noises when you scrape the last bit of food from the breakfast bowl? (Come on, Daddy, you can do it!) A lot of diet therapy is more art than science, so list any tricks you've found that work for your child. Then take a final check to make sure they have all the necessary meal plan ingredients on hand, and relax. They'll do just fine. And if not, at least you know they're really going to appreciate you when you get back.

Emergency Prep

Before you get too smug feeling that you're ready to take on any emergency just because you've got a freezer brimming with ready-to-eat food, consider this: if the electricity goes out, all your carefully prepared meals will be melted mush in a matter of days or less. We've all seen the crisis scenarios on the evening news—think hurricanes, earthquakes, floods, fires, tornadoes, blizzards, and civil unrest. Let's hope it never comes near your or my door, but common sense dictates that it's smart to be prepared. You will want to have on hand the supplies you need to continue your child's diet therapy uninterrupted in case:

1. The power goes out.

2. The stores are closed.

3. You have to quickly evacuate your home.

If you have the *Basic Equipment for Travel* listed earlier in this chapter, it will serve you well in case evacuation becomes necessary. Your travel/emergency supplies should include scales, measuring cups, as well as a cooler and other basic equipment. You will also want to include a small camp stove to boil water or heat food if necessary. Keep a pantry or closet stocked with canned food and non-perishables, as well as water (clean drinking water is often the first service to go in a public emergency). It doesn't hurt to keep non-perishable foods stored in your travel cooler as well, ready to go at a moment's notice. Some basic supplies to consider stocking up on are:

■ Bottled water

■ A clear meal plan listing the food you have on hand and their carb values (you may not have access to the Internet to use the KetoCalculator or to check food values)

■ A small portable stove and matches

■ Fat sources that you know work for your child, such as oil, mayonnaise, coconut cream, canned butter, UHT cream, etc.

■ Canned meat, tuna, chicken, etc.

■ Canned vegetables

■ Powdered eggs

■ Dried meat such as jerky, as well as dried vegetables and fruit

■ Sausages that do not require refrigeration

■ Canned nuts

■ Sweeteners, salt, and a few regularly used dry spices or herbs

■ Disposable cups, plates, and cutlery (if water is off you will need them)

It is also a good idea to have ready to travel:

- A written description of your child's diagnosis and treatment as well as the contact number of your neurologist, pediatrician, and family member who is familiar with your child's diet treatment (in case something happens to you, whoever is caring for your child will need this)
- An emergency supply of any prescribed anti-seizure medication
- A first aid kit stocked with Keto-friendly products and fever/pain medication
- A flashlight
- Toilet paper

Now that you've had a crash course in how to practically travel the world on a ketogenic diet, you're ready to learn how to march into your child's school and advocate for a seamless implementation of your warrior's diet in the classroom, which we discuss in the following chapter, "Warriors at School."

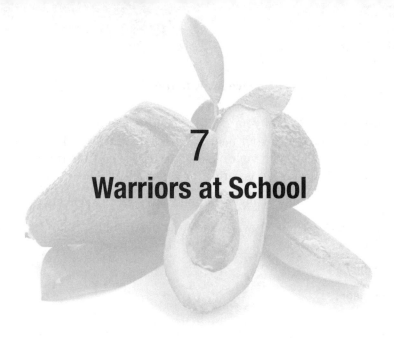

7
Warriors at School

Even before you send your young warrior off to class with a well-packed lunch bag, one of the first tasks you'll have to tackle is getting everybody at the school—teachers, aids, school nurses, administrators, and classroom peers—on the same page regarding your child's new diet. The younger the child, the more oversight and work this will mean on the part of the school, so good communication with your child's educators is essential. First, they will need a clear understanding of their role in the diet therapy. Then, you can create a step-by-step plan together to ensure your warrior stays on course while at school.

How Can I Work with the School to Accommodate My Child's Diet?

Children with epilepsy in the United States have several formal options when planning how to ensure they get the care they are entitled to receive at school. Understanding how to access services is an important step in becoming an effective advocate for your child, so it's good to become familiar with any and all departments and programs catering to your child's specific needs. Perhaps like most parents of school age children with seizures, you are already familiar with the terms IEP, IDEA, and 504 Plan, but if not, here's a quick review.

IEP. Children who need special education classes are steered into developing an IEP (Individualized Education Program) that falls under the IDEA

(Individuals with Disabilities Education Act) umbrella. An IEP's purpose is to help children reach educational goals more easily than they otherwise would. It is a document that helps teachers and related service providers understand the individual student's disability, how the disability affects the learning process, and how they can help the student learn more effectively.

504 Plan. Children with disabilities who do not need specialized classes are usually steered into creating a 504 Plan (formally called "Section 504 of the Rehabilitation Act"). This document ensures that students receive accommodations that provide them proper access to the learning environment. The individual plan gives educators information about the specific needs of the student and practical strategies they can incorporate into lesson planning.

IDEA. Technically all children with epilepsy are accommodated under IDEA (Individuals with Disabilities Act). This act addresses the educational needs of children from birth to age 18 or 21 who fall under 14 specified categories of disability. While most children with epilepsy are of normal intelligence, even without developmental delays or other disabilities, they still fall under the "other health impaired" category of this act. However, the 504 Plan is less complicated than IDEA's IEP and requires less documentation of measurable goals, so most kids who are not in Special Ed use the 504 Plan.

Your school will advise you on whether an IEP or a 504 Plan better suits your child's needs. These plans can be written to include the school's responsibility in overseeing the diet and how to respond if your child has a seizure, as well as all other issues affecting your child's education. For example, if your child needs to arrive later in the morning due to frequent morning seizure activity, or if he needs help from an aid when frequent absence seizures cause him to miss teacher instructions, it can be accommodated under those plans. For the sake of simplicity we will only talk here about creating an IEP, but most of the information can be used in developing a 504 plan also.

Baking the Diet into Your Child's IEP

Parents are entitled to work together with the school and teachers to develop an IEP designed to meet the unique needs of each child. Every IEP has a medical/health section that should outline in detail a plan of what to do in case your child has a seizure, as well as how to comply with any needed medical therapy such as the diet. Federal law stipulates that all school employees MUST follow any medical directions in your plan, so it is important that the diet is included in the Health Plan section. The school must provide the oversight needed to make sure your child is not given food forbidden on the diet, and steps can be set up (usually daily signed communication books) to make sure all staff including substitute teachers, volunteers, and teaching assistants know the procedure and follow it to the letter. Part of the measurable educational goals of the IEP can include educating your child (depending on his age and cognitive abilities) to understand what foods he can and cannot eat and how to respond appropriately when forbidden foods are offered. Staff compliance and age-appropriate oversight of your child is the school's legal responsibility.

Despite the fact that you and your child have federal rights, this is the time to remember the wise old adage that you catch more flies with honey than with vinegar. If you are used to advocating for your child you may already be in fight mode. However, we suggest you bring it down a notch when arriving to discuss diet therapy with your child's school, and remember that you and your child's educators are a team. What you are trying to accomplish in your first meeting is to open a line of communication and cooperation, and help the school and teachers reach the logical conclusion that having your child's diet therapy succeed is in THEIR best interest, despite the extra work. They may HAVE to do it legally, but helping them WANT to do it is a very smart move and will ensure better care for your child in the long run.

Besides a winning smile, you should also come armed with explanations and documentation about the diet, a letter from your doctor, and a suggested step-by-step plan of what the school and teachers need to do to make it work. Take into account that the hard-working teacher you face may initially feel overwhelmed at the thought of all this, particularly if your child is young. (Remember how you felt when you first heard about the diet?) While the school is legally bound to accommodate the diet, helping a busy engaged teacher feel confident about it will require a lot of reassurance on your part.

The battle plan is simple, really: NO FOOD or drink other than that sent from home will be given to your child at ANY time, no exceptions. The tricky part (especially for a very young child) is ensuring that everyone at school follows the rules, and that your child eats all the necessary food sent in each day. This is essential if on Keto where all food must be eaten, but even on the more flexible Modified Atkins Diet (MAD) you may need school staff to encourage your child not to leave too much uneaten food in the lunch box. The school may be very much on board with helping your child stick to the plan, but they may need your help thinking through all possible situations to cover. For instance, one parent described how the staff at her very supportive school had overlooked the fact that they were expecting her developmentally delayed daughter to handle foods she liked, but was not allowed to eat, in art projects, gluing raisins to the letter "R." The teachers did not allow her to eat them, but had not taken into account that seeing and handling these forbidden treats would be upsetting for the girl. We asked several educators with experience in overseeing children on diet therapy for their input and here are the ideas and suggestions they generated.

Step One: The Introductory Letter

Wendy, the director of a charter school who also has a daughter on MAD, suggested that a good starting place for parents and schools working together is delivering a letter to the school before the first scheduled parent-school meeting in which you'll discuss the diet. This gives the school time to gather more information and prepare for the coming change. A general template for such a parent's letter can be found below:

Dear <Teacher> and <Administrator>,

To help manage <child's name> seizures, we are beginning the <Ketogenic diet/Modified Atkins Diet/Low Glycemic Index diet> for her on <date of diet initiation>. There's compelling research and data to support the effectiveness of this diet to manage seizures. After discussing it with our neurologist, there is agreement that the diet is the next best step. You can learn more about the diet under the F.A.Q section of the Charlie Foundation website at www.charliefoundation.org. After beginning this medical therapy, <child's name> intake of food and drink will be completely controlled by us. It is crucial that she not be given anything to eat or drink at school. Her neurologist has warned us that even a tiny change in her diet could bring on severe seizures, hospitalization, or worse. We will be sending her to school with her lunch, snack, and bottled fluids. (Optional: We would also like to discuss arrangements for the diet to be explained to our child's classmates so they understand <child's name> cannot share any food with them.

Studies have shown that it is not unusual for this diet to be more effective in managing seizures than medication for many children with difficult-to-control seizures. You may have heard or seen the movie, First Do No Harm, starring Meryl Streep in 1997, that deals with a parent's experience using the Ketogenic diet. In this true story, a child becomes seizure free after using diet therapy. Many other people have seen similar results or have experienced improved seizure control, and we are hoping for good results for our child as well.

We will call to schedule a meeting with you and the school nurse to discuss our mutual understanding of the significance of the information we've shared, and then work out a plan together to ensure that it will be carried out. We are both very grateful for your steadfast support of <child's name>.

<Parent's names>

Step Two: Developing a Clear Plan for School Staff to Follow

You'll want to arrive at your scheduled school meeting prepared, so the next step is to do your homework:

- Compile a list of guidelines for the school to follow, involving all aspects of your child's care related to the diet.

- Bring a letter from your neurologist stating the need for your child to be on this diet. Writing this as an actual prescription makes it "doctor's orders," which the school must follow.

Obviously, each child's situation will vary and it may take time and a lot of back-and-forth communication to get everyone agreed on how to get it all running smoothly. We asked Heather, a parent of seven-year-old Abbie, who is on the Ketogenic diet, as well as Amy, Abbie's teacher, to explain how they made it all work. They provide a great example of parents and teachers working together to find solutions.

From a Parent's Perspective

Q: As a mom and teacher, what suggestions do you have for creating a successful IEP?
Embedded in Abbie's IEP is her Health Plan. Her IEP is her education plan, and the Health Plan contains everything necessary for her to feel safe in school, and especially how to respond if she has a seizure. To make the Health Plan successful be completely honest about the diagnosis, the medications, the restrictions, and outline every possible

incidence that a Keto Kid would come in contact with any substance that could cause a seizure reaction.

Q: What should a parent going into an IEP meeting bring along in order to be armed for success?
To be prepared for the Health Plan meeting, come with a letter from your neurologist stating that a ketogenic diet is used in place of (or in addition to) a drug regimen for epilepsy and should be treated as if administering medication. Your neurologist should include the times that the food ("medication") should be administered, monitored, and checked. The neurologist should also include how and why the food needs to be scraped and checked (if on Keto) to make sure every single piece of food or drop of oil is given to the child. At Abbie's school she is walked to the Health Room/Nurse's office and they check her food containers, document it in her book that is carried home, and checkit every night.

Q: What guidelines did you suggest to the school for Abbie's Health Plan?
Abbie's Health Plan has taken two years to run almost 100% fool proof. It has been successful because, as parents, we are able to see daily that Abbie's containers are checked and documentation shows that this has occurred. It also protects Abbie if she comes in contact with any substance and makes the school liable if this contact occurs. Here is what is included in the plan.

1. All food and water will be provided from home. Abbie is not to be given any food in school that has not been provided from home.
2. A refrigerator is placed in her classroom to keep her milkshake cold or any other water bottles, food, snacks.
3. Abbie will have lunch every day at 11:00 a.m.
4. After lunch Abbie will be walked by a member of the school to the health room. A member of the health staff will scrape with the spatula provided from home any and all containers. Containers that have liquid will be filled a quarter of the way with water (provided from home) swirled in the container and Abbie will drink this liquid
5. Abbie's notebook will document that the containers were scraped. This notebook accompanies her from home to school.
6. A document is attached to this Health Plan that outlines what substances Abbie can NOT come in contact with. She is to wear purple latex gloves provided by the health room/nurse's office if she or anyone suspects she may come in contact with any substance during art or her regular classroom instruction.

7. A walkie-talkie will accompany Abbie everywhere she goes. This is in case a seizure occurs and the nurse can be contacted immediately, or to check to see if she is allowed to come in contact with certain substances.

8. An emergency plan is also attached that includes what to do if the paramedics are called because of a seizure reaction. This explains any and all medications, prescription and over the counter, as well as what intravenous solutions can be administered. It is signed by a neurologist.

9. The rest of the health plan outlines how to respond if Abbie has a seizure.

Q: In conclusion, are there any specific DO's and DON'Ts that you'd like to share with parents who are creating their own child's IEP?

- DO advocate for your child.
- DO call any agency that can offer suggestions or advice.
- DO have an advocate attend an IEP or Health Plan meeting
- DO have all doctor's letters, recent reports, or concerns/questions prepared ahead of time.
- DO know the laws and your child's rights.
- DO join the Yahoo group and ask questions or ask to see other plans.
- DO research all you can find about schools and the Ketogenic diet.

From a Teacher's Perspective

Q: What were your fears and concerns when you first learned that you'd have a child on the Ketogenic diet in your class?
When Abbie first came to me as a beginning third grader, she was having her first "snack" at 9:30 a.m., which fell right in the middle of our Language Arts block. My biggest concern was that I would somehow lose track of time and forget to give her the snack. We were able to alleviate this pressure by having the school nurse call me every day to ensure that the snack had been given. Still, even with that in place, I purchased an alarm clock that went off every day and I also used to set my cell phone alarm as a backup.

My second concern was about the amount of the snack administered. I would worry that I'd get her snack and her lunch mixed up or forget part of a snack if it was more than one container. Initially, her food was kept in either the daycare refrigerator across the hall or in the health room refrigerator. It was quickly determined that this was ineffective because I was not able to leave the room to get the snack myself and ensure that we got all the correct containers. The school then purchased a small refrigerator to keep in our classroom for all of Abbie's meals. This was extremely helpful and Abbie's parents also did a great job of making sure that each container was clearly labeled with the time and whether or not there were multiple containers. I also made sure that Abbie was seated at a table to eat in order to minimize the risk of spills. That year, I was responsible for making sure that she finished <u>all of her snack</u>, down to the scraping of the container. That also made me a little nervous because I was always afraid that my idea of being finished might somehow be incorrect or inadequate. It was eventually established that Abbie would go to the health room to have her containers double-checked by the nurse, which was a very successful addition to her health plan, in my opinion.

For part of third grade, Abbie's snack schedule changed and she began eating just a lunch during the day. Unfortunately, her lunchtime fell at a different time than the rest of the class. We had to have another staff member come and pick her up when it was time to eat. Then, when it was time for the rest of the class to eat, Abbie had to go with them and watch them eat, though she couldn't eat herself. I'm sure that this was difficult for her and she told me that she didn't like it because it made her feel different. This year, I followed Abbie to fourth grade and our schedule worked out to be much easier. The school administration was able to plan our schedule such that Abbie's lunchtime was at the same time as her classmates and that her afternoon snack came at the end of the day in daycare or her mother's classroom. This took a lot of the pressure off me, but also was great for Abbie because she was able to feel more like everyone else and eat with her friends.

Q: How did Abbie's mom help you to understand how the diet worked?

Heather did a fantastic job of explaining how the diet worked, both to me and the health staff. At times, I think I was overcautious, as I was so afraid of making a mistake and causing Abbie to have additional seizures, so I bugged Heather constantly with questions and clarifications to make extra sure that we were all on the same page. Heather did a great job of not only telling me what needed to be done, but she also told me "why" it needed to be so.

Q: What have been the biggest challenges of having a child with the Ketogenic diet in your class, and how have you addressed those challenges?

We have to be very careful about what Abbie comes into contact with, as some chemicals, sugars, lotions, and so on. can be absorbed through the skin. For that reason, she has special soap that she has to use and sometimes has to wear gloves if we are handling any substances that might cause a problem for her. We cannot have tissues with lotion in them and I have to be careful about what I put on my hands in case Abbie touches me. We are careful about what we put on her desk and even about things such as using sunscreen on Field Day so that it doesn't get on her skin. I also try to advocate for Abbie to ensure that other staff members remember to consider all of these constraints when planning school-wide behavior incentives and other activities.

It is difficult for Abbie when we have classroom parties and when parents bring in "surprise" treats for the class. I try to always keep little non-food prizes on hand and to think ahead to upcoming events to make sure that she has something to make her feel special and not too different, even though she can't eat the treat. Sometimes she has been able to have a treat that is approved by her parents/doctors, such as frozen ice or a "sizzle" water, but most often, I try to plan on a non-food reward that she will enjoy. Luckily, she is a very joyful and appreciative kid, so she doesn't allow it to get her too upset. I try to give her choices whenever possible, so she feels like she has some control over what she would like to do or have.

I have found that we have really minimized the use of food items as rewards in my classroom as a result of Abbie's diet, which is great for all the kids because it is far healthier for everyone. They seem to enjoy extra recess or a game of Freeze-dance more than the treats anyway. For holiday parties, I limit the amounts and types of foods that are brought in so it doesn't make Abbie feel too badly about not being able to eat them.

Q: How long did it take you to feel comfortable with the responsibility of dealing with the diet?

It honestly took me about four months to feel really settled and comfortable. Part of the reason for this length of time was that there were some changes to the health plan and schedule during this time, so it took a bit longer to get everything straight. I was fortunate to have the school staff and health room staff to help me so that I didn't feel as if I was singularly responsible for Abbie's care. I think that is the best advice I could give any parent…don't put all the pressure on one person. It truly does take a village to raise a child and it is so much easier if you have several trained staff members to share in the responsibility of caring for a child on the Ketogenic diet. By the time we got to fourth grade, I felt extremely comfortable with everything and was able to relax a lot more.

Q: What tips can you offer to help a parent work together with a teacher to create an effective and practical plan for supervising the diet at school?

I think the most important thing is for the parent to make sure that school administration, teachers, health staff, and any other staff who come into contact with your child are trained on his/her health plan before the school year begins. This will take some pressure off the classroom teacher and make sure that a system of checks and balances is in place.

I have also found that it is important to designate someone who will step up and take over if the teacher is absent to make sure that the Health Plan and diet are still followed by trained school staff and that the substitute knows exactly what to do. The first few times I was out sick, I was nervous about what was happening in my absence, but our school manager did a great job of making sure that Abbie's Health Plan was followed.

In addition to making sure the health plan is in place (parents should):

- Be receptive to questions and concerns so that the teacher and the child will feel as comfortable as possible during the school day.
- Request a classroom refrigerator and label all your containers, making sure that they seal properly and the teacher knows which containers go with which meal.
- Thoroughly explain what your child cannot use or come into contact with, including but not limited to lotions, markers, glue, hand sanitizer, band-aids, soaps, etc.
- Provide any special soap or water that the child needs to use during the day.
- Let the teacher know how you want classroom parties or treats to be handled and whether you have any specific concerns about your child's welfare and happiness during the school day.
- Also, make sure your child is aware of the procedures and plans that you have made with the school so that he/she understands what the teachers and staff are doing and why.

The last bit of advice I can give is to make sure that you talk to the school staff about how you want your child's dietary needs to be handled with the rest of the class. We held a class meeting on the first day of school to explain to all my students how Abbie's diet worked so that they could look out for her needs without treating her differently. Work with the teacher and health staff to find the best way to make sure the rest of the class is on board.

From a Special Education Preschool Teacher's Perspective

Overseeing a very young child on dietary therapy in a classroom setting comes with its own set of challenges. Heather, teacher for Noah, the preschool son of one of the authors of this book, Erin Whitmer, shares her feelings and experiences about making the Ketogenic diet work in her classroom.

Working with Noah

When I first found out that I had a student coming to my class that was on the Ketogenic diet I really didn't know what to expect. Previously I had students with other dietary concerns, including gluten free, toxic metal diets, etc. I enjoy having my students learn and explore materials in many different ways. My students learn through cooking, hands-on experiences, music, play, etc. I have found it difficult to adapt cooking lessons for my students with dietary needs, so when I found out Noah was coming to my classroom on the Ketogenic diet, I was a little concerned.

Noah's mom did a great job teaching us about the diet. We had a meeting before Noah came to school and she brought a PowerPoint that explained the diet in detail. Noah's mom also explained the importance of us sticking to the diet. I appreciated and studied the information in detail to learn as much as possible about the diet. I also asked lots of questions to make sure what we were doing in the classroom was acceptable for the diet.

After our meeting and receiving the PowerPoint information I began to get a lot more nervous about the diet. In Noah's Individualized Education Plan it stated that he put everything in his mouth so I was thinking we would constantly have to follow Noah around to make sure he didn't eat anything. I was so worried that he would eat something he wasn't allowed to eat and then have a seizure. I would have felt so horrible and guilty if this happened so I literally was thinking that Noah needed a teacher to constantly be right beside him! After our meeting Noah's mom also came to our classroom and took home the paint and glue that we use in class to research more about it. She wanted to make sure Noah could use these materials without it affecting his diet. After she left I was thinking, "Oh my gosh, I'm going to have to come up with completely new art ideas, cooking ideas, etc. Aww!" I was so nervous!

Noah came to school soon after the first meeting and my paraprofessional and I kept a very close eye on him! We watched everything he touched, put to his mouth, etc. I think that we were probably more protective over him than anyone else in the classroom. Noah brought breakfast to school with notes on what he needed to eat and in what ratio he needed to eat it in. There were many times that I needed to call Noah's mom to confirm the notes she wrote or make sure I was feeding Noah correctly. The food and ratios were sometimes confusing so Noah's mom suggested that she would start sending in "all in one foods" so that I won't have to worry about the ratio demands. I would suggest that if the child is very young and doesn't know what they should be eating for the diet that the "all in one foods" are best to send in when providing a snack or small meal.

Luckily, Noah is not extremely sensitive to touching art supplies including paint, glue, markers, etc. However, I sometimes get very nervous when we decide to explore different art supplies in class. For example, one day we decided to use dot markers in class. Noah absolutely loved using the dot markers and got it all over his hands. Noah's mom had told us previously not to worry if Noah got art materials on his hands, just wash it off immediately after he was done. Well, after he was done creating his art with the dot markers we helped Noah scrub and wash his hands. The ink did NOT come off! I was scared to death! My stomach was literally hurting when I called Noah's mom to let her know that the ink was stuck on his hands. I had to leave a message and by the time it was

*time for Noah to leave I hadn't heard anything back. Needless
to say at this point I was freaking out! I thought for sure
Noah's mom was so upset with me! I heard back from Noah's
mom by e-mail soon after Noah went home and she said that
she was sure everything was just fine! What a relief! Learning
from this experience I would suggest that teachers plan ahead,
send home art materials that you are thinking about using,
and make sure that these materials are approved on the
Ketogenic diet before you use them!*

*I believe that I was finally comfortable with the diet after Noah
was in my classroom for a couple of months. Noah is such a
joy to have in the classroom and it is not hard to accommodate
for his dietary needs. Staying in constant communication with
Noah's mom and family has made it very easy to accommodate
for the dietary needs and ask questions about the diet. The more
information I have about the diet the more comfortable it is educating Noah. So, I would suggest if you are a parent, educator,
or related service provider, educate yourself, ask questions, and
make sure you are prepared to make accommodations if needed!*

What to Do When It's Just Not Working at School: How to Advocate for Your Child

We can scarcely express how wonderful it is when children are blessed
with dedicated, caring schools that work closely with parents and are willing to explore solutions to make diet therapy work. If your child attends
such a school, you might want to throw rose petals at the feet of the teacher,
principal, and staff! Let them know how much you appreciate their efforts
and hard work, and support them at every step. But what do you do if,
despite numerous attempts at communication, negotiation, and meetings
with teachers and the principal, the diet therapy aspect of your child's IEP
Health Plan just isn't being followed properly? Then it's Warrior Time.

First, understand you aren't the first one who has had to fight for their
child, so learn from others who have gone before you. Laws will vary in
each state, but a good summary of the legal steps to follow if your efforts
to negotiate with your child's school are not successful can be found in a
publication put out by the *Disability Rights Network of Pennsylvania,*
offered for free download at www.drnpa.org/File/publications/how-to-
resolve-special-education-disputes.pdf.

Also, some very helpful suggestions can also be found on the Talk About Curing Autism website (www.tacanow.org) and their "Tips for Including Dietary Restrictions in Your Child's IEP" page. We've summarized some of their advice here:

- If the school district is refusing to implement some aspect of your IEP, request prior written notice. This means the school district must explain in writing why they are refusing the parent's request. Gaining the district's position in writing is the first step in overcoming the obstacle.

- The district must give prior written notice if they A) Propose to begin or change the identification, evaluation, or educational placement of your child or the provision of a free appropriate public education to your child; or B) Refuse to begin or change the identification, evaluation, or educational place of your child or the provision of a free appropriate public education to your child. Your request for dietary accommodations is part of "free appropriate public education."

In some instances when the teacher was not able to properly oversee the diet, the parents won approval for a one-on-one aid to be assigned to assist and oversee their child at meal and snack times. Being your child's advocate means knowing your child has a right to a great education as well as the right to follow his medical diet therapy while at school. Keep knocking on doors until you get the results that meet your child's needs.

Keto in the Lunchroom

After all you've learned about preparing meals at home, packing up a lunch for school is easy if you have the right equipment and a few tricks up your sleeve. Here are a few tips to make lunchtime go smoothly.

- Start with a good insulated carry case and food containers. Girls like tote bags in pretty colors, so some great lunch box ideas for girls can be found at Fit & Fresh on their website: www.fit-fresh.com/. They have reasonable prices and you can find all sorts of stylish designs (even zebra stripes!).

- Then you need some containers with tight fitting lids. Chapter 4 had several small container options, but Fit & Fresh also sells containers with removable ice packs and *Kid's Healthy Lunch* and *Lunch on the Go* sets in bright colors. Try to include a wide necked thermos in your purchases for soups.

■ If your child really wants to have hot lunch on a tray like the rest of the kids, see if you can arrange with the cafeteria for him to give his lunch to the staff each day and then get in line to receive it on a tray just like the other kids. Some parents report the staff was very willing to accommodate this.

■ Try to keep your solutions simple if possible. One mom wracked her brain trying to find a diet-friendly replacement when her preschooler sobbed that he could no longer have a juice bottle at snack like the other kids. She was having all sorts of mommy-guilt pangs about him feeling left out. The answer? She simply bought the coveted juice, dumped out the contents, gave the bottle a good washing, replaced it with a diet-friendly version of "juice" (water colored pink with a few frozen berries and a dash of allowed sweetener), and then labeled it clearly with his name. He was delighted and she learned not to sweat the small stuff.

■ Find out if your child's school is willing to reheat food in a microwave, or even cook food already weighed and sent from home in clearly labeled containers. School policies vary considerably on this. The school would need clear instructions for heating and serving, as well as clear directions on scraping all the ingredients from the pan if your child is on Keto.

School Lunch Ideas

With the proper containers you can send almost any hot or cold meal to school with your child. Here are a few ideas to start you off:

■ 100 Ways Egg Soufflé (see recipe section)

■ Keto pizza (there's a great recipe in *The Keto Cookbook*)

■ Cheesy Bread with Dipping Sauce (see recipe section)

■ Dips and veggies

■ Corn Dog Poppers (see recipe section)

■ Cold meat and cheese roll-ups on romaine lettuce with mayonnaise

■ Tuna or egg salad with lots of mayo

- Faux "nutella" (ground hazelnuts with cocoa powder and Stevia) on a muffin, such as the muffin in a mug from the Charlie Foundation

- Keto cheesecake

- Wonder Waffles (see recipe section)

- Tangy Waldorf Salad (see recipe section)

- Summer Muffins (see recipe section)—or any other all-in-one muffin recipe

- Yogurt

- Hot dogs

Having a great plan, good communication with teachers, and some well-packed lunches and snacks on the menu should ensure that school time is a Keto-friendly experience. You can then send your warrior off to school without worry, knowing everything is going to be just fine.

8
Marching Across the Globe

If you've managed to make it this far through this book, you've surely realized by now that we're passionate about making diet therapy understandable and available to those who need it. Considering epilepsy is the most common neurological problem on the planet, and nearly a third of people suffering from seizures cannot get full control with medication alone, it astonishes us that more money is not being poured into promoting this effective treatment. Once two or three medications have failed, a ketogenic diet is more likely to do a better job of controlling seizures than any other medication currently on the market, yet, sadly, it still remains unavailable to most children and adults in the world who need it.

As unsettling as that is, there is comfort in the fact that there are more Keto Clinics available now than ever before, particularly in North America, which is comparatively a "land flowing with milk and honey" when it comes to Keto access. At present, only seven states in the United States., located mainly in the Midwest region, do not have Keto Clinics to our knowledge, yet many large metropolitan areas have more than one. In the rest of the world, however, there are still areas that need more Keto Clinics, especially in the developing world (Central America, Africa, and Southeast Asia). It is true that the diet is increasingly gaining worldwide recognition; several decades ago the Ketogenic diet was available in only a handful of hospitals, but the 90s brought a renewed interest, and currently over 150 hospitals in 50 countries offer the therapy. As wonderful as that statistic sounds, it is nevertheless sobering to realize that the remaining 145 countries in the world do not yet possess even a single hospital that offers the diet. Families in those countries are forced to travel abroad to seek treatment if they are to find any hope for their children:

I gave birth in Dubai, one of the emirates of United Arab Emirates (UAE). After two and a half months my son, Yousuf, started having seizures. I kept on seeing doctors from different hospitals and clinics, but everyone failed to discover what had happened to him, so I was forced to go back to my country, Nepal, for further treatment. Since the medication was expensive I came back to Dubai and started working. But medicines seemed to have no effect on him. Searching online helped me to know about the Ketogenic diet, but unfortunately no doctors are practicing it here. So I am seeing a doctor from India and applied the diet for my son. The diet seems to be effective and hopefully his seizures will be stopped completely soon. —Sabira

After communicating with Sabira, we helped her search online and discovered that there actually are several hospitals in Dubai that offer the diet, and more in Abu Dhabi and Al Ain (UAE), so we directed her toward them. Sabira's plight illustrates what many frustrated and overwhelmed parents have encountered while wandering in the desert of misinformation that can surround and isolate ketogenic therapy. Families of children with refractory epilepsy in countries outside the United States are frequently *not* informed by their physicians about the benefits of the diet or which hospitals offer it locally, and instead are simply given medication after medication after medication, without being told of an alternative.

While some desperate parents go to the extreme of traveling the globe in search of treatment for a beloved child, sadly, that option is financially out of reach for most of the world's population. Making dietary therapy for epilepsy available to all who need it is imperative. Interestingly, the driving force motivating much of the diet's current global awareness campaign and expansion is the parents of Keto kids. Foundations established by thankful parents have formed websites and support groups, networked, and organized international symposiums to educate doctors and dietitians about current research and the benefits of a ketogenic diet. This parental grassroots lobbying is a curious phenomenon in the medical world, where information about new therapies is generally disseminated via substantial marketing campaigns funded by pharmaceutical companies. However, as

Donald Shields, head of pediatric neurology at the UCLA Medical Center, stated in an NBC *Dateline* TV interview:

> *There is no big drug company behind the Ketogenic diet and*
> *there probably can never be, unless somebody starts marketing*
> *sausage and eggs with cream sauce on it as a drug.*

One would think that pharmaceutical companies would applaud the diet and donate to campaigns promoting it. As naïve and utopian as that statement may sound, there are actually credible reasons why it would be in the best interest of corporations to endorse it. No genuine competition for corporate profits exists when patients use the diet, since those turning to it have usually found medication alone does not control their seizures. However, the diet often works in partnership with medication, rather than in competition with it, thus making medication more effective in many difficult-to-treat cases. Diet therapy and medication may appear to be strange bedfellows at first glance, but in truth they often are compatible mates. Patients weaned from the diet are often advised to remain on medication, and they continue to maintain the benefit of seizure control they gained while on the diet, a benefit that medication alone did not achieve. One major exception to the pharmaceutical rule is the company Eisai, which makes rufinamide. They offer information and free copies of the book *Ketogenic Diets* (5th edition), by Dr. Eric Kossoff et al., on their site: www.livingwithlgs.com.

At the very least, seeing large pharmaceutical companies promote and encourage diet therapy would be a gesture of goodwill akin to the scene in the film *Miracle on 34th Street*, when Macy's department store Santa sends a mother seeking a treasured toy on her child's Christmas wish-list down the road to another store because Macy's stock was sold-out. Santa didn't want a child to be disappointed at Christmas. When the miracle of medication isn't enough, how much more should we strive not to disappoint children with a chance at a seizure free life?

Parents Moving Mountains

Mobilizing the Troops in North America: The Charlie Foundation

Never underestimate the power of parents to move mountains to find answers for their children and then, out of gratefulness, attempt to pay the miracle forward. A prime example of this parental force at work is the case of Jim and Nancy Abrahams, parents of Charlie, a young boy with profoundly debilitating seizures who failed most then-available anti-seizure medications, as well as brain surgery. He became seizure-free within 72 hours of starting the Ketogenic diet. Jim, a Hollywood film producer, questioned why he had not been told about the diet much, much earlier in his son's illness. In a 1994 NBC TV *Dateline* interview Jim Abrahams said this: "*It doesn't come in a pill form. It cannot be administered with a scalpel. And the only people who profit from the Ketogenic diet are the patients.*"

He managed to bring the diet to the attention of the general public with his release of the 1997 touching television film, *First Do No Harm*. Starring Meryl Streep, a personal friend of the Abrahams family, the film mirrored their own experience of having a child with catastrophic epilepsy who was helped by the diet.

The Abrahams established the Charlie Foundation in 1994, a charitable organization that promotes awareness of ketogenic diets by focusing on education and encouraging research. With the foundation's support, medical consensus guidelines regarding the diet's use and implementation were first published in 2008. Beth Zupec-Kania, the foundation's consulting dietitian, developed the KetoCalculator, a tool that has brightened the lives of many families cooking with the diet. She has traveled to such diverse locations as Saudi Arabia, the Dominican Republic, and Germany to conduct training in Ketogenic diet therapy.

Since the Ketogenic diet and Modified Atkins Diet (MAD) are now both widely available in the United States and Canada, and numerous published studies document the efficacy of these diets, one would think North American physicians would routinely endorse diet therapy and recommend it to patients with difficult-to-control seizures. Surprisingly, there is still considerable reluctance to do so, though the reasons for this are not entirely clear. In a summary published after the International Symposium on Dietary Treatment for Epilepsy and Other Neurological Disorders was held in 2010 in Edinburgh, it was noted:

> *A study of neurologists from South Carolina in 2008 found that only 36% used the diet frequently after numerous anti-epileptic drugs had failed (Mastriani et al., 2008). Of the remainder, 16% "never use it," 24% "rarely," and 24% "only as a last resort."*

Things are much better now in the United States per a recent study. They found that about half of families surveyed rated their neurologist as a

10 out of 10 in terms of recommending the diet, even when they had to refer them to another Keto Clinic. It appears that more and more neurologists are realizing the diet is helpful.

England and Beyond: Matthew's Friends

Across the Ocean, a similar grassroots parental movement took place after Matthew, the son of Emma Williams, a child with Dravet Syndrome, suffered years of uncontrollable seizures. After being diagnosed with epilepsy in 1995, Matthew failed numerous medications, and his desperate mother describes on her website how physicians discouraged use of the diet, telling her it would "limit the quality of her son's life." She says, *"I was fobbed off and told that there was no real evidence that it worked and that it was very difficult to manage and 'drugs are the better option.'"* It was not until nearly five years had passed, and her son had endured 10 to 20 seizures per day, that Emma was finally able to enroll him in a clinical trial of the diet in London. Matthew now has, on average, three seizures per week and Emma says, *"If anyone tells you that miracles never happen, please tell them from me that they are wrong."*

Inspired by the Abrahams' work in the United States, she formed her own website and charitable group, Matthew's Friends. Since 2004, the charity has become a leading voice in the Ketogenic world, providing support, education and training in dietary therapy for both professionals and families. In 2011, Emma's dream of seeing her charity's own specialist clinic became reality when the Matthew's Friends Clinic opened at the Neville Childhood Epilepsy Center in Surrey. They employ a neurologist, dietitians, and ketogenic assistants, and they offer care for children and adults in the classic Ketogenic diet, Medium Chain Triglyceride (MCT) diet, Modified Atkins Diet, and Low Glycemic Index Treatment (LGIT) diet.

South Africa and New Zealand: Matthew's Friends Go Global

Matthew's Friends charity has since spread its wings and flown abroad. When we asked Emma about developments in their expanding international work, she informed us that they have taken root in both South Africa and New Zealand:

> ***Matthew's Friends South Africa:*** *The Matthew's Friends South African project is small, but we do have a Matthew's Friends-linked dietitian based in Johannesburg who does training throughout South Africa and treats patients, as well as a few*

key parents, who support others. We offer a child sponsorship program (if funds allow). Any money raised in South Africa will be used in South Africa to treat patients and help support families and professionals. The Matthew's Friends website has a section devoted to South Africa and the Ketogenic diet.

Matthew's Friends New Zealand: *The CEO is Susan Hill. They have registered the charity in its own right and it has a section of the Matthew's Friends website. The charity is currently raising funds to place ketogenic dietitians within hospitals around New Zealand as well as providing support to families and all those interested in ketogenic dietary therapies.*

The Middle East

Israel: Oliver's Magic Diet

As dietary therapy continues to circle the globe, it is being modified in interesting ways to suit the culture of each country. Adapting a dietary regimen in this way can be a complicated business. In Israel, for instance, certain religious restrictions may need to be taken into account when initiating the diet. If the father of the family is a descendant of a priestly lineage and forbidden to enter a place that may hold dead bodies, the diet may have to be started outside of a hospital on an outpatient basis. Some Jewish families keep kosher and observe religious dietary restrictions that forbid the use of pork and shellfish, and do not allow the mixing of milk and meat in meals.

As in other countries, parents in Israel have come to the fore to help spread awareness of the diet and to encourage its use. Eli and Talia Berger created the Hebrew website Oliver's Magic Diet after their son saw great improvement on the Ketogenic diet several years ago. In June 2012, as part of Israeli Nutrition Week, they helped organize and raise sponsorship for a training event, which brought Dr. Eric Kossoff and dietitian Zahava Turner from Johns Hopkins Hospital to Tel Aviv.

Talia Berger:

Upon first hearing about the diet, we only heard "bad" stuff: "the diet is too hard to actually succeed on," "it mimics starving, therefore you need to starve your child," "the portions are tiny and your child will cry and whine all day that they are hungry and eventually you'll give in because there is no food to give them"—to say the diet had a "bad" reputation was an understatement!

Even now, after two years of trying relentlessly to change the "press" and give the diet a good, confident, easy-to-accept spin, it still amazes me how differently a parent who hears about the diet objectively accepts it, in comparison to a neurologist—who might also be a parent—trying to pretend they had to put their healthy daughter/son on the diet. They realize that it wouldn't go down well at home! But we're not talking about our healthy, happy, well-adjusted, even medically-balanced children. We're talking about our other special ones—the ones who are seizing most of the day and don't respond well enough to drugs, who are running out of options to offer a better quality of life...

The first order of business: a website. We chose www.oliversmagicdiet .com, because that's exactly what it was in our house, MAGIC. We built the site up constantly, looking at it from a newcomer's perspective, which was easy since the site went up by the time Oliver was four months on the diet. We added essential tips and advice from our experience and heaps and heaps of translated medical material about the diet in Hebrew, so that there is easy and direct access to the amazing statistics that show the diet is better than any of the drugs' statistics after failing two or more. Our phone number went up on the site as well, and business cards and silicon bracelets were distributed by us at all the main national centers, mostly through neurologists whom we made a point of meeting at national neurology conferences. Once we introduced the website as a helpful tool, and the fact that we are happy to support them once they're at home with recipes, tips, a listening ear, etc. (all, of course, approved by their dietitian), they started to "use" us!! Yippy!

There have been times during the past two years that we've had four or five new families a week calling, asking questions, and sifting through our webpage and Facebook page with a fine comb! We welcome them, and I'm never turned off at having a long phone conversation, reassuring them that if the neurologist has suggested the diet, there's a pretty good chance some improvement might come. It can be pretty intense—and to each child there is a world of history attached. But all our fears are common and we all want is to try and improve our children's lives as much as we can. Furthermore, from our experience, we're in touch with most of the families four to five times a day at the beginning of the diet. By the end of the first month they are happy, busy, and adjusted to life with the diet. Usually we'll hear from them only once in a while and on holidays!

Upon setting up the website and talking to families, we knew we needed to somehow put together a package that could help both the dietitians when initiating the diet, as well as the families once they got home. We're very proud that we've managed to put together the first Hebrew My Ketogenic Diary *with Nutricia and Megapharm funding the print. This is a tool, not a cookbook, to be used by the dietitians to explain the diet in a comforting, good-looking fashion! The diary has room for the dietitian to add notes and recipes as well as existing recipes that the dietitian can check to see if they are suitable to the child in question. It is not a "stand-alone" book—it MUST come from the medical team looking after the patient. Every photo in the Diary (photographed by Ms. Yula Zubritsky, a fellow Keto mom and professional food photographer) is 4:1 ratio and all are things Oliver can eat (!) as well as having over 20 tips for the Keto kitchen! The diary is printed on very thick paper so it's suitable for spills and use in the kitchen!*

We hope the Berger's story will inspire other parents to try to make a difference in their own communities, and find creative ways to share their experiences with diet therapy with other families starting out.

Persian Gulf Countries

Interest in Ketogenic diet therapy is also spreading rapidly throughout the Mideast. At least one hospital in Saudi Arabia has been using the Ketogenic diet for many years and recently hospitals in Kuwait, Iran, and the UAE now offer the diet as well. Dr. Eric Kossoff from Johns Hopkins, and Beth Zupec-Kania, consulting dietitian for the Charlie Foundation, have visited countries in the region several times to conduct training, and they commented on the high level of excitement and interest they found among doctors, dietitians, and families.

In a report written for epilepsy.com after a trip to Saudi Arabia, Beth Zupec-Kania noted that, though there is a difference in the use of herbs, sauces, and spices as compared to western cuisine, many local foods are similar to western favorites, and local high-fat food preferences include heavy cream, cultured cream, butter, safflower oil, and olives. She described a local dietitian's efforts to create a low-carbohydrate coconut biscuit, to replace the high carbohydrate version children in the region commonly eat. The MAD also shows great promise in a region where enjoying food together with family and friends is an important cultural tradition.

Asia—Advancing Across the Eastern Front

India: Curry's on the Keto Menu!

When renewed interest in the Ketogenic diet was sparked back in the early 90s, the Keto Team at Johns Hopkins became busier than ever training visiting neurologists and dietitians from around the world. Dr. Janak Nathan attended such training in 1996, studying under Dr. John Freeman and dietitian Millicent Kelly, with the intention of bringing the therapy back to his home country.

India is a vast nation that abounds with a variety of regional food preferences, cooking methods, and languages. Additionally, it is a country with diverse religions, each having their own set of dietary restrictions. Dr. Nathan and his team from Shushrusha Hospital, Mumbai, have successfully modified the diet to suit the unique needs of patients on the sub-continent.

Dr. J. Nathan, Shushrusha Hospital, Mumbai, India:

The first problem was the difficulty in using American recipes in India. So, to Indianize the recipes a team of dietitians prepared recipes using different caloric and Keto ratio values. These were carefully weighed, prepared, and tasted by the team. Slowly, a bank of 100 recipes was fashioned and a book prepared with basic instructions included. However, as India is multilingual we had to translate these into at least three Indian languages. A few of our patients were so illiterate that they could not read numerals in Roman figures and, therefore, this had to be taught before they could use the weighing scale.

There was, however, a lot of negative feedback from other physicians initially. In fact, one family physician convinced the parents to stop the diet after the child developed an incidental urinary tract infection, convincing the family that the ketones in the urine were the cause. Luckily the child's infantile spasms had already stopped and there were no more seizures after just four months on the diet.

There was also a lot of resistance to the use of fasting in the initial phase of introduction of the Ketogenic diet. This was more from the parents than the children who went through this phase without much fuss. However, we soon realized that hospitalization also entailed a fair expense to the parents, especially as most Indians do not have medical insurance. So, in late 1997 a short carbohydrate washout period was introduced during which very low to zero carbohydrates were given. As there was no fasting phase we stopped hospitalization. Thus, we reduced initiation to two days. Since 1998 we have been using a total outpatient approach.

India has a large number of vegetarians and even some who will not eat anything that grows below the ground, like onions, potatoes, garlic, etc. Also, culinary practices vary every 100 to 200 kilometers. Therefore, recipes have to be tailor-made depending on the region of origin. The protein content of vegetarian food is low and therefore we started using soy as a source of vegetable protein. The advantages are many. Compared to the Western Ketogenic diet, where protein is mainly of animal source, the Indian Ketogenic diet's protein is largely from soybean products. Soy is associated with a decrease in the risk of coronary heart disease and is a rich source of lecithin. Lecithin has been used as a treatment for high cholesterol. In bile, lecithin acts like a soap to dissolve fat for digestion and absorption, and is a major source of choline. As choline increases the fat metabolism, it can thus lower blood cholesterol. Soy also contains soluble fiber, which interferes with the absorption and metabolism of cholesterol and thereby decreases serum cholesterol. Soy is also a good source of minerals like iron and calcium, which are deficient in the KD.

There is probably much the west can learn from the Indian version of the diet; the more international research continues, the more all nations will benefit from shared discoveries. For instance, in order to address the problem of high blood lipid levels, a common side effect of ketogenic diets, patients in India are encouraged to limit saturated fats and use a combination of groundnut oil (MUFA, or mono-unsaturated fatty acids), corn oil or saf-flower oil (PUFA, or poly-unstaurated fatty acids), and ghee (clarified butter, a saturated fat), which has helped keep cholesterol levels down. Dr. Nathan's team also encourages the use of spices, a very important component in Indian cuisine, and he notes recent evidence points to several advantages of doing this. Two recently published studies involving extracts of cumin and saffron, both commonly used in Indian cooking, have shown them to be effective in significantly decreasing seizure frequency. A study of curcumin, the active ingredient in turmeric, a bright yellow powder used in curry, suggests that it has potential to both prevent seizures and to protect seizure-induced memory impairment.

In a country as large as India, the job of training Keto Teams to serve in hospitals throughout the country is a daunting task, but much progress has been made since Dr. Nathan first introduced the diet. From 1996 until 2006, even after several presentations at national level conferences, physicians still did not train in the use of the Ketogenic diet. In 2006, 21 doctor and die-titian teams received training. Then in November 2012, Dr. Nathan joined forces with Dr. Helen Cross from London Children's Hospital, and Dr. Eric Kossoff from Johns Hopkins Hospital in the United States, to train over 60 doctors and dietitians from various parts of India and Sri Lanka. The team in India has proven that patient, steady progress wins the race against seizures. Dr. Janak can be contacted at: www.ketogenicdietindia.org.

China: The Long March of the Ketogenic Diet

Interest in the Ketogenic diet in China dates to the 1960s when it was first investigated as a therapy for refractory epilepsy, until the Cultural Revolution interrupted research. During the tense decade of political upheaval that engulfed the country from 1966–1976, all research came to a screeching halt and doctors were forced to abandon the project. A very different social climate exists in China today, and the medical community has once again actively embraced ketogenic research.

The Ketogenic diet was reintroduced to China by Dr. Liao Jianxiang, who admitted the first two patients using the therapy to Shenzhen's Children's Hospital in October, 2004. The diet is now being offered at 24 hospitals across the country, though only ten have a significant number of patients on the diet. Over 600 patients across China have used the diet to date, and the image of the Ketogenic diet being used as a "last-resort-only" therapy is slowly changing. The MAD is also gaining ground and has been used with patients since 2010 by Dr. Deng Yuhong in Guangzhou, who is currently studying the use of the diet with MCT oils. A beta version of Chinese software used for calculating the Ketogenic diet is now being tested, and in May 2012, meetings were held among members of the China Medical Association's Pediatric Branch of Neurology, revolving around plans to standardize treatment recommendations and further promote the use of the Ketogenic diet and MAD in the country.

Though the Asian diet has a strong emphasis on rice and noodles, there is also a great fondness for meat and vegetable dishes, particularly stir-fried low-carbohydrate green leafy vegetables generously laced with oil, which makes the diet adaptable to local cuisine. At celebrations and feasts, particularly in the countryside, foods prepared with lavish amounts of oil are perceived as a sign of prosperity. Chairman Mao, the founding father of the People's Republic, was a great advocate of the benefits of fatty foods. His favorite dish was Hong Shao Rou (fatty pork belly stewed in sweet soy sauce) and he always requested to be served this food during strenuous military campaigns, believing that the fat in the meat helped him somehow think more clearly in battle. Knowing what we do now about the positive effects of fat on the brain, he just may have been on to something!

MAD made its debut in China after Jeanne Riether, one of the authors of this book, used the diet successfully with her son Jordan in 2009 while living in China, as related in Chapter 1. After seeing what it could do for her own child, she approached Chinese neurologists to discuss ways to work together to bring this valuable treatment to mainland China.

The Healing Young Hearts MAD Training DVD

I e-mailed Eric Kossoff from Johns Hopkins who kindly offered his help reviewing any material we would put together about MAD. We made a Chinese PowerPoint covering the how-to's of the first three months of the diet and began showing it to different neurologists in a few different cities. We quickly realized that there were definite obstacles to introducing MAD in China.

For one, there is no unified cup measurement system used in China to measure food by volume. Recipes here commonly use general amounts—a "handful" of greens, for example—or they use rice bowls to measure food or liquid and these often come in varying sizes, so teaching patients to estimate net carbs by volume was tricky. Also, there are no easy online resources or handy pocket-size booklets in Chinese that list the net carbohydrate values of common foods. No one could quickly Google a food to check the net carb count unless they spoke English, which most families don't, and even if they could understand English, the net carb counts of foods on most Western websites are measured in cups, anyway. Then there was the problem of the shortage of dietitians. In Western countries, patients starting MAD usually work with a dietitian who helps them plan menus and choose foods. However in China, dietitians do not generally see individual outpatients (though this is changing in some cities) but usually only work in hospitals and schools to plan menus. Many families have no knowledge about nutrition, so instruction would need to be quite thorough if they were going to be able to use the diet on their own at home.

To further complicate things, neurologists in China already see a high number of patients each day, so taking on the additional time-consuming job of training individual patients to understand and use MAD was—well, let's just say it was unrealistic of us to expect it of them. We realized that instead of helping things, offering MAD to patients would actually create a huge headache for the already overworked doctors, and give them an extra job. Obviously that wouldn't be well received, so we went back to the drawing board to brainstorm solutions.

We realized that what would be most helpful for neurologists and patients alike would be to create a DVD tool that would do the training for them. If a doctor thought a patient could benefit from MAD, all he had to do was check the patient's blood work, and then copy the DVD to give to the family to view at home. Voila! (Or, as they say in Chinese, "Wa!") Again, Dr. Kossoff helped us review scripts, and working with Dr. Deng Yuhong and Dr. Liao Jianxiang, we filmed training sessions that walked patients through everything they would need to know to begin.

Our Healing Young Hearts Modified Atkins Training DVD includes the diet's history, patient success stories, and step-by-step instructions so families can plan meals that are high fat and low carbohydrate. To get around the problem of measuring cups we have them weigh foods on a gram scale, and compiled a list of the net carb content of 100-gram weights of common foods to include as a printable resource on the DVD. We even filmed a professional Chinese chef demonstrating how to cook simple, great tasting MAD meals. Dr. Kossoff helped us arrange funding with the Stroup Kids-for-Kids foundation, a wonderful organization that helped us cover part of the cost of the project. The China Association Against Epilepsy is helping us distribute this free tool to neurologists in the country.

At the time of the writing of this book, our MAD Training DVD is nearly ready to launch in China. Our Healing Young Hearts Project is also offering free copies of the English version of the scripts to hospitals in the developing world that would like to use it to produce a similar training tool in their own country. We hope this will further promote the use of MAD as an outpatient therapy throughout China and beyond. —Jeanne Riether

We Are the World...

To cover everything that is happening in the 50 or more countries of the world that currently have hospitals offering ketogenic diets would take far more space than this book allows. Below is a brief news summary of some of the dietary developments in various corners of the world.

Europe: Western Europe is one of the fastest growing areas of the world regarding use of the Ketogenic diet. Many different countries are currently conducting research, and Germany, Denmark, Poland, and the Scandinavian countries have all organized ketogenic symposiums in recent years. Parts of Eastern Europe, however, still lack the therapy, so patients must travel to surrounding countries to receive it. The diet is only used sporadically in Russia.

South America: The Ketogenic diet has been used in Argentina and Brazil since the 1970s (with many publications in the last few years), and in recent years it has also been introduced in Uruguay, Ecuador, Chile, and Colombia. Both the Ketogenic diet and MAD are being used, and there are plans to expand diet therapy services to surrounding countries.

Australia: Physicians in Australia first used the Ketogenic diet with patients in the 1960s at the Royal Children's Hospital in Melbourne. Currently it is being used at all the major pediatric teaching hospitals throughout the country, and several are also using the MAD. However, due to limited dietetic resources, the diet is usually reserved for children with refractory seizures for whom surgery is not an option. Increased funding for dietetic resources would allow the diets to be more widely used in Australia. Interesting work is being done in Brisbane with offering ketogenic diets via telemedicine (due to the very large distances in the Queensland region of Australia).

Korea: The Ketogenic diet has been used in Korea since 1995, and physicians claim that adapting it to the local culture has been an important step in helping it gain acceptance. Studies report that families often showed considerable resistance to the therapy initially, as the Korean diet is traditionally high in carbohydrate-rich foods, so patient education is important. The MAD has been well received, as it allows patients to use small amounts of rice and also makes sharing food at meals easier. Several research studies from Korea have been published and the diet has been discussed at several Asian scientific congresses. They are probably the world experts on mitochondrial diseases and the Ketogenic diet.

Japan: Both the Ketogenic diet and the MAD are currently being used in Japan, and Ketogenic diet websites in Japanese and parent support groups are available. Results from a number of research studies have been published, including a study on the successful use of the MAD with non-convulsive status epilepticus.

The Empty Spaces on the Map

Looking at a map of the world from a ketogenic perspective, there are still many blank spaces where no services exist. Nearly the whole of Africa, apart from the southernmost tip, lacks access to diet therapy for epilepsy. Mexico and much of the Caribbean are still without Keto Clinics, and a number of countries in South America have no hospitals that offer the diet. Parts of the Middle East, Central Asia, and Southeast Asia lack access, so patients must travel to surrounding countries. Even countries that are fortunate enough to have a hospital offering dietary therapy may only have one or two that serve a huge population; Indonesia, the fourth most populous country in the world, has, to our knowledge, only a single hospital in the capital that offers the Ketogenic diet.

Is it unrealistic to hope that every family, in every country, at every corner of the globe, should have access to diet therapy for seizures? Perhaps we will not see it happen in our lifetime, but some impossibly difficult goals are still worth fighting for. We hope by the time a second edition of this book is published, that many more spaces on the map will no longer be empty.

To the Unknown Soldier...

We realize there are a great many dedicated physicians and enthusiastic parents across the globe who have not been included in this chapter, who are working hard to bring the miracle of diet therapy to their own corner of the world. These unsung heroes are changing lives. You know who you are. Please write us, for we'd love to hear what you are accomplishing. Rest assured that even if you have not been included in these pages, we salute you!

9
Warriors of All Shapes and Sizes

Take a walk down any street in New York City and you are instantly reminded how unique individuals are. You will see people of every shape and color, you will hear different languages and accents, and you will see people wearing items of clothing in ways you never would have thought possible. It's an incredible testament to the human spirit and to the uniqueness inherent in all of us. While you might not have a fearless fashion sense, you are no doubt fearless when it comes to you or your child's well-being. After all, you are reading a book that has dedicated dozens of pages to telling you how tough diet therapy is, and here you are, on Chapter 9!

Within this chapter we have culled advice from all over the world—literally—and we have come up with simple tips and tricks to help guide you through the different developmental stages of children (and adults) who are pursuing diet therapy. After all, the challenges you will face with a toddler on the diet are nothing like the challenges of a teenager's father. We understand the differences of these age groups, and we've put together tips that cover some of the bigger issues; but of course, we can't possibly tackle them all.

Our favorite element of this chapter is the collection of personal stories written by young warriors in which they are utterly candid about their experiences on diet therapy. Never before in a book have we been able to look into the minds of the children who are deeper in the trenches than their parents. For those adults who are considering diet therapy, we also have several stories written by adults across the spectrum of ages.

Infant Warriors

Of the parents we interviewed for this book, the overwhelming majority of parents with infants on the Ketogenic diet remarked that the diet is actually fairly simple with an infant. For starters, most infants are either on an easy-to-mix formula such as KetoCal, which is given through a bottle, or they are fed via G-tube. Formulas require little thought and creativity, and babies tend to transition nicely from standard formula to a ketogenic formula. Babies are also not notoriously picky eaters.

The challenges often arise when Baby is beginning to transition to solid foods. Of course, this obstacle comes with developmentally delayed infants or children as well, just a little farther down the road. Thankfully, making pureed fruits, veggies, and meats Keto friendly is as simple as adding a little oil, butter, or cream.

Risking the Allergies

First-time parents typically go by the book and follow the standard protocols for introducing new foods to Baby. Dairy such as cheese and yogurt is usually left out of the diet until around nine months, whole milk until 12 months, and egg whites, nuts, and other big allergens are also avoided until at least 12 months. Chances are, if you're reading this book, you've been dealing with epilepsy, and so trying to get those seizures to stop has overshadowed the little things in life—like when to give your child cheese for the first time. The question, then, is how do you move forward on a diet that has a lot of allergens as staple ingredients?

Here's the good news. There is a little more leniency when your child is on a ketogenic diet; however, the approach is still the same: add one new ingredient at a time and keep a food record to track any potential allergic reactions. Don't add another ingredient for at least three to four days. To play it safe, stick within the basic guidelines of food introductions (i.e., cheese around nine months), and ask your dietitian about when you can add those riskier ingredients. The only real restriction, unless your child has known allergens or there is a history of allergies in the family, is the use of cream—best to keep that off the menu until around a year old.

For more ideas on how to create foods with different allergies and sensitivities, refer back to Chapters 4 and 5.

Transitioning to Solid Foods

*It's hard to practice finger foods like Gerber Puffs, Cheerios, etc.
if your kids won't drink the right amount of cream or oil to balance it out.*—Bethany

Bethany is just one of many parents of an infant who finds the idea of
transitioning from pureed foods to finger foods tricky terrain. Take a walk
down any baby aisle in your local grocery store or super store and you'll
find dozens of options of yogurt bites, a variety of puffs, cheese curls, and
fruit snacks—all of it full of sugar and chock full of carbs.

You want your baby to make as many developmental milestones as
possible and eating with her fingers is one of those big milestones. We've
come up with a few suggestions to help you get through this challenging
phase; after all, how will your baby eat all those fun toddler-friendly Keto
meals if she doesn't get the chance to learn how to chew?

■ **Stick with all-in-one ratios:** It's tough to take a chance on your infant
taking a bite of food if you end up fighting him to get the appropriate
amount of fat. Take the stress out of the situation and create something
that is all-in-one. Luckily, our Baby Puffs and Yogurt Melts recipes are
both all-in-one, and they melt in the mouth nicely.

■ **Behold: the avocado:** In Chapter 4 we taught you that the avocado is the
perfect ketogenic food. It is also a perfect food to give Baby as a first finger
food. For some infants the texture can be hard to get used to, as it's soft
and slippery and can sometimes slide down the back of their throats. Try
picking an avocado that is just ripe, but not overly soft yet. A ripe avocado
is black instead of green. If you can push on it and it gives just slightly, it's
ripe; if you push on it and you can make an impression, it is too ripe.

■ **Try flaxmeal:** Ever heard of the trick to roll slick foods in infant oatmeal
or rice cereal to make a texture that is easier for Baby to grasp? Instead
of cereal, use flaxmeal, which is full of healthy Omega-3 fats and is high
in fiber. If you wanted to try a little cooked apple rolled in flaxmeal, you'll
also be able to create an all-in-one ratio that way. Flaxmeal is also a great
first cereal. Mix the flaxmeal with butter, ketogenic formula, water, and
a little sweetener and you have a tasty first cereal. For lower ratios, mix
in a little chunky pureed fruit.

■ **Make your purees chunky:** Baby foods come in several different
stages. As you continue to work with your infant on chewing skills, you

can adapt your homemade Keto purees to suit your infant's needs. Make your own apple sauce by simmering apple chunks and a little water. Mix the apples with a mild-flavored oil and you have a Stage 2 or 3 food. This idea can be transferred to any fruit or vegetable.

- **Calculate small amounts:** When you are first trying to get your infant to eat solid foods, you're only going to introduce small amounts at a time. His formula and pureed foods are still going to account for the majority of his calories, so when creating a first finger food meal in the KetoCalculator, think small, maybe 25 calories. This way there's less pressure on finishing the food, making the whole transition as natural for Baby as possible.

The following are three stories written by moms about their personal experiences having an infant on the diet:

A Warriors' Story: Carson, Ketogenic Diet, Five Months Old at Diet Initiation

Carson was a perfectly healthy five-month-old until January 29, 2007. She was in her high chair and I noticed something strange, similar to someone motioning "I don't know." Her arms went up and out to the side, and both eyes rolled up to one corner. Every time I would ask her what she was doing, she would then motion "I don't know" again. Something that I thought was funny at the time turned out to be a momentous and critical turning point in our lives. Carson had just had her first seizure.

Carson was diagnosed with Idiopathic Infantile Spasms on February 3rd at Johns Hopkins Hospital after having an EEG. We were given the choice of four different treatment options, including the Ketogenic diet because of the quick diagnosis. We decided to try the diet, as recent studies had found that trying the diet before anticonvulsant drugs had a high success rate for infantile spasms.

Carson started her fast in the hospital on Sunday around noon and began KetoCal on Monday. Her final seizure was on Tuesday, February 6th. Within two days of starting the diet, her seizures had ceased.

Two weeks into the diet, I noticed a marked difference in her behavior. She had stopped rolling and making sounds once the seizures started. She woke up on the morning of Valentine's Day and was cooing in her crib. When I took her out and laid her on the floor she starting rolling all over the place. I knew something had changed. After eight weeks on the diet, her EEG brain scan had completely normalized.

She continued on the diet for eight months and officially finished on October 5, 2007. The weaning process was terrifying. I would have kept her on it for ten years if it had been my choice! I fully admit that when she went off the diet, I still stayed with low-carb meals, not full Keto meals but it took about a year to cave in and give her a big piece of cake and ice cream at a birthday party or something along those lines.

We were very lucky that Carson was only five months old when she started the diet. Giving her a KetoCal bottle every three hours was really no different than the formula she had been on prior to the diet. When we introduced snacks and meals a few weeks later, she absolutely loved them. The only tricky part was coming up with foods for her to pick up on her own. I would make Keto cookies and break them up into small pieces. I tended to rely on all-in-one meals so that I knew she was getting exactly what she needed. She loved picking up chicken pieces but getting canola oil in her or butter was a challenge! So I would make a Keto casserole, so to speak, where it was an all-in-one meal!

I know that we were very fortunate that she was an infant. She did not know any different at that point, and I did not have to worry about her sneaking food, someone else giving her food, etc. It really was not much different with other babies who are on a regular diet.

Honestly, the only challenge I personally faced with Carson being on the diet was that I felt very alone and isolated from my friends and their children who were the same age. I just did not feel like I could relate to anyone at that point in my life. Carson was delayed physically the first two years, was eating special foods, and I lived every minute in fear of another seizure.

Carson continues to be seizure free and has developed completely normally both physically and mentally. She is about to finish kindergarten and is absolutely perfect due to the diet. Everyday, I look at this intelligent, beautiful, sensitive, thoughtful, incredible little miracle and I know that I have the diet to thank. There was nothing harder than watching her have a seizure, so the effort and level of difficulty of the diet were worth every second.—Gerry

A Warriors' Story: Drue, Ketogenic Diet, 21 Months Old

My son Drue, who is now 21 months old, was diagnosed with Hypoxic Ischemic Encephalopathy at birth from an accident with his cord during delivery. He also was diagnosed with Hydrocephalus at ten months old. At two months old, a few days after retuning from the NICU, I noticed him doing some weird repetitive movements. He was diagnosed with Infantile Spasms at three months old. Our first neurologist wanted to put him on vigabatrin even though we didn't feel like that was the best option for us. We switched doctors and started the KetoCal 3:1 formula when he was eight months old. Drue's seizures increased the first day, and then he became seizure free on day two of the diet.

One of the biggest problems we had with the diet early on was that the oiliness of the formula made the connectors of the Y port of his G-tube not stay together, and food and stomach acid would pour out all over him, and me, and sometimes our bed. It also made him nauseous towards the end. He stopped tolerating the formula, and he threw up all the time. The doctor said it was a side effect, and we'd just have to deal with it. We had to have his labs checked often to make sure he wasn't acidic or his electrolytes were stable.

Doing the diet with Drue was great because he was able to go seizure free without putting him on drugs. Having him G-tube-fed felt easier at times because I could measure out his food and set the rate, and I knew he was getting the amount of food he needed. But it was challenging that he couldn't have sugar in anything. Family outings weren't much different on the diet because he'd be on a formula anyway; we just had to plan how much food he'd need for whatever we were doing—easy to manage.—Ashlee

A Warriors' Story: Oliver, Ketogenic Diet, Two Years Old

We started the diet just a few days before Oliver turned one year old. It was bittersweet for us because we knew that our baby would never get that first birthday experience of trying birthday cake and being super messy. On the other hand, we were anxious to start the diet as quickly as possible once we decided to go through with it.

Oliver responded pretty well to the diet at first. He didn't really fight us on his meals (baby food like carrots or peas mixed with butter, plus cream to drink in his bottle). I think this is because he was so young and just used to eating jarred baby food anyway. The first couple of months we saw the same frequency of seizure activity but his clusters were only lasting 5 to 10 minutes instead of 30 to 45. Sometimes we didn't have to use Clonazepam (our rescue med) to break them up.

The biggest challenge with having an infant on the diet was that Oliver was never on a set feeding schedule. A lot of people say the key to success with the diet is consistency. Oliver is just now starting to get into more of a routine with meals at the same time each day, and he's been on the diet for over a year and a half. Another challenge is feeding him. If he doesn't want to eat, he won't. Because of his severe delays with development, he's not independent at all. He can't feed himself and we have to make sure all of his meals are all-in-one. We also have to make sure each meal is pureed into an applesauce-like consistency so that it's easy for him to eat. Because he can't sit on his own, it's difficult feeding him out and about. He's never been able to sit in a restaurant high chair.

The easiest thing about feeding an infant on the diet is that they're too young to be picky. Another advantage is that he still drinks bottles very well and we've been able to use the KetoCal liquid for easy meals on the go, or when he's sick or not feeling well. We'd be lost without that ability. The number one takeaway from this is that Oliver has not been on daily seizure meds during the ages when a baby develops/learns the most. While Oliver is severely delayed, both physically and cognitively, due to a genetic disorder (Congenital Disorder of Glycosylation), we can only imagine how much further behind he'd be if he were still on the medications that made him groggy and out of it.—Bethany

Toddler Warriors

Eating in Front on Your Toddler: Do You or Don't You?

The choice of whether or not to eat in front of your toddler depends on the cognitive level of your child, and of course, your personal parenting style. There are parents who advocate that you should not bend your life to avoid eating in front of your child, but for some families avoiding the family mealtimes is easier.

Consider, first, your child's level of understanding. Toddlers under the age of three are below the age of reason, meaning they simply can't be reasoned with. When you eat in front of your toddler and it's a food she can't have, your child has absolutely no way of comprehending why. Sure, we say no to many things when our children are toddlers. No to touching the lamp, no to throwing food, no to hitting. Yet, when children are below the age of reason, distraction and redirection are often our only reliable discipline tactics. We want to show our toddler what they are capable of instead of what they can't do. By eliminating the family food, you're at least taking away one massive challenge in dealing with the diet with a toddler.

> *We didn't eat in front of Noah while he was on the diet. Previous to the diet Noah loved going from plate to plate and stealing bites. Because he couldn't understand "No" and we couldn't reason with him, we tried to protect him from some of the hurt and disappointment that off-limits food could potentially bring him.*—Erin Whitmer

Of course there are families who can't do this because of other children. If you have a toddler in a bigger family, or you simply refuse to not eat "normal" meals around your toddler, try this:

- Put bites of your toddler's meal on your plate so she can enjoy sharing with you.
- Try to make your toddler's food look like the family's food.
- Find creative ways to shift the focus away from the food when the family eats together.

Battling Picky Eaters and Food Strikes

When toddlers hit that stage when they become picky about everything, it is often that they are learning to assert their independence. Being a picky eater is common for children around two to four years old. The fact that their food is their medicine just makes this age-appropriate phase a tremendously frustrating time. Your child might chipmunk his meals by holding his food in the side of his mouth so that he looks like a chipmunk, his cheeks full of nuts; he might throw his food onto the floor to test your reaction and see what he can get away with; and she might clamp her mouth down firmly, not allowing you to spoon-feed one bite of food.

> *I could have screamed daily because of Noah's food strikes and picky eating. Most days I was somehow able to keep my cool, and other days I displayed embarrassing and juvenile behavior by throwing perfectly good—albeit rejected—food in the kitchen sink.*—Erin Whitmer

Even typical toddlers with no dietary restrictions will drive their parents mad with their unpredictable eating habits. The stress factor is certainly increased when you've added a ketogenic diet into the daily grind, and while we can't guarantee an end to your frustration, we can at least provide you with a few tips we hope will make coping with your toddler warrior a little easier.

- **Rely on all-in-one meals:** Trying to get your picky child to eat a meat and a veggie (which he may have decided he hates today) in addition to a fat source—all in a finite amount of time—is guaranteed to send you straight to the nuthouse. By preparing all-in-one meals you have the peace of mind that your warrior is getting a perfect ratio with every bite. This way, when your stubborn son eats only half the meal, you can just give him the rest later so he gets his full calorie count.

- **Keep it simple:** It's fun to be creative, but many toddlers don't have particularly refined palates. We certainly encourage adding seasonings and exotic tastes to your child's food, but do it sparingly and only one new ingredient at a time. Toddlers love to use their hands, so consider simple chopped foods, thinly sliced hot dogs, waffles, muffins, and pancakes.

- **Foster her independence:** Toddlers are in the Autonomy Versus Doubt stage so they are building their confidence through their independence. While it might be tough to give your toddler independence where mealtime is concerned, you can still find ways to encourage this important developmental stage and perhaps encourage better eating habits. We provide you with several ideas throughout this list.

- **Start by offering a choice of one or two meals.**

- **Load her up with choices, such as plates, cups, or silverware:** "Would you like to use your blue plate or pink plate? Your Elmo spoon or your princess spoon?" Choices give her a chance to build confidence and feel a part of the process.

- **Stick with foods she can feed herself:** If she's confident using her hands but not her spoon, stick with meals that don't require you to feed her. While some fats just have to end up in a bowl with a spoon (i.e., ice cream, yogurt, or guacamole), you can try making a game out of spoon-feeding her, or you can encourage her growth in this skill by helping her use her spoon.

- **Pick your battles:** This is old advice that will never go out of style. No toddler wants to hear NO all day long, and many of them do. If your toddler is having a tough day, try bending on some of the other potential battles so that meal time can be a positive instead of a negative.

- **Have a back-up plan:** There will be days when you have tried everything you can think of to get your child to eat a meal. When all else fails, have a back-up meal lined up. In fact, it's a good idea to have a freezer full of back-up meals when you have a picky eater.

- **Know when you've lost:** You can still win the war against epilepsy even if your warrior misses a meal here or there. Trust us. We know it's tough to give in, but force-feeding your child will be a terrible experience for everyone and it will cast a shadow over mealtime for days and weeks to come. As long as you keep your warrior hydrated, everything will be fine.

Lori has a toddler son on the Ketogenic diet. Here is what she has recently learned about finding success in feeding her son:

> *I have had a hard time not feeding my son because of messes and spills, but I am realizing he really needs to have this independence. What I have done recently is to try to make his meals less messy. For example: he was eating a turkey salad meal that was chopped turkey and cheese mixed with mayo and then cream to drink, with some blueberries on the side. The mayo*

always ended up smeared everywhere on his face and the table.
To make this meal less messy I changed it to be a slice of turkey
rolled up, with a slice of cheese and the blueberries on the side,
and then I added grapeseed oil to the cream for his milk. This
way the meal is comprised of all finger food and then a drink.

Keeping Hydrated

The significant risk of kidney stones and dehydration on the Ketogenic diet (less-so with Modified Atkins Diet [MAD]) makes hydration an essential element to your child's health. But getting your little warrior to drink around 30 to 40 ounces of water a day can be tough. Some children are natural drinkers, while other seem to completely lack interest. When it comes to hydrating your toddler, you might need to get clever. Here are a few tricks we picked up along the way.

■ **Ice:** Young children love ice. Give your little warrior small cups of ice throughout the day as a fun snack and a way to keep hydrated.

■ **Popsicles:** Get yourself a popsicle mold and freeze sweetened or flavored water. If you use any of the low-carb drinks on the market, you can also freeze those. Our personal favorite is the simple combination of a little flavored Stevia and some natural food coloring. Zevia sodas (www .zevia.com) or Hint Naturally Flavored water are also great choices (www.drinkhint.com).

■ **Flavored water:** You can opt for one of the low-carb, zero calorie drinks that your Keto Clinic has approved, or you can do your own thing with a little Stevia. For a Keto-friendly lemonade, add one or two drops of lemon oil and some plain sweetener for a refreshing twist on the original sinfully sweet beverage. A drop or two of peppermint oil and sweetener is also perfect for a summer day.

■ **Fun drinking containers:** Try out different cups, bottles, sippy cups, sports bottles, twisty straws, or any colorful combinations of drinkable fun. Kids are easily bored, so the more variety you can give them, the more inspired they might feel to take a nice long guzzle!

Making Mealtime Fun

This is your chance to be creative. If you're not naturally creative, do a little research online and see what clever ways you can present food. When kids are in preschool programs they often have cooking activities when they make food into shapes, animals, insects – anything. You can do this too. Dawn Martenz, author of *The Keto Cookbook*, once made an adorable penguin out of black olives, cream cheese, and a little carrot for the nose. This intense level of creativity is time consuming and might be best left for special occasions, but in everyday life you can jazz up mealtime with:

- Colorful plates, cups, and silverware
- Natural food coloring
- A special theme such as princesses, trains, or farm animals
- A fun lesson wrapped into mealtime
- A "mealtime is video time" theme
- Taking the food out of the kitchen and opting for a picnic or dinner at the playground

Out and About

When you take your toddler out, be prepared to be an on-duty lifeguard the whole time. Playgrounds, indoor playrooms, children's museums—they are a landmine of hidden, dangerous carbs. Behind every rock or toy there always seems to be a Goldfish cracker or a crushed Cheerio, and your toddler, like every toddler out there, will want to put it in his mouth. The key is to always be on the lookout, and you'll be fine.

- **Be prepared—and never leave your house without a snack for your toddler warrior:** Regardless of where you go, you will likely find another toddler or child with a snack that looks dangerously appealing to your toddler. Since most toddlers are still too young to reason with, you won't have a chance to explain the nature of his diet, and you certainly won't want another meltdown. When you have a snack of your own, you can at least redirect your toddler to whatever tempting treat you pull out of your bag.

   There have been times when Jack sees other kids with something that he wants and just can't have. It's heartbreaking to see him throw his fit and I can't really blame him for being upset about it. If I plan ahead properly, I can usually avoid the meltdowns by either having something prepared or distracting him with some activity when the food comes out. —Sheryl

■ **Whenever you can, explain your warrior's dietary needs:** If you're just going to a playground, you're obviously not going to walk up to every parent and explain that his or her child's snack is kryptonite to your child. But when you're at a playgroup or somewhere with adults where you can have a conversation, be up front in the beginning. This way you can avoid the situation of the nice mom giving your child a food he can't have.

A Warriors' Story: Max, Ketogenic Diet, Three Years Old at Diet Initiation

Max started having seizures at 25 months old and started the diet at three years and eight months of age. He has intractable seizures due to prematurity and static encethalopathy. Before the diet he presented with tonic clonics and partial complex as well as many startles a day, like 50 to 60. His tonic clonics were every four to six weeks and would last hours and hours. He was always life-flighted to our children's hospital.

After starting the diet his speech improved. He has pretty significant Cerebral Palsy, couldn't sit on his own or tell me when he needs to go to the bathroom, but 18 days after starting the diet he was potty trained! He was just more aware of everything around him in general! He has not had a tonic clonic since he has been on the diet. He has had several times when we will see break through, but these are very short partial complex, maybe 45 seconds. His startles have all but stopped—maybe once or twice a day.

Having a tube-fed kid is really not a problem for the diet except for the mixing of three different things to make up the formula. It's just time consuming, and you can't just make a batch for the week; you have to make it every day. Max does eat by mouth too. We use RCF formula with polymers and micro lipids. For outings I always make sure I have an oral snack with us so he is not left out.

Max never transitioned to a bottle, but he will take pureed foods thickened. Without the thickener I think he would never have been willing to eat. Table food is a bit difficult for him in the chewing.

We had an instance at Whole Foods when I turned my back to get stuff off of the salad bar and the sample lady poured this green drink in his mouth. I freaked out! I had to go to the store manager and ask what their policy is for giving children samples without the parent's consent. I went into depth with that poor man, but he needed to understand that there are so many people out there with possible allergies and things like this cannot happen. To educate our friends and family, I always encourage them to ask as many questions as they want or need to ask in order to understand this crazy life Keto puts us in!! With preschool I gave them info from Charlie Foundation. The problem was that they thought that the list of things that can't be played with/touched were the only things that he was restricted from. It took me a bit to help them understand that it was just a simple list of some basic things—so school is the most difficult!—Shannon

A Warriors' Story: Jack, Ketogenic Diet and Modified Atkins Diet, Three Years Old

Jack was diagnosed with infantile spasms when he was five months old. He went through another battery of tests and was diagnosed with Tuberous Sclerosis Complex (TSC for short), a rare genetic disease that causes benign tumors to grow in all of the major organs, epilepsy, and potentially a host of developmental delays. Somehow we are the lucky ones and despite seizures for the majority of his life, his only delay is about a four to six month speech delay.

We got the spasms to stop with anticonvulsants when Jack was 10 months old but he continued to have simple partial seizures. When he was 14 months old he was having up to 17 seizures a day, some with head drops. He had failed five different drugs and we had to switch doctors to get him started on the Ketogenic diet. On the fifth and final day of our hospital stay Jack only had one seizure all day. I was amazed at how quickly we started to see results. By the two-week mark he was down to having only one seizure a week and at one point we think he went 63 days seizure free.

Keto gave us a lot of the freedom to do some "normal" toddler things. We could actually go to playgroups because he wasn't completely wiped out from seizing all morning. Of course, playgroup presented a whole different set of problems and the first big play group we went to some "kind" mother handed Jack a piece of dried fruit that I had to dig out of his mouth. After that, I found a very small play group, and the first few times I had to just hover over him.

*Getting a toddler to eat, even one not on a special diet, can be a
challenge. I am actually really lucky that I have a good eater, but
he still went through his picky phase. I remember days when
I would feed him three bites and then he decided he was done.
I also remember several days when I would go to my bedroom,
shut the door, and scream into my pillow before returning
calmly to the kitchen. It was usually lunchtime that was his difficult meal so I started only making all-in-one meals for lunch.
We would let him watch TV while he ate and if worst came to
worst we would let him run around and we would follow him
with the food. Usually if he could play and move he would take
a bite here and there.*

*After about 12 months on the diet we tried to tweak some things
to get his one pesky seizure a week to go away. The doctor
thought that he might be a good candidate for surgery, so when
Jack was two and a half he had resection surgery. Medically he
did well after surgery and was then weaned from the Ketogenic
diet to MAD. I think my husband and I both cried when the doctor told us we could start weaning.*

*Jack is now on MAD and loving it. We still have some of the
same challenges, but one huge change is that we all have
family meals now. Jack loves getting a bite of what is on our
plate, even if it's the exact same thing he is eating. He can
now have a cheese stick in the grocery cart, which is much
cheaper than the balloon I used to get him while he was on
the Ketogenic diet. Unfortunately Jack is not seizure free, but
his seizures now are only about 20 seconds. I don't regret one
moment of having Jack on diet therapy. Knowing that I can
make a difference in my kitchen, using my own hands and
creativity gives me a way to fight back. And I will never stop
fighting.*—Sheryl

Kid Warriors

Empowering Your Warrior and Avoiding Food Strikes

Just like toddlers, kids can be picky eaters and subject you to painful food
strikes. Believe it or not, some of their motivational factors are also the
same as toddlers: the desire for independence and seeking control. Low
and behold, though, sometimes they might just not be hungry and would

rather play than eat. That's a tough concept to wrap your head around once food becomes the center of the universe.

Regardless of the motivation behind the behavior, here are a few tips to help you when you find yourself in the midst of a power struggle with food in the center.

- **Create an open dialogue:** Thankfully, your school-age child can be reasoned with. Unless he's developmentally delayed, you can explain the importance of his magic food and encourage him to talk about why he's not interested in eating. It could be any number of reasons, but the reason often matters less than the conversation itself. The simple act of sharing a conversation and of strengthening your bond with your warrior might be enough to get him back to the dinner table without a fight.

- **Learn to negotiate:** When your child is looking for ways to assert her independence and gain a little control back, look for ways that you can bend, even if just a little. If your child absolutely refuses to eat a meal, learn when to stop pushing and see if you can come up with a negotiation. For example: "You can skip this meal, but why don't you eat a snack of your choice?" or "You finish your whole breakfast and you can choose what you want to eat for lunch."

   Now after one and a half years on the diet, if Oliver puts up a fight, we talk it out with him. There is A LOT of negotiation in our house—we don't always "win" the negotiation, and we'll sometimes agree to "skip" a meal—but it will only be ONE meal and a promise to eat the next.—Talia

- **Offer endless choices:** The best way to empower your warrior is to allow her to make as many choices in her daily routine as possible. When possible, offer those choices in relation to food, such as "Do you want Keto pizza or corn dog poppers for dinner?" "Would you rather eat inside at the dinner table or on the back porch?" When a choice about food isn't possible, find other ways to let your warrior make decisions. The more power of choice your warrior is given on a daily basis, the more she will feel in control; this confidence will improve her compliance with the diet.

   We've tried to empower him in other activities big and small; for example, we try to let him choose his clothes, what color plate he'd like to eat on, which of his menus he feels like eating, and we've also made an effort to give him back his "rights"—as *he is our eldest son—we let him stay up later than our two younger children, and he gets first choice on non-food related decisions with the kids, etc.—*Talia

■ **Teach by example:** Chances are, when your child began either the Ketogenic diet or the MAD, he gave up some his favorite foods. Why not try giving up a food you love? You can show your warrior that food doesn't define you, and it doesn't have to define him.

*When Oliver started the diet, we [my husband and I] both decided that we'd give up sugar and sweets and one of our favorite foods. So for me it was no desserts, sweets, or granola, and for Eli it was no desserts or sweets and no pizza. I lasted around ten days and then started cheating, and Eli is still sugar and pizza free a year and a half after Oliver started his diet.—*Talia

The Cheating Factor

Cheating is a topic that comes up quite often on ketogenic forums. Usually the cheater is new to the diet and having a tough time transitioning. Cheating can be as small as stealing a piece of food off a sibling's plate or it can be monumental, such as eating an entire box of cookies from the pantry. The greatest risk of cheating is losing ketosis and seizure control, though they are not always linked. There are children who have come out of ketosis and their seizures have worsened as a result, and we've also heard of occasions when there were no obvious repercussions of the cheat. No matter what, cheating is an issue that needs to be dealt with, and it can be tough for you not to feel guilty about the entire situation. (This is one of those key moments when you need to re-read Chapter 2 and learn to get rid of the guilt of depriving your child of food and take action.)

■ **Eliminate the temptation:** While this is not always practical depending on how many children you have, consider getting rid of the off-limits food—at least in the beginning. Boxes of cookies, granola bars, potato chips, etc. are all superfluous foods that no one really needs. You should absolutely keep the house free of your warrior's favorite food items that are now off-limits. Once your warrior is on the diet a while and has become accustomed to her new way of eating, you can add some of these items back into the pantry, or you can just continue on without them.

■ **Out of sight, out of mind:** What you aren't willing to go without, make sure to keep out of sight. It might sound drastic, but visual reminders of food we want will always get us in trouble.

■ **Offer an award system:** Don't misconstrue this with bribery. It's not *quite* the same. You are rewarding your child for doing something incredibly difficult, and if you have taken our advice and given up something you love, you know it's *really* tough.

> *We took our warriors to the toy or dollar store every week for the first month. I literally tried to keep the kids out of the house and away from food or the kitchen until the diet became a habit. After six months we went to one big party, celebration, shopping trip, etc. per year.—April R.*

■ **Get the family involved:** For some reason, a compliment seems more significant when it comes from someone other than Mom or Dad. This mom had a great idea on how to empower her warrior with the help from family:

> *Another thing we did during the first few months was have family members send her cards/notes in the mail about how important it was to be on this diet and how strong she was during this hard time. Each person found a different way to encourage her...and this was just the cost of a stamp and a little time.—April R.*

■ **Be a little sneaky yourself:** This dad is pretty clever. Here's how he combatted his child's desire to cheat:

> *I build in cheats. It's the whole reverse psychology thing. I make cookies for her that she can only have on "special occasions." But I actually work them into her diet for the day. This way I can use them as a reward or if she needs a pick-me-up. Now after two years on the diet, she doesn't really have the need to cheat.—Phil*

■ **When all else fails, lock up the food:** When your tactics aren't working and you're desperate for the diet to work despite your warrior's numerous efforts to sabotage it, go to the baby supply store and get some childproofing gadgets. Try the Tot Lok by Safety 1st. It's a magnetic locking system that requires a special key. The best part is that if your child's cheating improves, you can keep the Tot Loks on your cabinets but don't use the key to activate them; if your warrior begins to cheat again, and if conversation and negotiation don't work, all you need is the magnetic key to get the cheating-proof system up and running again.

The Fun Factor

These are just a few ideas to keep the fun rolling. Look through magazines, books, and ask teachers and friends to help you come up with additional ideas. If you implement at least a few of these, your ketogenic journey will be far less bumpy.

- **Reuse familiar containers:** Applesauce containers (even the squeeze ones), yogurt containers, small ice cream cartons, Lunchables boxes—anything you can clean out well and replace the contents with a Keto version. This allows children to feel less "different," especially when around their peers.

- **Be creative with presentation:** We've mentioned fun plates, cups, silverware, and straws. Feel free to think beyond the children's aisle at the store. One mom found bud vases and serves her daughter's cream in them (perfect for small amounts). Try wine or champagne glasses for sparkling cream drinks. A drop of natural food coloring here or there always brightens up a meal.

- **Pack a small toy in a meal:** Check out a local dollar store and see what little tokens or toys you can add to the occasional bagged lunch. Pulling a surprise out of a bag will put a smile on your warrior's face.

- **Add a dip:** This one is simple enough, and with these diets, the dip is often another way to hide fat, whether you're making a mayo-based dip or adding oil to low-carb ketchup.

    Adding a dip is always a huge hit in our house, simple but I limit it to only occasional usage, so when we hit a rough patch with not wanting to eat, I pull out the dip.—Dawn

- **Call food by silly names:** Kids love to laugh, so be silly and have a little fun. Make an avocado smoothie and call it "green slime"—anything that might elicit a laugh.

■ **Play around with appliances:** While we don't recommend you fill your kitchen with superfluous machines, a kitchen gadget here or there can make a big difference. Try out ice shavers; snow cone makers; waffle makers; pizzelle makers; or mini pie, cake, or doughnut machines.

■ **Take the meal out of the kitchen:** This advice is sprinkled throughout the book, and that's because it can work with any age group. Take the meal out of the kitchen and you have an adventure, whether at home, outside, or in a restaurant.

Eat somewhere other than home, like the park with the promise to play after the meal...make a fort in your house and have an in-door picnic with your kids during the winter. —Dawn

We go out to eat a few times a month. Abbie loves it! She sometimes orders the appetizer she would want for us all to eat, or she gets to pick the dessert for us. We bring everything she needs with us to eat and we have never had anyone question us. Restaurants go out of their way to make her feel special and normal. —Heather

■ **Plan a themed meal:** Base food off of themes from favorite books or TV shows. Have a tea party and dress up. Get your warrior in on the meal planning.

In a Warrior's Words: Oliver, Ketogenic Diet, Six Years Old

Oliver is six years and ten months old and lives in Israel. He has absence seizures, drop seizures, and many varied seizures (arms up to the sides, head drops, jaw drops, night seizures). He started the diet at the age of five, exactly one year after diagnosed with epilepsy and after failing eight anti-convulsants. Below are the questions *Fighting Back with Fat* asked him, as translated by his mother from Hebrew to English. The text in the parentheses following Oliver's answers is his mom's further explanations of his answers.

Q: What was it like starting the Ketogenic diet?
A: I had seizures and I was "confused." ("Confused" was our code word for seizures before we called them seizures!)

Q: What emotions and fears did you have?
A: I was "confused" but my pooh-bear looked after me. (Pooh came with us EVERYWHERE, every hospital visit, etc.)

Q: What do you think of the foods you get to eat on the Ketogenic diet? Do you have a favorite food?

A: I feel good with my food. I have three: bacon omelet, tuna salad, and focaccia.

Q: Do you sometimes find it hard to be on your magic diet?

A: NEVER EVER—I'll never give up on the diet. Mom makes me food and I feel better.

Q: How have your parents helped make this diet easier on you?

A: They make me food and let me play on the computer by myself!

Q: What's the hardest thing about being on the diet?

A: Nothing bothers me (!)

Q: What is it like being on this diet and being in school with other children who aren't on this diet?

A: Half/half—happy and sometimes sad. Happy because I have lots of friends to play with at Kinder and sad cause I'm hungry.

Q: What do your friends think about your magic diet?

A: We don't talk about it, but I think they think that the diet is special and that it's dietetic and that I have a doctor whom I visit.

Q: What would you say to a child who is supposed to start the diet?

A: "Hi, how are you? You ok?"

Q: If you could offer advice to a child starting out on this diet, what would you tell him?

A: I would tell him it's worthwhile for him to start the diet, because the diet is a GOOD thing—they give you food and you can ask your mom and dad if you can watch TV while you eat and NOBODY bothers you!

Q: What's the most important thing about the diet?

A: It makes seizures stop and the diet helps me.

Q: What is the best thing about the diet?

A: It makes me feel good and not "confused" and I get to watch TV.

In a Warrior's Words: Abbie, Ketogenic Diet, 10 Years Old

It's okay to have epilepsy. It just makes you different and special because nobody else has epilepsy in my family or classroom. Just me, and that makes me awesome. Some of the stuff I get to do is cool and if I didn't even have epilepsy it never would have even happened. I got to go in a helicopter because of epilepsy and go to Johns Hopkins and meet famous doctors, like Dr. Kossoff. I got to play all kinds of games in the helicopter and in the hospital. Also, I got an IV. It was so interesting to watch them put it in my arm. And guess what? It didn't even bother me. It was just fascinating to see them do that. I am used to needles now, and because of my diet I get my blood tested every couple of months and have to have nine tubes filed. At the hospital they taught me how to swallow pills. I now swallow up to 13 pills a day. Some of them are really big ones!

When I am going to have a seizure it feels like I get all tingly or like it's just a feeling I have that it is coming. I don't know how to explain it. I just lay down on my side and wait, sometimes I don't move but I can feel the seizure in my head and other times—look out—because I am going to get crazy wild. My hands, legs, and arms all shake and move. It just makes me so mad about having a seizure because I can't make it stop. Not even my Mom or Dad can make it stop.

Medicines didn't work for me so now I am on a special diet, called the Ketogenic diet. I have to eat and drink a lot of fat, heavy cream, and meats. My Mom and Dad have to weigh and measure my food so it will stop my seizures. I am not allowed to have any sugar! That is the worst! I really miss eating C-A-N-D-Y and J-U-N-K-F-O-O-D! But I can eat all the salt I want...so that is good. I have a secret box where I am keeping things that I am not allowed to eat right now, but when I am off my diet, look out! I am going to eat all the Halloween candy, Easter candy, and the IOU's from birthday cakes and pies in the last two years. I can't use some arts and craft stuff and have to wear purple gloves so my skin doesn't touch the chemicals or ingredients in the glue and paint and other stuff. It's not as hard as it was when I first started.

Here are ten things I worry about now because I have epilepsy:

1. *When I get nervous about staying at someone's house because I might have a seizure. I have never had a sleepover at someone's house.*

2. *I hope my seizures go away because I really want to drive a car when I am older.*

3. *I really don't like it when I have a seizure in school. It makes my friends worry about me and I just want them to think I am just like them.*

4. *I am scared to grow up and go to college because what if I have a seizure in college!*

5. *If I get nervous about school or a test sometimes it makes me have more seizures.*

6. *I can go swimming, but someone has to be right next to me or really close because I don't want to have a seizure in the pool and drown.*

7. *Someone always has to be with me! Even to walk me to the bathroom at school. It makes me feel like a baby not a 4th grader!*

8. *I have to have a baby monitor so my mom and dad or Miss Ashlie can see me in case I have a seizure at night. A monitor for a baby…I am not a baby!*

9. *What if my friends don't like me anymore because I have epilepsy? It looks scary when I have a seizure. I don't want them to be afraid of me.*

10. *What if some people think I am weird because I have seizures? I can't help it or make it stop and I really, really want to!*

Teen Warriors

Getting Everyone on the Same Page

Navigating these diets with a teen is a very different story than attempting them with a young child. With little ones you pretty much call all the shots, but with a teenager securing their cooperation is essential. A lot of change happens over the teen years, from 13 to 19, so the advice on these pages is not necessarily one-size-fits-all. The goal is the same, however, at any age: motivate your teen to stick with the therapy. Reminding a teen of all they stand to gain is an important part of the strategy. Chris, mom to Liam, shares her opinion:

> *I think this is critical that the teen/tween is involved and understands why they are on the diet! They want some control and involvement, and I believe this helps tremendously. The*

problems come when they want too much control and that's when I have to remind my son why we are on the diet and what we hope it does for him! This diet is hopefully going to reduce/eliminate seizures so that he can go to his friend's house more often, play sports, go to movies, swim, dances, etc. These seizures keep him from being able to do many of these things on a regular basis because of his fear of having a seizure. So it's a lot of conversations especially when I see him get frustrated with it.

The teen years are all about a young person's struggle to take control of his own life and establish independence. Like a building when it's first going up, small children need strong scaffolding, your parental nurturing and control, to support them initially. As they develop, they become more and more capable of standing on their own. During the teenage years much of the parental scaffolding is incrementally removed, and it can be a nerve-wracking time as parents adjust to this new role and the seeming loss of control they have over their child. The anxiety factor tends to double when your child's seizure control is at stake. You may fear she will make unwise decisions that could seriously affect her health.

One of the best tactics we can advise if your teen balks, threatens to quit diet therapy, or you discover he is cheating, is to remind him (and yourself) that, "The decision to do this diet is entirely up to you. You can continue having seizures or you can take control of your epilepsy." Gently explain that you'll be there to support him and encourage him, but the actual choice belongs to him. Most kids will opt to stay on the diet, but feeling forced to do so can actually encourage rebellion and cheating. Emotional blackmail and high-pressure tactics tend to backfire and usually make a teenager more resistant than ever.

Try to take into account all your teen is going through. Dealing with epilepsy in adolescence can be exhausting emotionally as well as physically. Besides the stress of seizures and side effects of medication, now your teen must also learn to take control of his eating, be constantly on guard against temptation and slip-ups, and risk being different from everyone else because of what he eats. It's no wonder some kids get frustrated and want to toss the diet and all it entails out the window. If they already feel their life is spinning out of control, the diet can seem overwhelming, and at some point they may want to quit.

So what can you do? Here are a few tips to help you offer the support your teen needs.

■ **Don't minimize her struggle:** Diet therapy is just plain hard at times, no way around it. Acknowledge how tough it is and how proud you are that she's been willing to give it a shot. Encouragement is important.

■ **Listen to his frustrations:** You have two ears and one mouth, so listen twice as much as you talk. You may not have an answer to all his troubles, but keep in mind that he may not even be seeking an answer in the first place. Sometimes all a teen really wants is to be heard.

■ **Let her know that you will be there for her; she doesn't have to do this alone:** Children of all ages look to the adults in their lives for cues about how to handle stress and problems. Let your teen know you care, and that together you're going to make it through this rough time.

■ **If your teen wants to quit, ask him to give it a week** (or a month if you can get them to agree) so they can seriously think it over instead of making a snap decision. It may only seem intolerable because he's having a bad day or week. Remind him that these diets usually take three to six months in order to see what they can truly do.

■ **Respect her choice to quit:** You can let your teen know that you don't agree with her decision, but if she truly insists on stopping, in most cases you'll have to let her make the call. If a major loss of seizure control results, hopefully your teen will realize the diet was helping more than she realized. Your teen may be willing to start the diet again at a later time if she realizes it actually was making a significant difference in seizure control.

■ If your child is struggling with his feelings while on diet therapy, consider arranging for him to talk to a counselor or therapist. Having someone outside the immediate family to talk to can sometimes help enormously.

Fitting in

Nothing is more loathsome to a teenager than being different, so finding ways to help your child fit in is helpful. Here are a few tips to give you an idea of your role in helping your teen continue to be part of the crowd.

■ **Make the food look "normal":** Creating diet-friendly foods like chicken nuggets, pizza, muffins, or even cheese crackers with peanut butter or cheese will help your warrior during mealtimes around his peers.

■ **Shift the focus away from food:** Find other activities and healthy distractions during public events, parties, get-togethers and sporting events.

■ **Encourage your teen to eat around friends who "get it":** This might be easier said than done, but chances are your warrior knows which of his peers will likely understand the limitations of his diet and which friends might criticize the diet. Surrounding himself with understanding peers, at least during meal times, can take away some of the pressure.

Owning the Diet

Empowerment is the key to owning the diet and making it work. Here are some ideas that may help your teen make the diet part of his life:

■ **Tap into the power of choice:** Having choices helps us feel in control of our lives, so let your teen make as many choices as possible when it comes to food. Sometimes just choosing what's packed in a lunch can be an inspiration boost. Get your teen involved in planning the menus and he'll be more likely to stay on course.

> *I offer a choice of two or three meal options and HE chooses (feeling empowered helps him). I learned this the hard way when he just did not like what I offered and as we all know he needed to finish it. It was painful and we fought the entire time. So now he chooses!! —Chris*

■ **Make food fun:** Food is a really fun part of life, and there are lots of teen favorites you and your child can learn to make so nobody misses out. Your warrior will no doubt tell you all the foods he's craving, and while you can't tackle some of those desires, you can come up with some delicious alternatives. If he's craving the classic all-American meal, ask, "Do you want fries with that?" (Turnip fries!) They go along great with a cheeseburger (hold the bun), or a Keto-friendly pizza and shake made with heavy whipping cream. Your options are only as limited as your imagination.

> *Once, when my son was eating lunch with some of his teen friends in the school dining room, he was digging into his MAD meal of fried chicken and cheese breadsticks, and his friends were eyeing their own school lunch. They all started complaining, "Hey! How come you get the good food and we have to eat this!" My son grinned and said, "Well, too bad. You only get this*

*good stuff if you have epilepsy." With that, one by one, each of
his friends at the table slumped to the floor. Then they popped
their heads up and asked, "Now can we have some?" My son
still laughs about it.* —Jeanne Riether

Keto carrot-on-a-stick: All of us love rewards, especially the proverbial carrot-on-a-stick types that are close enough in sight that we're motivated to keep trotting along in pursuit. Keep rewards frequent and fun. A
reward doesn't have to be food centered. It can be something as simple as
a funny card, or as elaborate as a weekend away together as a family. The
important thing is that you recognize your wins together and do what you
can to make your warrior feel special. Here are a few reward ideas:

- **Have friends over for a fun celebration.** Your warrior and her friends
  can just hang out and watch movies, or if she's up for it, you could do
  what one parent does and throw a Friday night pizza party.

- **Offer small incentives:** You know your child best, and you can gage by
  her personality and interests what small tokens you can present as a way
  to encourage her. Notes and cards, a bottle of nail polish, an iTunes gift
  card, a new book, or a monetary award system. The incentives don't have
  to be items than can be bought, but they should be valuable to your teen.

- **Make a day of it:** Let your teen pick a place he'd like to go for a day with
  you or the whole family. It could be something as low-key as hanging out
  playing ball at a local park or you could go all out and do an amusement park
  (of course you'll have to pack some great Keto-friendly snacks for the day).

*There are times he needs fun so the way I can make it fun is to
take the focus off the food and make other things fun! Like going
to a "fun" restaurant where the food isn't the focus. He eats his
food that I bring with no complaints.* —Chris

Personal Hygiene

Tackling the issue of personal hygiene (especially for the boys) can be a
challenge for every parent of a teen, but sometimes there can be a few
extra concerns when your child is on the diet. Here are a few ideas:

- **Keto breath control:** If your teen is concerned about the strong breath
  that heralds ketosis, a few drops of peppermint oil on the tongue can
  help. (Check with your dietitian, of course.)

- **Oily skin and hair:** A high-fat diet coupled with puberty might mean more frequent bathing is in order. Encourage your warrior to hit the showers regularly and remember to use personal care products approved for the diet, such as those listed on the Charlie Foundation website.

- **Creative solutions:** Anyone who's ever parented a teen girl knows the importance of the make-up right-of-passage and shopping for just the right shade of lip color. One teen girl was heartbroken when she realized the sorbitol in her lipstick was causing problems with seizure control. Her very creative mom came to the rescue by experimenting with berry juice and Vaseline. She produced some sensational and original lip-gloss and packaged it in cute little containers. It was such a hit that all her daughter's friends wanted some as well.

Keep Your Eye on the Goal

Young people tend to live for the moment. Doing something difficult today in order to reap the benefit of future rewards does not come easy for most, which is why hearing inspiring stories of success from those who stuck with these diets is such a strong motivational factor. Before our teen warriors share their personal stories, here is an inspiring story about Lindsey, a teen whose life was turned around when she started MAD nearly five years ago. If you're wondering why the story below is written by Lindsey's mom, rather than Lindsey herself—like the other stories in this section— it's because she is a very busy lady, preparing for her upcoming wedding!

> *Lindsey has been battling seizures since she was about 10. She is now almost 23. At the age of 11 she had her first tonic clonic seizure. We tried one med after another and at the age of 13 she completely fell apart due to meds and 1,000's of absence seizures per day. She was almost catatonic and had no life. We continued this way with some occasional good days, but mostly she was missing in action. We had lost our precious daughter.*

> *I begged for dietary therapy. I was told numerous times, "No, it would be too difficult..." We continued to watch her slip away. She had very few friends and was a prisoner in her own body. She could not write or process information, so she was unable to learn or do schoolwork. I tried to keep her busy by listening to Mozart, crocheting, beading, folding laundry—anything to keep her mind from wasting away.*

When she was 18 her seizures began to morph again and she started having focal seizures that lasted for hours. I watched the movie, "First Do No Harm" and became a warrior mom. I collected all my information about MAD in a three ring binder and we went to see Lindsey's neurologist. The first thing her doctor wanted to do was put her on Keppra, the only drug she had not tried at this point. I began my appeal for MAD. I began to cry and beg the doctor to let us do the study that Dr. Kossoff at Johns Hopkins had offered. She agreed to let us do the study and said, "As a neurologist I cannot recommend this diet, but as a mom, I see your need to try it."

In August of 2007 we began MAD. Immediately, Lindsey began to have more clarity and ability to speak. She began to play the piano again. Within two weeks, Lindsey was 85% seizure free. We kept tweaking, purifying the diet, and continuing on. We had good times and then some difficult times as we continued to try and adapt things for her body. Right now, she is on reasonable doses of Zarontin and Zonegran as well as MAD at about 65 to 70 grams of low glycemic carbs per day. I am not happy about the meds, but I am thankful we have them if she needs them. We tried to wean a couple of times and things did not go well for us. So, even though she is not med free, the diet has been an amazing miracle for us.

Lindsey's brave spirit and willingness to work on her own health has been amazing to watch. She is my hero!!! —Dorene

In a Warrior's Words: Liam, Ketogenic Diet, 13 Years Old

Starting the Ketogenic diet was terrible. The food was bad and it gave me stomachaches. I always felt sick to my stomach but it got better after a couple weeks. In the beginning I worried about how long I had to be on the diet and if I was going to ever have food I liked again. It got better once my mom found more meals that I liked. I also was hungry at first but not anymore. The food actually fills me up. I don't miss the normal food as much anymore. My mom says I was a picky eater and didn't like to eat much of anything anyway. At dinner I look at what my sisters are eating and am often glad I don't have to eat what they do.

Now I think the food is good, and I don't mind it anymore because I ask my mom to only make the things I like. I even don't mind drinking the cream and oil since my mom flavors it. Sometimes I get sick of certain things and we have to find new ones. She also gives me a couple choices so I pick what I have a taste for.

I don't cheat because I know that if I cheat the seizures will come back. That keeps me from wanting to cheat.

The hardest thing about being on the diet is that I don't get to eat whatever I want whenever I want!!! That's it! I miss pasta, donuts, and chips the most. I also miss Subway. It was my favorite. Best part of the diet is the rewards that I get for being on the diet. It makes it a little easier knowing I get special things my sisters don't. I also get to come home for lunch and eat with my mom.

If another kid were starting the diet and I could give them some advice, I'd say: If you try the diet it just might take some seizures away. It has taken away many of mine and made them shorter too. So give it a try and just remember it's just food.

In a Warrior's Words: Jordan, MAD, 15 Years Old

When I was 12 years old, I had my first noticeable seizure, a drop seizure. I didn't know what it was, and neither did my parents, teachers, or doctors. Over the following period of nine months I had several different types of seizures including drop seizures and tonic-clonics. Then we heard about the Modified Atkins Diet.

At first, it sounded crazy. Somehow, meals consisting of high fat, low glycemic foods, and extremely low carbohydrates were supposed to stop my seizures. To top it off, I was used to a diet of low fat, medium protein levels and fairly high carbohydrates, so starting MAD was a big and frustrating adjustment. At one early point in the diet, I actually considered secretly going off it, but I soon decided against that option, realizing that cheating would only ruin my already fragile health.

For the first two weeks of the diet it was hard. Maybe it was carbohydrate withdrawal, maybe it was that I wasn't used to the food. But once I got used to it, I realized pretty much that eating that food was better than having seizures. Having a life with seizures is a lot worse than a life without bread or noodles. My life became better after I started the diet.

Once I adjusted to it, the diet just became routine. I would have little twinges of nostalgia about certain foods but it wasn't a big deal.

Mom discovered and invented dozens of low-carb recipes for foods such as cheesecake, bread, pizza, fried rice (believe it or not, we used cauliflower as a substitute for rice!), cookies, hot chocolate, milkshakes, soda, and tons of other dishes and beverages. My personal favorite was a special pudding-like dish made from blueberries, whipping cream, cream cheese, and Stevia.

I had a normal life, but I would not have been able to lead the same kind of life if I hadn't gone on the diet. I would say that going from a wheelchair to being a fencer is a pretty big change. Becoming a fencer was not an overnight change and it took me about a year before I could start fencing, even though my seizures stopped right away after going on the diet.

Truth be told, I was overjoyed when I heard I could get off MAD. After two years of having a pleasant, but strictly controlled diet, who wouldn't want to eat normal food again? But, although the diet may seem to be frustrating at first, if you have a chance to gain control of your seizures it's a chance worth taking. So I say, "suck it up, buttercup" and try it. It may just work.

In a Warrior's Words: Jenn, MAD, 19 Years Old

I've had Juvenile Myoclonic Epilepsy since age 13 and was diagnosed around 17. I've had basically every type of seizure out there. I started MAD for epilepsy when I was 16. I heard about it from my mother and was expecting having to give up everything from food to makeup and hygiene products in case they had sugars in them. Luckily the diet wasn't as strict as I was scared of, which helped it seem a lot more manageable. Anything to help control my seizures was an option—at that point it was our only hope left.

I started at the end of my sophomore year in high school as the oldest person to ever attempt MAD. Besides me the oldest patient was a seven-year-old, quite a difference in age, but through self-control I was able to become more successful than ever imagined.

I started on 10 carbs a day for three months. Before I started I had a major sweet tooth and had been weaning myself off of it until the day I started the diet, rather than going into a sugar coma. I gained 15 pounds from the meds I was on, which also benefited from Atkins by losing the excess weight I was unable to lose before. I ate the same meals for the most part, eggs and bacon for breakfast, bacon cheeseburger pre-packed for me to bring to lunch, with a high-fat dinner when I came home. With time we found and made more and more recipes from home-made no-carb high-fat ice cream to quesadillas. Life is what you make of it, and the diet proves that mantra true every day.

Most people I went to school with knew about my seizures because of their severity, and they were all supportive when I started my diet. They were shocked when they gradually saw my seizures become less and less frequent.

Whenever I think about cheating on my diet I look back to videos I recorded when I have my seizures and remember that I never want to go back to having seizures for 12 hours a day three times a week, knowing that eating can control that, I don't have the urge to cheat. I have more dreams for myself than letting epilepsy consume me.

The best way I explain my diet to other people is it is similar to diabetes. When I control my sugars and fats I am stable, when I don't I'm not and go back to twitching and seizing. You realize that as humans we eat to live, not live to eat as many people have it lodged in their brains.

My parents are always looking for new recipes and ways to add the foods I enjoy into my diet. We were slowly able to add more carbs and lower my medicine. We have even held MAD friendly parties for my birthday parties. We serve diet sodas, pizza, a vegetable platter, popcorn, and other snacks. Without realizing it, my friends were also on MAD for a day or so when they would eat at my house.

It can feel isolating at times but you have to know that everyone has challenges to face in life. As people with epilepsy we don't have many options in our treatment plan besides medication or surgery. I was not a candidate for surgery and medications didn't work. I would choose to change my eating habits any day over having one more seizure than I have to.

Now I'm almost 20 years old, on the amount of medication a six-year-old is started on, able to attend college, and only have seizures once every few months. It's not a cure...but I have taken back control of my life.

Adults

Most online forums and support groups are geared for parents of children with epilepsy (though they usually welcome adults as well), but being in the minority can feel isolating and lonely. Adults may be reluctant to ask for support, or feel they should be able to figure things out entirely on their own, but if that were the case this book would cease to exist. We can all benefit from the help and support of others, and as more adults pursue diet therapy, the need for connection, encouragement, advice, and confidence-boosting support is also increasing. While we haven't been in your boots before, we have fought a similar battle, and we hope the tips in this section will answer some of your questions and concerns, and the stories from our prolific adult contributors will fill in the rest.

Attitude Is Everything

Most adults starting diet therapy have seen a lot of action in this war, and after failing a number of medications you may be reluctant to risk being disappointed once again. While it's important to have realistic expectations when starting out, it's equally important to keep hopes high and give the diet your best shot. Having the right attitude when starting is essential, otherwise it's far too easy to quit when the going gets rough. Give the diet time to work and pace yourself; in the process you'll learn the art of patience—and maybe even happen upon a miracle.

Explaining the Diet—to Everyone

A challenge that never seems to quite disappear is the need to educate other people, everyone from family to co-workers, and even the guy at the grocery store who remarks on how much coconut oil you're buying. Wherever you go, people will be baffled by your diet, especially because it goes against every modern concept of healthy. Count on a good laugh—silent, perhaps— when you say to a co-worker, "I'm on a diet" and then smother your lunch with oil and butter, or you dive into a heaping pile of egg salad. Her utterly dumbfounded expression could keep you chuckling for at least a day. Once you stop laughing, consider thinking of this never-ending food education class as a positive step in accepting your diet. With a little practice, you'll have your own mantra down, a practiced speech that you give to everyone who asks about your diet. Usually by the time you have this little speech down pat, you're well on your way to adjusting to a diet full of fat.

Wartime Rationing

Everyone loves life's little pleasures, and sometimes it can hurt to give them up. If you're tempted to indulge in some dietary no-no's however, a good point to remember is that by trading in something good that you enjoy, you stand to gain something better that you want: seizure control! Be prepared for some "wartime rationing" of some common adult pleasures:

- **Alcohol:** Chances are you've already given this up, or perhaps you never had the chance to indulge due to a seizure history, but this will definitely be off the table now.

- **Coffee:** Some people can handle coffee fine, with or without caffeine, but unfortunately others can't. However, for Heidi, one of our adult contributors, her switch from caffeinated coffee to decaffeinated coffee actually increased her seizures dramatically:

> *I absolutely love coffee and could drink it all day. When I started I didn't believe that caffeine was an issue so didn't cut back on the coffee. My seizures were drastically reduced within a couple of months. After I suffered from a severe concussion during a seizure my neurologist wanted my caffeine intake stopped, so I switched to decaf coffee. I discovered that during those four months my seizures actually got worse. I am probably sensitive to something used to decaffeinate the coffee. Switching back to regular slowed my seizures down again.*

While you might have no negative reaction to caffeine, keep in mind that you might need to alter your coffee habits once on the diet.

■ **Soda:** Soda, like coffee, is loaded with caffeine, and unless you're drinking zero calorie soda (which is full of questionable ingredients), soda is
loaded with sugar. Our advice is that you eliminate all zero-calorie soda
in the beginning, at least until you have improved seizure control, then
you can decide whether or not to add it back in. (Remember: the less
ingredients to track, the less sleuthing you will have to do.) Try carbon-
ated water with a splash of lemon juice, and perhaps some Stevia sweetener, for an additive free alternative.

■ **Fast food:** While there are some items you can get at a fast food chain
(see our suggestions in Chapter 6), for the most part quick, high-carb
food will be a distant memory. With a little planning, however, you can
make delicious, MAD-healthy foods that travel easy, for those moments
when you previously would have headed to the drive-through.

Restaurants

Eating out in restaurants is easier if you have a plan to fall back on. Here
are a few tips to help your restaurant-going less stressful:

■ **Know before you go:** Eating out is easier if you know what your choices
are before you arrive. Take a little time to know where you're going and
what your potential meal options are. There will be some restaurants
that are diet-friendly, and others where ordering a low-carb meal will be
tough. Go online, read the menu, and learn whether or not you should
bring your own meal or snacks with you.

■ **Question everything:** Restaurant food can be challenging for diet warriors, as the only thing more abundant than hidden carbs is salt. When
possible, stick to the simplest menu items, asking for no sauce or seasoning. Salad dressings, gravies, sauces, and even low-carb-sounding options
such as pecan-crusted tilapia could use white flour or sugar in them.

*I have discovered that a lot of the waiters do not know what
is actually in the food. So they have to make trips back to the
kitchen to find out for you. You have a right to know this information but it does annoy them sometimes. I encourage you to
ask what is in the food because burgers will have seasoning (and
sometimes even bread crumbs) added that have carbs, steaks
and chicken breasts will be marinated in things that have carbs.*

*One of my favorite menu items to order at a restaurant is a plain
chicken breast or steak but then order some sautéed mushrooms*

to go with it and a side salad with bleu cheese dressing. If it's a place that serves breakfast 24 hours a day I will order a mushroom and cheese omelet and a side of butter. —Heidi

Out and About: Handling Social Gatherings

By all means, your social life shouldn't halt when you stop eating high-carb foods. This diet is meant to enhance your life, not limit it, so don't be afraid to participate in get-togethers with family and friends while on the diet. Here are a few tips to help you confidently navigate social occasions:

- **Shift the focus away from food:** Whether you are hosting a party or attending as a guest, remember that people are the real focus of the party, and the food is not really what it's all about.

- **Eat before you go out:** It's hard for anyone to stick to a diet if you are hungry and can't eat anything that's being served. Eating beforehand will ensure you don't arrive ravenously hungry only to discover that the diet-friendly pickings are slim.

- **Practice the art of making conversation:** If you are stuck at a function where everyone but you is eating, try to focus your attention on interesting conversation with the other guests. You might just become the life of the party, thanks to your new diet.

I have discovered that by walking around with a glass of water in my hand and talking to people it really opens you up to meeting more people and learning more about people, than when you are so focused on snacking. —Heidi

In a Warrior's Words: Heidi, Modified Atkins Diet, 32 Years Old

I have Juvenile Myoclonic Epilepsy. I have tonic clonic, myoclonic, and absence seizures. I started the diet in October of 2010 when I was 30.

When I first started the diet I had some cravings, as my body was looking for all the carbs it was used to having. It was a rough two weeks in the beginning. I spent a lot of time looking for different foods that I would love. And some time crying at night because I wanted something to snack on that tasted the same. In the beginning I was scared that the diet wouldn't work;

it was this or I did have Felbatol left to try but I don't like the listed side effects of that medication so I didn't want to try it.

I have an awesome support system. A friend came over and helped me clean out my cupboards and fridge when I started, and she helped me donate the food that I couldn't use at all. She then took me shopping to restock with only appropriate foods for the diet. It made starting so much easier. That friend also makes sure there are diet-appropriate foods at her house for me all the time so I always have food to eat when I'm there. All of my friends understand that when we go out to eat we have to go to certain places that offer types of food I can eat, and they are ok with it.

One of the biggest challenges is when people don't understand the diet. I've been accused of having an eating disorder, because people think I'm trying to lose weight using the Atkins Diet when I'm already skinny. They don't take the time to ask, they just assume.

The best thing about the diet is the seizure control that I have gained. For the most part I have had gained very good seizure control. I still have a tonic clonic every couple of weeks and some daily absence and myoclonic seizures, but they are so few compared to before that I celebrate the enormous progress that I have made.

In a Warrior's Words: Mike, Ketogenic/MAD, 46 Years Old

My story starts when I was 34 and running Fitness Services at a UK university, when I had my first seizure. I cannot recall anything. Doctors subsequently told me that I'd had a tonic-clonic seizure. They sent me away with anticonvulsants to prevent a recurrence. I had more seizures and then went for an MRI and an EEG, which identified a "lesion immediately deep to the rhinal sulcus in the vicinity of the left uncus" and was told this meant I had left temporal lobe epilepsy and that it would never go away.

Over the following eight years I was prescribed different anti-convulsants. I experienced increasing memory, endocrine, immune, and digestive problems. This included food intoler-ances to dairy, wheat, sugar, yeast, red meat, soy, citrus, and nightshade vegetables (potatoes, tomatoes). I had developed chronic fatigue syndrome and insomnia. Epileptic seizures continued—they were unpredictable and severe. I could no longer work. My parents needed to look after me. It was abysmal.

My consultant told me that if I reduced the amount of anticonvulsants I was taking, the effect would be fatal. They told me that they'd no longer treat me if didn't follow their instructions. I honestly believed that I was slowly dying anyway. I wanted to say goodbye to family and friends in a lucid manner. So I chose to die: I stopped taking anticonvulsants and medical appointments stopped. I believed that I was facing the end.

Thanks to the Internet, I had conversations with a bodybuilder that I knew only as "Dom" who lived in Florida. I discovered later that Dom was actually an eminent neuroscientist, investigating metabolic and nutritional therapies for neurodegenerative diseases. He suggested that I try the Ketogenic diet—which he knew had been used with success for children—to assist my situation. Dom was aware that adult bodybuilders safely use ketogenic diets when preparing for competitions. Hence, Dom and I worked with a UK bodybuilder called Adam to adapt Adam's competition diet in a manner that could support not only my food intolerances but also continue indefinitely to maintain a ketogeic metabolism. That way, we argued, I wouldn't need anticonvulsants to stay alive! So with their help, I devised a hybrid diet, which I started on July 15th, 2008. I have not stopped since. It has involved not eating more than 20 grams of total carbohydrates on a daily basis. I've also weight trained regularly.

The first result that I recognized was that my seizures decreased: after starting the diet, I didn't have any tonic-clonic seizures for nearly three months. My quality of life rocketed: my short and long-term memory improved, my sensation of appetite and thirst returned (these had disappeared while taking anticonvulsants), regular sleep returned, and I began to dream again.

I've recorded every gram of every ingredient I've eaten during this time. It all gets analyzed in spreadsheets daily. I also have regular blood tests that record cholesterol and ketone levels. My body gradually adapted to certain elements of the diet, and best of all, mental clarity and lucidity returned. On the rare occasions that I do have a seizure, I find that they are not as intense and recovery is quicker than when I used anticonvulsants.

I handled starting the diet in pretty much the same way people approach giving up smoking: I saw it as giving up carbs. The day I started, I threw out any food that contained carbs—the whole lot—because I knew I'd sneak in trips to the fridge to snack if I didn't.

It is a very isolating experience. Eating is social—it's one of the main times when we connect and share with others around us. We naturally eat in groups—sharing food around tables. Controlling seizures through very strict eating does not fit in with this approach. In the past I'd experienced full seizures when eating out, so when I started the diet I initially didn't feel left out when not invited. As the diet's benefits escalated I occasionally attempt eating out...It works out easiest if I prepare food in advance and bring it with me.

Thanks to suggestions from bodybuilders, I've learned to prepare food in advance and put it into airtight containers. I take them with me, whenever I'm away from home. If I'm away from home overnight, I keep a small set of digital scales and a writing pad on me at all times.

In a Warrior's Words: Wanda, Modified Atkins Diet, 43 Years Old

I was diagnosed with a seizure disorder at age 20 following a grand mal seizure while driving. My first seizure resulted in a wreck causing a broken jaw and totaled car! This was followed by 16 years of living a life full of seizures. Most of my seizures were focal seizures, which resulted in me blacking out. I had a demand pacemaker put in when I was 21 years old. I had several generalized tonic clonic seizures through the years in addition to the absence seizures. A neurologist in my hometown, Roanoke, Virginia, diagnosed me. I still have contact with him periodically to keep him updated. He tried me on many medications and combinations of medications, to include Phenobarbitol, Tegretol, Depakote, Mycoline, Neurontin, Dilantin, Topomax, and Lamictal. These medications trials continued until I reached age 31. I was very fortunate to have a baby girl when I was 29 years old. My daughter was born healthy and has no delays whatsoever. (She is currently 14 years old.) When she reached age two, I was tired of not being able to safely drive her places and have the independence of going wherever whenever I wanted to go.

I decided to pursue other options by going to a doctor at University of Virginia (UVA) to be evaluated for surgery. I spent two weeks in the hospital under continuous EEG monitoring and was taken off some of my medications. The doctors found the spot on my left temporal lobe that the seizures were stemming from in my brain. They presented me with the opportunity for a partial temporal lobectomy to remove the part of my brain that was causing my seizures. I agreed and gave consent for the surgery. It worked for approximately six months and I almost had my driver's license back in hand! The seizures returned sending me back to the hospital for further testing. The doctors found that the seizure stem location had jumped during surgery causing the seizures to return. I was evaluated for a second surgery, which they performed a few months later. I had a second major brain surgery! This surgery stopped my seizures for a couple months. At this point, the doctors added more medications and told me there were no other options.

Afterwards, I went home totally depressed and disgusted! I immediately started researching other options on the computer. I found the doctors at Johns Hopkins Hospital and e-mailed them immediately. They returned my e-mail and asked me to schedule an appointment. I met with a doctor a couple months later. He experimented with newer medications. These trials continued for approximately a year. At an appointment I asked, "Can it have something to do with what I eat?" He said, "Let me get a coworker to talk with you about diets." He brought in the wonderful Dr. Eric Kossoff. He explained the Modified Atkins that was being used on a trial basis for pediatric patients. I agreed to give it a shot! I decided that I would look at my plate like a steering wheel. He explained that I would be limited to 15 grams of carbohydrates a day and no sugar. I said, "Let's do it!!"

The adventure began in February 2005 when I was 36 years old. I have been seizure free since starting the diet. I am now 43 years old. All of the seizure medications and depression had caused me to gain weight through the years. At the time of starting the diet, I weighed 290 lbs!

In the first year [of the diet], I lost 100 pounds and continue to keep this weight off. I have never cheated on this diet through the past seven years. My carb intake has gone up to 20 to 25 grams of carbs a day.

My tastes have changed to the point that I rarely crave the foods that I had to stop eating. The toughest times are parties, family gatherings, and holidays. Everyone is eating all kinds of home-made foods FULL of carbohydrates!!

I reach out by going online to find new recipes. The Atkins for Epilepsy website has been great! I can e-mail with others who are on the diet. We share recipes and success stories to help other people start the diet.

This diet has made me believe that the expression "You are What You Eat" is very truthful.

In a Warrior's Words: Georgia, the Ketogenic Diet, 50 Years Old

At 49 I chose to try the Ketogenic diet because I am already coe-liac and read somewhere that many coeliacs also have problems with grains of all kinds, so I cut those out too. Simply by doing this I realized my seizures were reduced. By researching it even further, I discovered that by following a low-carb diet, this could help control seizures more. It was scary starting the diet, but I found my seizures were reduced even after only two weeks!

At first I was totally lost as to how to go about this diet, as my "carb brain" was telling me all that fat was wrong! I was also concerned that my doctor would not be happy about it and I wouldn't get the support I felt I needed. I was also scared I would have a heart attack from all the fat and I would get enor-mous! The opposite seemed to happen, which really surprised me. My first week was wonderful but then the "carb flu" kicked in and I felt dreadful for another week before it eased off. I had eaten low fat for so long that my body seemed to object to so much fat and made me feel quite sick. Thankfully, that did pass quite quickly and I now have no problems at all.

I have found great support while on the diet. I'm lucky that my doctor is surprisingly supportive even though he admits he knows nothing about ketogenic diets for seizure control. I have joined online Keto groups and forums that have been a wonderful support. However, one of the main obstacles has been that the majority of support is for children with epilepsy, not adults, so finding a Clinic in my own country that would support me has been a Godsend.

10
When You Want to Go AWOL

We have written countless pages in this book on how to overcome the obstacles you will no doubt encounter during your diet therapy adventure. We have been honest with you about the emotional landmines, the pressure you can potentially feel when healing power is now in your own hands, and we have provided you with time-saving tricks and advice on how to make this uphill march a little easier. We believe in the power of information, and we believe that while some of these chapters might be a challenge to read because of the enormity of information they present, we have given you a book that will accompany you through all the different stages of this fat-fisted war against epilepsy. This chapter is specifically meant to strengthen you when you're in the midst of this fight, when you might need reassurance, a confidence boost, or just a simple, "We get it. You're tired, and this is tough." For those of you who have been in the trenches and aren't finding the seizure control you want, or maybe you're just out of steam, or, wow, it's already been two years and it's time to talk weaning, this chapter is for you.

Feeling Defeated

There were times when I ran out of the house crying, my husband left with the kids and knowing all too well Mommy had reached her limit. I walked back into the woods once and just stood there for a solid 10 to 15 minutes surrounded by trees, and

*knowing that sooner or later I'd have to go back in and face my
son—and his temperamental eating habits.* —Erin Whitmer

Should we say it again? Or have we made it clear? These diets are tough.
You'll have moments when you'll vent to a friend or a neighbor about your
warrior refusing to eat and they'll likely say something like, "He'll eat when
he's hungry," or "It's just a phase." While the likelihood that it's just a phase
is high (especially if you're dealing with a toddler), we don't have the pre-
rogative to just wait until our kids get hungry. Ketosis suppresses the appetite so the longer your child goes without eating, the tougher it will be to
get back into an eating routine. Part of what makes these diets so challenging is the simple fact that the diet is our child's medication. The non-stop
essential nature of these diets increases the stress factor and, sure, at times
you'll just want to run into the woods and consider living with nature for a
while. After all, fighting an angry squirrel for a nut would probably feel like
a vacation after watching your child fill her cheeks with food and keep it
there for hours.

Regardless of where your stress originates from you will likely consider waving your own white flag at least once. We've all been there,
throwing our own adult tantrum when we just want to give up. What's
important to learn when you're dealing with a ketogenic diet is *if* and
when it's OK to quit. And equally important is learning how to find the
strength to keep going.

Stephanie, whose son is on the Medium Chain Triglyceride (MCT) diet,
had a tremendously tough time in the beginning:

*Cobey blamed me for putting him on the diet and he became
very angry and resentful towards me. I found his anger and
resentment to be harder on me than weighing and measuring
the required six meals a day. Thankfully, after a few months of
being seizure free on the diet, I was able to help Cobey understand that we had finally found something that worked and
reminded him of what it used to be like when he was having
seizures, and how we didn't want to go backwards! His anger
eventually softened and he began to trust that I only wanted him
to be happy and healthy, out of my deep and unconditional love
for him.*

We guarantee that Stephanie had days when she was full of hurt and
frustration over the diet, and perhaps she had moments when she wondered

whether the diet was worth the pain she was feeling and the resentment her son was displaying. Those moments were likely short-lived, however, as anyone who has a seizure free child on the diet seems to quickly snap back; after all, seizure freedom is a rare gift.

Feeling defeated can come at any point in your journey: in the beginning when you are hoping for seizure freedom but have to learn to adjust your expectations to seizure improvement; it can come when you were hoping to make adjustments to medications but side effects prevented that option; and there will be days when you will feel defeated just because you wish you had a more normal life—either for you or your child. You will have a day or two when you wish you could just toss a granola bar at your warrior and not worry about the consequences. But of course, this kind of desire is as useful as wishing you could rub a genie out of a lamp. When the tough threatens to get the better of you, we encourage you to reread Chapter 2, "Boot Camp," and the battle tactics you were taught.

■ **Target your dysfunctional attitudes:** Don't fall into the trap of mindsets that will encourage you to fail. Remember that you are strong. If you weren't, you wouldn't be on this tough road to begin with.

■ **Rely on your allied forces—your family and friends:** You've gathered the troops, given them marching orders, and allowed them to be a part of this journey. Be honest with them when you need a little additional help or comfort. They will likely feel honored to support you.

■ **Take care of yourself:** If you forget to put yourself first, you'll crash fast. Getting through the tough days takes stamina so don't forget to do the simple things: eat, drink plenty of water, get a good night's sleep, and whenever possible, take some time for yourself.

■ **Empower your warrior:** Sometimes you're feeling challenged because your warrior is having a tough time with some element of his diet. If that's the case, schedule some one-on-one time or a fun family outing to help lift his spirits. You'll be surprised how much easier it will be for you to trudge forward when you have a smiling companion to rough the terrain with.

While we can ensure that you will have tough days, we are also confident that by following the simple advice laid before you in Chapter 2, you will learn how to power through the mud instead of feeling like you're sinking in quicksand.

When You're Tempted to Quit: Battle Tip from a MAD Warrior

Diet therapy isn't easy and there will be times when you will want to go AWOL. What can you do when you feel you've had about all you can take? Here's a tip from Heidi, a battle-seasoned veteran:

Cry it out, laugh it out, beat a pillow, do whatever you have to get through it. On that third day when that greasy plate of food is staring up at you and your stomach is churning and you feel like you just can't do it anymore, know that you have a whole world of people who have been there before and done it and are cheering you on. I have walked where you have walked. I have cried the tears you have cried. It will have its ups and downs but it will get easier. You can make it through this journey.

Journaling for Strength

Journaling is a great outlet for the myriad raw emotions that come with dietary therapy and epilepsy in general. While we aren't all writers, we can all benefit from the clarity and perspective than can come with writing down our thoughts and visiting them later.

There have always been days here or there when I'm just sad: sad to have a child with epilepsy, sad that his seizures stole so many of his early gains, and sad that he can't do things his little brother can do. On those days when I really just want to curl up in bed and cry, I take out the journal that I keep. I've written down all Noah's gains since starting the diet, and when I think about how far he has come, I have something to be proud of and grateful for. It doesn't take all the sadness away, but it makes moving forward much easier.
—Erin Whitmer

Journaling is not second nature to everyone, and it's not always easy to know what to do or how to start. Here are a few tips so that at least journaling is one less thing you'll think of as a time-killer.

■ **Record the date:** Sure, it's obvious, but we're stressed people and have a tendency to forget things, and without dates, we lose our frame of reference and our ability to gain perspective.

■ **Write down all minor gains:** When you have a child with epilepsy, your gains are often smaller, but they deserve just as much praise. Every time your warrior does something new, write it down. If you get your journal out nightly, this will only take moments.

■ **Jot down what you're thankful for:** When you're fighting hard in life it's easy to focus on the challenges and forget all the good things. You might simply be thankful that you were able to drink your coffee hot instead of cold today.

■ **Add an image when you can:** Most of us live with a cell phone tethered to us, and we have pictures of nearly everything. Why not add a picture every now and then to your journal? It can be a photo of a happy moment or it can be a photo of your child before the diet, allowing you to see how the diet has transformed her.

By doing this, you are helping yourself cope with the tough days in two ways:

1. **When you journal, especially if you can write what you are thankful for, you are training yourself to become a more positive person.** The simple act of writing down positive moments in your chaotic life allows you to take a moment of quiet to yourself and meditate on the good instead of everything else you have going on.

2. **When you're having a tough day and you take the time to read what you have written, you are empowering yourself.** You have a visual reminder of every positive step of this journey, and when you can look back and see the amazing progress—be it little or large—you are fueling yourself with the knowledge that you have the strength to keep going.

Do I Surrender?

For some people, the desire to quit the diet is less about not being able to handle the strain of the diet, but whether or not the diet is overall worthwhile. There are individuals for which these diets just don't offer significant enough improvement to make the challenges worth it. For children who aren't finding seizure improvement, or for adults who are finding that anticonvulsants are offering equal protection against seizures, the diet becomes more hassle than benefit. For those people, the desire to quit the diet is a little more obvious. But what about the rest of you? What about those of you who have seen seizure improvement but not as much as you had hoped, or your children are struggling with serious constipation or reflux issues? How do you know when to power through and when to surrender?

Here is what we believe you should do when trying to figure out whether to step back into battle or retreat.

- **Reference your list of expectations:** We suggest you first go back to the list of expectations you created before initiating one of these diets. If you or your warrior has accomplished even one thing on that list, this diet has worked for you. Consider if that gain is worth losing if you quit.

- **Talk with your doctor:** It's important to talk with your doctor whenever you're thinking about quitting. Trust us, she's either seen or heard it all, and maybe she can offer some suggestion on how to get you back to the frontlines of success.

- **Fall back on your comrades:** Whether you rely on close family or friends or an online support group to keep you in check, definitely weigh this decision with them. Parents in the support groups have all encountered a moment when they thought about going AWOL but most get over it. Their feedback and advice is invaluable.

- **Trust your gut:** Parents too often don't trust their own instincts. If you want to quit but you feel something pulling you back and you just can't make that call to the neurologist, chances are you know it's not the right step. Just make sure to only trust your gut after you've had a good night's sleep and taken enough time to evaluate the situation fully.

If you are hitting a wall for some reason, or have questions that you don't think your doctor is able to adequately answer, it doesn't necessarily mean it's time to thow in the towel and walk away from diet therapy. Instead, you may want to consider seeking a second opinion from a specialist clinic in order to fully understand your options. We asked Dr. Eric Kossoff of Johns Hopkins Hospital to share the most common questions he sees in his Second Opinion Clinic. For many of you, this section may be enough to get you thinking about how to go back to the drawing board with your current Keto Clinic and how to continue striving for success on one of these diets.

From the Front Lines: The Dietary Therapy Second Opinion Clinic at Johns Hopkins, by Eric Kossoff, MD

About ten years ago I started to notice a subtle shift in e-mails I would receive from parents. Instead of getting e-mails asking me if they should start the diet (and why no one would recommend it), I'd say that most of the e-mails today are asking me which center (out of several possibilities) is the "best" and whether they should try more medications or surgery first. This amazing transformation is difficult for parents in some regions of the United States or countries to believe, but it's the truth. As I tell most parents, there is a Keto center now on nearly every corner (at least in every major city in the USA).

As a result of this explosion of ketogenic diet centers, we have also noticed an increasing desire for "Keto second opinions." These requests are typically from parents, but occasionally from neurologists and dietitians at these ketogenic diet centers. Of course, most of these parents have children who are not doing as well as desired on the diet, and they want to make sure they're doing the right thing. Approximately three to four years ago I started seeing children for one-time second opinions, as long as the families realize it was a single hour visit and their care would not switch to our center afterwards. The vast majority of the cases I've seen in the three to four years I've offered this service are being very well managed and I have only a few things to add.

When Erin Whitmer asked me to write a section in this new book about some of the frustrations that parents have on the diet, and how I handle it from a medical perspective, this "Keto second opinion" clinic seemed like the perfect way to start. Many of the questions parents ask are quite similar to each other. In this section, I will for the first time ever, share my list of the most frequently asked ten questions of parents of children at the Ketogenic diet "second opinion" center. For many of you starting the diet, this may appear initially to be not relevant to your family situation. I can assure you, within a few months on the diet, many of these questions will be very important.

1. **Is the diet working? How and why do you think so (or why do you say "no")?**
   The analogy I like to use, as a big fan of the New York Mets, is that assessing the response to the diet is like baseball. There are four outcome measures we look at: getting one would be a single, two a double, three a triple, and all four a home run! For some families with very difficult situations, a single may be enough. For others, only a home run will make the diet worth the trouble.

These outcomes are: 1) seizure reduction (or improvement in intensity), 2) medication reduction or elimination, 3) brighter, more alert children, and 4) improvement in the electroencephalography (EEG). I tell families that all of these outcomes are important, and all will get the family one additional base around the infield equally. If a child has a homerun, then it's obviously working (and most of these families are not coming to see me for a second opinion!). If a child has none, then it's a strike out and time to stop and try a different treatment. If a child is better cognitively and on less medication, despite no change in EEG or seizures for example, then I'd consider that a "double." Other neurologists might not agree, so that is where the analogy comes in handy.

There are other ways to get a sense if the diet is working, which usually is clear by three to four months on the diet. Does cheating lead to seizures? Sometimes we'll test the waters with some "controlled cheating" to find out. What's happened when medications were lowered? Did seizures get worse? That might suggest medications are playing more of a role in seizure control than the diet is. Sometimes the only way to know if the diet is working is to take it away and find out. More on that later in this section.

2. **Should I switch from MAD to the Ketogenic Diet (KD) (or vice versa)?**

Some of our families come to see us on the Modified Atkins Diet (MAD) and their child is 90% better. Is it worth a switch to the full KD? That comes with extra work and weighing/measuring foods, plus often a hospital admission. We studied this question a few years back by combining our patients with those at three other epilepsy centers and found surprising results. First, no child with zero improvement on MAD improved on the KD. Second, about a third of children had an additional reduction in seizures. Was it worth it? For some yes, for others no (and they switched back). Lastly, the only children who became seizure-free with the KD after the MAD was started were those with myoclonic-astatic epilepsy (Doose syndrome). Perhaps that means higher fat and ketones are important for that condition (on occasion). It also means that if your child doesn't have Doose syndrome, the chances of becoming seizure-free with the KD after the MAD is slim.

We know that many children long-term on the KD can successfully switch to the MAD over time. In fact, that's mostly how we figured out the MAD worked (parents had done this on their own). There are exceptions, so if the MAD is not as good as the KD was, consider switching back.

3. **Should I be checking blood ketones? Urine ketones? Blood glucose? Anything?**

This is a hot topic in the Ketogenic diet scientific community. The data is really just not there that ketones (or glucose) matters. We call it the "Ketogenic" diet because the body burns fats into ketone bodies, which can be measured in blood and urine. But is that how it's working? The data would say that probably not—ketones tell us that the child has made the metabolic shift to burn fat, but like a blood level of a medication, it may just be a marker of how much fat. Like some drugs, we check levels once in a while and the level doesn't always correlate with improvement. The diet is probably similar. For that reason, we are placing less and less importance on ketones, and many of our families stop checking after 6 to 12 months. Considering that tidbit of knowledge, I feel strongly that blood ketones are equally not important and unnecessary to stick children to check. If a family does notice that the level of urine ketones does correlate very closely with seizure improvement (although these families are rare…), I will then keep a close eye on ketones and perhaps check a blood ketone result once in a while. Many families who come to our Keto second opinion clinic are surprised that we don't care much about ketones.

4. **Are there medication adjustments (up or down) I should be doing?**

In general, you don't have to change the dose of anticonvulsants when the diet is started. Recent data has shattered that myth that levels change on the diet. However, we do have to sometimes adjust medications for weight (both up and down), and at times change the dose necessarily because a tablet form has a different strength than a carb-containing liquid.

After about a month on the diet, we will typically pick a medication and try to slowly wean it over two months. For some children on many medications, it's hard to choose. For some children on one drug, it's a bit more tricky to make that tough decision. It certainly is not mandatory and many families have no problem with the anticonvulsants and don't want to "rock the boat" if things are going well. I tell many families that drugs and the diet are a "partnership" that often continues throughout the life of the diet: they are NOT mutually exclusive. Some data would suggest that zonisamide may work well in combination with the diet and phenobarbital less well.

5. **Do you have any ideas on ways to tweak the diet to make it work better?**

This is the toughest question, and the number one reason the families come to our Keto second opinion clinic. It is most heartbreaking when a child is seizure-free initially on the diet, then the seizures come back.

We know this can happen with medications, but it's harder and perhaps more personally devastating when it happens with the diet. Answering this question is beyond the scope of this section, and we have devoted chapters to this in our *Ketogenic Diets* book, but here are a few tips to try.

We will sometimes change the calories and ratio (not usually by 0.5:1), but if a child is on 3:1, then try 4:1. If a child is hungry, more calories might mean more fuel and better control. Contrarily, cutting back from KD to MAD can help on occasion. We will look for hidden carbs in medications and supplements. Adding carnitine, MCT oil, and polyunsaturated fatty acids has helped other children when all else has failed. After a month or two of changes, it may be time to move on and stop the diet, sadly.

6. **What about all those supplements? Do I really need them?**
   It depends. Critical supplements include a multivitamin, calcium, vitamin D, and (in our opinion) Polycitra K. Others have advocated carnitine, extra selenium, and salt, but there's no proof it's required (above the other supplements). Many children end up on stool softeners, anti-reflux medications, and these can be helpful.

7. **If I decide to stop, how should I do it? What might happen?**
   We studied this in the last year and were surprised how many ways there were to come off the diet. It can be stopped immediately (over hours), relatively quickly (over one to two weeks), or the traditional slow method (over months). It turns out that it really doesn't matter. For that reason, we now use the "quick" method: cutting down the ratio every two weeks until the KD is over in two months. For the MAD, I'll go up 20 g/day of carbs every week until it is over in one month. Kids seem to do fine when you stop quicker than we used to.

   What happens also is relatively well known. If a child is seizure-free, the odds are 80% that he/she will stay seizure-free off the diet. A normal magnetic resonance imaging (MRI), normal EEG, and not having tuberous sclerosis complex increase those odds. Children who are at the most risk of having more seizures off the diet are those with 50% to 90% seizure reduction and on more anticonvulsants, which makes sense—they are tougher cases with more possibly to lose (than those with no improvement). It is very important to stay in touch with your neurologist throughout this weaning process.

8. **If I decide to stop, are there any other options left???**
   The diet is NEVER the last resort. I know it may seem that way, but it's not. Every year new anticonvulsants come on the market. Only about 1% will become seizure-free with these new medications…but if your child is that 1 in 100 case, how great is that!? In addition, there is VNS (vagus nerve

stimulation) and new stimulation technologies (to the brain and thalamus) in clinical trials. Surgery may be an option as well—it's always worth a look with video EEG even in the toughest cases when doctors said years ago that surgery was not a choice. Lastly, we'll sometimes try medications that were tried years back in new combinations. Never give up and don't feel that your child failing to respond to the diet means you have to.

9. **I feel frustrated—I can't get a hold of my neurologist and dietitian. What should I do?**

As a busy neurologist, and parent of two children, I can feel your frustration and understand why this may seem to be the case. Remember that most neurologists have hundreds if not thousands of patients—there aren't enough child neurologists to go around (especially in the Midwest and South). Most dietitians (including mine!) are not full-time for the Ketogenic diet; they have other responsibilities.

All that aside, if you feel like your questions aren't being answered within a couple days, keep calling. Once you get through, ask your neurologist and dietitian how best to reach them. For some, it's e-mail. For others, an epilepsy nurse. You might not have realized that. The diet is a lot of work for parents, it's also a lot of work for neurologists and dietitians: be persistent but also patient!

10. **I want to help other kids on the diet. How can I do this?**

Wonderfully, I get this question more often than some would believe! There are many ways to help. One would be to ask your Keto Team if there are support groups you can participate in. We have current (and former) families at Johns Hopkins come back and teach new parents each month. There are several great charity Ketogenic diet support groups all over the world like The Charlie Foundation, Matthew's Friends, Carson Harris Foundation, Epilepsy Cure Initiative, and Oliver's Magic Diet (to name a few!). All of these groups are looking for help, blog and website support, and of course donations. The authors of this book have taken a great approach in order to help thousands of families out there who need more help! You can write for your local newspaper or community blog, too!

As I've told many Ketogenic diet families who are now very active in groups such as those I've previously mentioned, perhaps there's a master plan out there (insert your personal religion and belief here). Although certainly no family wants their child to have epilepsy, and no family wants to be on the Ketogenic diet, maybe there's a reason your child needed the diet. That reason might be to help others get the help and support they need.

—Sincerely (and good luck!)—Eric Kossoff, MD

Seeking Tales of Victory

Have your ever spent time on the Charlie Foundation website and read all the stories about the children who have had amazing success on the Ketogeic diet? If not, we encourage you to do so, especially on the days when you are struggling to march forward.

Even if you aren't doing the Ketogenic diet and are doing MAD instead, these stories provide the perfect resource for inspiration. Sometimes when we're feeling overwhelmed by the nitty gritty of everyday life we forget about the big picture, and for many children on these diets, the big picture is astounding. When you've read the Charlie Foundation stories over and over again, thumb through this book again. With more than 50 contributors, you are bound to find stories that encourage and inspire you, especially within Chapter 9, "Warriors of all Shapes and Sizes," where even children and teenagers share how diet therapy has healed and strengthened them. Below is just one more story that started out tough and had its fair share of ups and down, but it ends with a miracle. Keep in mind that Sam is a real mom, and she's been in your boots before: scared, frustrated, and ready to fight. Just as you will no doubt find inspiration in her story, your story might someday be the inspirational catalyst in another desperate parent's jump into a ketogenic diet—and maybe a miracle.

Landon was born into this world on May 24th, 2007. He is our second child, first born son, and our special gift all wrapped into one. Despite minor delays as a baby, his early days were typical and filled with laughter, joy, and spunk. At the age of three, Landon received, what seemed to be, a devastating diagnosis of epilepsy after enduring two tonic-clonic seizures over the period of three days. It came quickly, unexpectedly, and uninvited. Pregnant with our third child, our lives abruptly changed and we now faced one of our biggest challenges. Our hearts were broken but our faith remained strong. In the begin-ning, Landon's neurologist gave us hope that medicine would be our best chance at facing this giant. Landon was prescribed Keppra due to it's "minimal" side effects when compared with other medications. However, we soon learned that anticonvul-sant drugs came with their own giants. Our once vibrant son, became aggressive, tuned out, fatigued, and irritable. Despite the overwhelming side effects, we believed we were on the right course and this was Landon's best defense against epilepsy.

After six months without a seizure, we had hope that this monster wouldn't return—that was until another type of seizure showed its face. At first we thought that Landon was falling asleep or nodding off due to the Keppra side effects; however, my motherly instinct kicked in and I soon realized that this was anything but ordinary. After a 72-hour EEG, Landon was diagnosed with yet another form of seizures called myoclonic drops. In order to control this new form of seizures, our neurologist prescribed opamax in addition to the Keppra. This mixture of drugs literally became a recipe for disaster in our lives. Landon was no longer interested in playing, his speech and sensory issues took a turn for the worse, and his little body became more fatigued then ever before. To make matters worse, Landon's seizures returned and they became more intense and more frequent. At the peak of Landon's epilepsy, he experienced up to 20 myoclonic seizures per day and up to three tonic clonics per week. We continued to cling on to hope that God would heal our son but our hearts became weak and we were waiting for a miracle.

Our breaking point came after a weekend of three tonic clonic seizures—we wanted answers. Landon was slowly slipping away into the world of uncontrollable epilepsy and we were determined to get our son back. My husband and I felt like the best and only option was the Ketogenic diet despite it's reputation of being restrictive and "hard to follow." In the matter of two weeks, our neurologist put us in contact with the Keto Team at Johns Hopkins. We were admitted a month later in May of 2011. The days leading up to our admittance were filled with anxiety and anticipation; however, this was our hope and our answer to continued prayer. Landon's initiation week was filled with highs and lows. We watched our son undergo fasting, monitoring, and sickness; however, we also experienced lessening of seizures, stories of hope, and a vision of the future. Within a few weeks, Landon's seizures decreased by 90%. He remained on both medications with the hope of weaning them after being stable on the diet. Within two months after Landon's Keto initiation, we started weaning Topamax under our Keto Teams supervision. Although Landon was not completely seizure free, it was our belief that Landon was making enough progress on the diet to go forward with the wean. In all honesty I was scared.

On one hand, I desperately wanted the drugs out of Landon's body; on the other, I was afraid of the unknown. Landon weaned from Topamax over the course of six weeks with only three myo-clonic seizures and one tonic clonic seizure. Beyond that, for the first time in over a year, we saw our son coming back to us. His clarity, alertness, and cognitive abilities were improving day by day. One month later, after remaining seizure free, Landon weaned off of his low dose of Keppra. Landon's last seizure to date was on September 5, 2011, two days before his last dose of Topamax. A date that I will continue to celebrate with a humble and faithful heart. Epilepsy has changed our lives; however, it's also given us a unique perspective on life. A life that is to be celebrated day by day. —Sam

Weaning the Diet

By the time you get the go-ahead to wean your child from one of these diets, you are likely either so excited you can't see straight or you're too terrified to drop the ratio even a little for fear that you might lose seizure control again. No matter whether you are weaning the diet because of seizure freedom over an extended period of time or whether you're weaning the diet after a couple years of improvement but not seizure freedom, weaning can be just as scary as starting a diet. You're coming back into the world of the unknown. Will the seizures come back? Will my warrior reject normal foods? Will I lose my mind without the gram scale and carb-counting books?

When to Wean

Weaning the diet is a decision that is made by you and your child's team. For the most part, it will be the decision of your neurologist, who will assess your child's success on the diet, how long your child has been on the diet, and the chances of whether seizures may return. In the past parents were told their child would be on the diet for two years, and many parents have also been told that only after a year of being medication and seizure free would they be able to wean the diet. In addition, the diet wean was *very* slow. As the ketogenic world grows by leaps and bounds, and research expands, we now know that the previous restrictions placed upon parents and neurologists regarding weaning the diet are no longer as relevant.

Many children are now on the diet for more than two years. Just take Abbie Ewing for example, our warrior featured in *Warriors of All Shapes and Sizes*. Abbie is doing so well on the diet that she may continue it for years to come, especially since there has been no other answer to seizure control other than the diet. There are some adults who have been on the diet over 20 years (and still going). Children can also be weaned from the diet after a period of time despite never achieving total seizure or medication freedom. Weaning is a very personal decision that is weighed heavily by everyone who has a stake in the warrior's care.

A study published in the August 2011 issue of *Epilepsy Research* journal reported that the speed of weaning the Ketogenic diet didn't necessarily have an impact on reoccurrence of seizures. This is exciting news for parents who don't want to take months to wean the diet, but it can still be disconcerting for some parents who have a hard time shaking the "what ifs." The article states that four to six weeks is often sufficient time to wean the diet without any repercussions. This journal article, however, points out that children's risk of recurring seizures during the wean is related to their current level of seizure control and the amount of medications they are on when beginning the wean. Children with a seizure reduction of 50% to 99% and who were on a higher level of anticonvulsants had the highest risk of seizure return overall. This probably suggests those children have more to lose versus a child with no improvement or, surprisingly, a child who is seizure-free.

We know that you can be on one of these diets for more than two years if the diet is working. We know that when we decide to wean it can be done faster that previously believed, or if you are fearful (as many of us are), you can still go slow. And we know that children at the highest risk for seizures coming back or worsening are those children who are between 50 and 99% improved and on a bit more anticonvulsants. So then...when DO you wean?

To help you understand where your medical team might be coming from when discussion begins about weaning the diet, here are topics that will be considered:

- **Time on diet:** If your child has been on the diet for two years and has either become seizure free or is greatly improved, this is the time that many neurologists will first talk about weaning. If the diet is working well, however, there will be circumstances that it might be better for your child to stay on the diet, if she is healthy and her blood work and urinalysis are good. However, it may, and probably is, worth a trial off the diet at this time.

- **Seizure improvement:** This is obviously one of the biggest factors and varies greatly with every child. What is significant improvement for one child might not be for another, so parents and the neurologist must really go back to the goals they set when beginning the diet, in addition to discussing potential risks of seizure return. Also, a normal EEG is a good sign that the diet can be weaned.

- **Parent participation level:** We hope this is not the case often, but we understand that everyone has a breaking point. If a parent is overwhelmed managing the diet, that is a big factor in determining whether or not to wean.

- **Negative health issues:** If your child has had medical trials including kidney stones, high cholesterol, bone fractures, nutritional issues, severe reflux or constipation problems, all these will be considered when weaning the diet is discussed.

- **The diet is not working:** For a number of children, the diet doesn't improve their seizures or their cognitive function to make the diet worth the commitment. If this is the case, weaning is probably the right answer.

Every parent can sense when the time to wean has come. You might be frightened, but you know. By the time the topic of weaning begins, you are likely close enough with your child's neurologist and his general attitude toward the big Keto topics—such as weaning—so you can likely judge when he's thinking a wean might be imminent. We've yet to meet a parent who didn't see the wean on the horizon. It's an exciting time, and a period when we all hope we can revel in our great accomplishment of helping to heal our child.

Battle Tips for Surviving the Wean

Fall back on the battle tactics we taught you in Chapter 2, "Boot Camp":

- **Share with your spouse how you're feeling.**
- **Talk openly with your warrior about how he's managing this transition.** Remember, that while this is challenging for you, it's a big step for your child. He might be over the moon about eating French fries again, but that new food comes with a big adjustment to his mindset and his body.
- **Allow yourself that extra time.** While weaning the diet, you'll be working harder to alter meals to lower ratios.

Wean Stories from Warrior Moms

*Rachel was just shy of six years old when she had her first
seizure in March of 2006. She had a ten-hour status, which
seemed to trigger the nightmarish roller coaster that is epilepsy.
Her diagnosis was Idiopathic Complex Partial Epilepsy. She
failed over a dozen anti-seizure medications before she was
referred to neurosurgery in October 2006. After two surgeries
her seizures were still not controlled. They began to increase
both in intensity and frequency. In November 2007 she was
admitted for the Ketogenic diet. They wanted to give her brain
a chance to "cool down" before they could go back in for more
surgery. She was on five anticonvulsants at that point. She had
26 seizures on the day I took her home, but the staff assured
me that she'd be better once she came home. I was doubtful, but
thankfully they were right. Within six months she was seizure
free! By the 1-year checkup we had weaned all but one drug.*

*In the spring of 2009 while at church, one of the Sunday school
workers who wasn't familiar with Rachel gave her a 12 ounce
cup of apple juice. She was watching the group while her regular
person ran out for a moment. When the mistake was discovered
they came and got me out of the services. I will be completely
honest. I freaked out! I snatched her up and took her to the car, sped
home (30 minute drive) and fed her a bunch of butter (trying to
counteract the apple juice)! But I was too late; she was completely
out of Ketosis. I was certain that all the seizures would return but
much to my surprise and happiness, they didn't. The e-mail I'd
shot off to Dr. K came back with a reply that perhaps it was a good
thing. I didn't see how it could be good. What good could come out
of it? It showed us that Rachel could come out of Ketosis without
having a seizure. We planned that at her two-year appointment in
November we'd talk about officially weaning the diet.*

*At first I was excited about the prospect of the imminent wean.
But then reality set in and I began to experienced a surge of fear
that would bring me to tears virtually any place and any time—
the "what ifs." What if we have to start over because the seizures
come back? What if the seizures come back and aren't controlled
by the diet the second time? What if they come back and I lose her?*

*At the two-year appointment we had completely weaned all of her
meds, been seizure free for over a year, and were ready to face*

the future. The plan was to go to 3:1 for two weeks, then 2:1 for two weeks, 1:1 for two weeks and then stop weighing.

The first lowering of ratio didn't seem very different than the 4:1 ratio. Ketones were still great, meals still pretty much the same. Second leg of the wean, 2:1, was a bit different. The meals looked considerably different! An ENTIRE slice of bread! Haagen-Dazs ice cream! It was going well. Rachel was handling everything like a champ! I was a nervous wreck! By the end of each two weeks I was pretty much used to the look of her new ratio on the plate. That was how it went. I'd get accustomed to the new ratio and it was time to drop again!

By the time 1:1 came, we were planning a trip to Mississippi to visit my family. Making a 1,200-mile trip by car with a child on 1:1 was much easier than our 4:1 packing. Rachel and I were both thrilled to see our family and to be able to partake of the big Christmas dinner at the party. I didn't have to prepare special things for her, I just weighed what was on the table and her plate looked much like everyone else's. And we did give her Christmas meal a LOT of leeway! As I watched her playing with cousins and enjoying her Christmas dinner I reflected back on how different it had been two years prior. Her "mashed potatoes" was a pile of Duke's Mayonnaise she ate from a special salad plate she had chosen for her "Magic Diet." She was still on several anticonvulsants then and was a bit lethargic. Now she ran around with the house full of cousins, aunts, uncles, and grandparents having a wonderful time!

1:1 was so comfortable. It felt safe. It seemed like we could just stay on 1:1. As a matter of fact, we stayed on 1:1 for four weeks instead of just two. I just couldn't seem to stop weighing the portions. I knew that weighing the meals wasn't magic, but it gave me such a feeling of security I had a difficult time putting the scale away. We waited until her big brother, Matt, was home from university and took Rachel to a family restaurant. It was a pretty big deal. She ordered chicken strips and French fries—a most decidedly normal looking meal. She ate it with gusto. I watched with relief. One of the fears I wrestled with was that she would reject the regular food. It was totally unfounded! She followed *up her meal with a giant piece of chocolate cake with vanilla ice cream! This was the beginning of a new era in our home. —*Ann

Ellen Summers is five years old. She was diagnosed with Doose Syndrome in February 2010 at age two, after experiencing myoclonic and tonic-clonic (grand mal) seizures for several months, following a history of febrile seizures. Soon after diagnosis, she began experiencing head drops and absence seizures as well. She was initially placed on Klonopin and Zonergran, a disastrous combination that didn't control her seizures but did make her a virtual zombie. Zonergran was replaced by Banzel, which worked slightly better, but seizure control was elusive. We started the Ketogenic diet in June 2010, continuing with both the Klonopin and Banzel. Her last seizure was July 7, 2010. We began weaning Klonopin in August 2010, and since it is such a difficult drug to wean, we took it very slowly. We were finished with Klonopin in October 2010.

After finishing the Klonopin wean, we switched Ellen from a 4:1 ratio to a 3:1 ratio, partly because Ellen was eating so poorly— she was always a picky eater and hated just about everything that was available to her. When we made the first reduction from a 4:1 to a 3:1, while she was still on one med and while seizure control was still a new phenomenon, I was VERY nervous. I asked if we could get rid of the last med before changing the ratio, because I so very much wanted for Ellen to be off meds. However, given her high cholesterol, Dr. Kossoff made the call to change the ratio, and I'm glad he did—her quality of life was greatly improved.

After moving to a 3:1 ratio, which allowed her a slightly more palatable diet, we weaned Banzel. We were done with medication before Christmas of 2010. Ellen had a normal EEG in June 2011 and was put on a 2:1 ratio then. We transitioned to a 1:1 ratio in September 2011, and her last day on the diet was December 31, 2011.

Our whole family had what I would call Keto-fatigue by this point, and we were ready to move on with our lives. We were ecstatic when the day came to stop, and having it be New Year's Day was a nice bit of symbolism.

Ellen's time on the Ketogenic diet was tremendously challenging for our family. The diet is equal parts logistics and emotion, and at any one time, you're not sure which will be overwhelming. But it was also triumphant, a real victory of the body over illness. Also, I will never forget what Dr. Kossoff said to Ellen at our last visit in December 2011: "You're cured. Have a nice life." It was one of the greatest days of my life. I wish for that moment for all families working their way through the Ketogenic diet. —Kay

In August 2011, after a normal 24-hour EEG and being 23 months seizure free while on the diet, 14-year-old Jordan got the go ahead to start weaning from MAD. That was a whole new adventure for us. Our progress was perhaps slower than most because I needed to travel regularly for my job and didn't want him to increase carbs during the times I was away from home. After being so very vigilant about every bite of food that went into my son's mouth for two years, lightening up was honestly, in some ways, unsettling. We were told to increase carbs by 10 net grams every two weeks, and to try out new foods we'd been avoiding. Testing whether your child will maintain seizure control while you wean the diet can feel a bit like sending your child out onto the frozen pond to test the ice, hoping he won't fall through. Though we were excited and I knew it was a necessary step, it was still a tense time for me as a mom.

We had a few crazy setbacks during our MAD wean that slowed our progress. We lived on the 17th floor of an apartment in China, and in a story far too long and involved to relate here, our elevator was out of service for nearly one month's time, much to the fury of all the building tenants. That meant hauling all food and shopping, let alone our own tired bodies, up 17 flights of stairs daily. Of course I worried about the possibility of my son having a seizure during this time, so we stayed at 45 net carbs until the power went back on. Jordan weathered it all just fine and by the end of the month he could take the stairs two at a time all the way up while carrying nearly 20 pounds of shopping. On top of it all, he went through a major growth spurt during the weaning time, shooting up two inches in two months, but still held his seizure control.

After we hit 60 net carbs per day we started replacing meals, adding one high-carb, low-fat meal at lunch for the next week. A week later, he ate two normal meals each day, and had a high-fat MAD meal only at breakfast. A week later we celebrated the end of the diet on Thanksgiving Day. We've decided to wait and not introduce highly refined sugars for a year, but other than that, he eats normal meals and all the fruit, rice, bread, and pasta he wants, loving every minute of it. —Jeanne Riether

We sincerely hope that no matter how you close your ketogenic chapter—whether the wean is fast or slow, peaceful or anxiety-driven—that you march forward without one regret, and that you cherish the knowledge that you did more than most people will ever do in order to save your child—and maybe even yourself.

Recipes

About These Recipes

We have divided the recipe section of this book according to age groups. While any recipe can be used by any variety of warriors, we wanted to group the recipes according to some of the dietary needs that are commonly associated with those age groups. Infants, for example, need pureed foods and transitional foods. Toddlers are notorious for being picky, so recipes that have an all-in-one ratio are going to keep Mom from losing her mind when her toddler tosses half his meal across the room. Kids' lives are so full of social functions such as birthday parties that we wanted their menu choices to be full of fun and flavor. Teens are active and busy, so it makes sense that their meals should be easy, and as much as possible, mirror what their peers are eating. After all, there's no tougher time to be on a different diet than during a period in life that's generally filled with hormonal fluctuations and angst. And finally, adults are more sophisticated eaters, and we wanted to cater to their more refined palates while providing meal options that will travel well and transition from home to work.

Because this book has been written for people doing any of the high fat diets (the Ketogenic diet, MAD, LGIT, or the MCT diet), we created the recipes using Ketogenic-diet ratios, accompanied by standard measurements so that each meal can be adapted, regardless of which diet you or your child is on. At the beginning of each recipe are basic meal facts, including the ratio, total calories, and the grams of fat, carbohydrates, and protein.

Because of our diverse audience, the ratios of each meal vary. Some meals have a 4:1 ratio, while others are anywhere from 1:1 to 3:1. When you find a recipe you like, you can use your KetoCalulator, if you have one, to alter the recipe according to the desired ratio, or if you are not on the Ketogenic diet but are using another high fat diet that doesn't require weighing the food, you can use the standard measurements as a guide to tweak the recipe. Just try to keep the original proportions of the meal, and you should be fine. Happy cooking!

Infants

BABY PUREE

KETO Facts	
Ratio 3:1	Protein 4.13 grams
Calories 201	Carbs 2.37 grams
Fat 19.49 grams	

This recipe is similar to a ratatouille and introduces you to the basic concept of making your own homemade Keto baby food. By using fresh produce that has been steamed and blended with fats, you have the perfect combination of healthful and healing. Stick with mild tasting oils that won't overpower the fresh veggies and fruit, and don't be afraid to combine fruits and vegetables in one meal.

raw zucchini, diced	20 grams
raw eggplant, diced	30 grams
raw tomato, diced and seeds removed	14 grams
grated parmesan cheese	8 grams
40% cream	20 grams
olive oil	9 grams

Instructions

ONE. Steam the weighed vegetables. While the vegetables are steaming, weigh out the cream and the Parmesan in a small bowl. Microwave on low until you've made a cream sauce. Set aside.

TWO. Add the steamed vegetables, including a small amount of water, to a small blender, Cuisinart, or baby food maker, and add the olive oil. Pulse until well blended. Add the cream sauce and pulse again. If the baby food isn't liquid enough, you can add more of the water from the steamed veggies—its full of vitamins.

Allergy Options
■ For infants under 12 months, skip the cream and stick with oil or butter for the fat. You can add a little high-fat yogurt to increase the protein of the meal.

Creative Alternatives
■ The options are endless for a Keto baby puree. Browse through your baby food aisle at the grocery store and use the food combinations as inspiration, paying particular attention to the ones with lower carb vegetables. If you use sweet potato and banana purees, you won't be able to use much due to the high carb content and your puree will be oily, but choosing spinach, green beans, and apples will work well. Stick to blander fats such as safflower oil, coconut oil, or butter, and work in natural sources of protein and calcium where you can—Greek yogurt is great for this.

Keto Bites

Wait until your infant is 12 months old to introduce cream.

The Vitamin A found in carrots helps your body fight off infections.

BABY PUFFS

KETO Facts	
Ratio 3.03:1	Protein 1.66 grams
Calories 100	Carbs 1.65 grams
Fat 10.03 grams	

Every baby needs a soft food that can melt in her mouth for that time when she's just learning to transition from purees to solid foods—being on the Ketogenic diet doesn't change that. These puffs are easy to make and easy on Baby's gums. Batch this recipe in order to have more egg whites to whip, making the process easier.

raw egg whites	15 grams
safflower oil	10 grams
Gerber's 2nd Foods Applesauce	12.5 grams
1 drop Sweetleaf Stevia	

Instructions

ONE. Whip the egg whites into stiff peaks. You should be able to turn the bowl upside down without the eggs moving.

TWO. Gently fold the applesauce and the oil into the whipped eggs. Do not overstir or your egg whites will lose their stiffness.

THREE. Using a spoon, make small circles by dropping about 1/3 of a teaspoon of batter onto a parchment-lined baking sheet. Repeat until you have finished the batter.

FOUR. Bake at 250 degrees until the puffs have slightly browned and are crisp. Do not undercook them or they will be soggy.

Creative Alternatives

- You can swap out the Gerber applesauce with any kind of baby food. Sweet potatoes, spinach, bananas, mixed berry, pumpkin—all are great options. Feel free to play around with seasonings too. Cinnamon, nutmeg, or pumpkin pie seasoning will all give a different flavor.

Keto Bites

Melt Baby Bell cheese and butter in a silicone up, firm in the fridge, and serve as a perfect all-in-one cheese snack.

Safflower oil is great for baked goods and helps to reduce cholesterol.

YOGURT MELTS

KETO Facts	
Ratio 3.02:1	Protein 1.17 grams
Calories 57	Carbs .66 grams
Fat 5.53 grams	

Yogurt melts are a great way to get Baby to adjust to finger foods. They are true to their name and melt quickly so keep them frozen until served, and only feed Baby one at a time or you'll have a mess on your hands.

Hershey's Unsweetened Cocoa	4 grams
Fage Total Yogurt	16.5 grams
coconut oil	4 grams
1–3 drops of Sweetleaf Liquid Stevia, any flavor	

Instructions

ONE. Weigh out the coconut oil in a small bowl and warm in the microwave on a low heat until it's liquid.

TWO. Weigh out the cocoa and Fage yogurt. Stir well. Add the Stevia and stir again.

THREE. Pour the warmed coconut oil into the yogurt and cocoa and stir it quickly to avoid the coconut oil from clumping.

FOUR. Pour the yogurt mixture into a small plastic baggie, making sure all the mixture is in one corner of the bag. Cut a small hole into the corner of the bag.

FIVE. Squeeze the bag gently, making little dots of the yogurt mixture onto a small baking sheet or plate lined with parchment paper.

SIX. Put the baking sheet in the freezer and freeze for about three hours before transferring into labeled bags.

Allergy Options

■ For a dairy free alternative, try coconut milk yogurt.

Creative Alternatives

■ Play around with different Stevia flavors to bring a little variety to this simple snack. Omit the cocoa and try a vanilla version. For lower ratios, you can use a flavored baby yogurt or add a little pureed fruit such as apples or peaches.

Keto Bites

Yogurt often contains more calcium than a glass of milk.

When making recipes that require whipped egg whites, save the egg yolks to use in a Keto ice cream or Keto custard.

Toddlers and School Age

100 WAYS EGG SOUFFLÉ

KETO Facts	
Ratio 4:1	Protein 6.1 grams
Calories 406	Carbs 3.83 grams
Fat 40.77 grams	

This is a great meal to cook in batches, as it freezes well. Just add the diced veggies to the mix after you've weighed out your individual servings. As the name suggests, there are no bounds to where you can take this soufflé.

cream, 40%	30 grams/2 Tbsp
group B vegetable	30 grams/¾ cup (spinach)
egg, raw and mixed well	27 grams/2 Tbsp
ground macadamia nuts, dry roasted with salt	10 grams/1 Tbsp, packed
olive oil	15 grams/1 Tbsp
cream cheese, Philadelphia brand	10 grams/½ Tbsp
dash salt and pepper	

Instructions

ONE. Chop veggies (with Group B veggies you can use any combination, but we used spinach for this recipe), or you can add other colorful veggies. Set aside.

TWO. Let the cream cheese warm to room temperature or warm it on low heat in the microwave. It will mix better this way.

THREE. Weigh remaining ingredients either in the same bowl or use smaller bowls and then mix all ingredients. Add your weighed veggies of choice.

FOUR. Pour into greased soufflé dishes or ramekins. Bake for about 45 minutes on 350 degrees, or until toothpick comes out clean. The soufflés will rise beautifully.

Creative Alternatives

■ The basic ingredients of this recipe are everything but the veggies. You can swap out the veggies for anything. Make it a Mexican theme by adding green peppers, jalapenos, and cheddar cheese. Go Italian with a little tomato sauce, hamburger, and Parmesan. Take this recipe to Greece by adding chopped spinach and feta. For picky eaters, keep it simple with a little cheese on top. This recipe will go as far as your imagination can take it.

Keto Bites

Switch out white onions for green onions, as they have fewer carbs.

Bacon will keep in the fridge for about two weeks.

WONDER WAFFLES

KETO Facts	
Ratio 2:1	Protein 9.58 grams
Calories 401	Carbs 8.67 grams
Fat 36.49 grams	

Let's face it: kids love waffles and pancakes, and they go hand in hand with Saturday morning cartoons. Sifting the flour out of your warrior's life doesn't mean skipping the waffles, and she'll be running for the kitchen after the smell of these delicious waffles wafts throughout the house.

40% cream	14 grams/1 Tbsp
finely-diced raw apple	50 grams/⅓ cup, packed
baking powder	0.5 grams/¼ tsp
egg, mixed well	39 grams/2 Tbsp + 1 tsp
ground pecans	15 grams/2 Tbsp
almond flour	13 grams/1 Tbsp + 1¼ tsp
melted butter	12 grams/1 Tbsp
cinnamon	0.5 grams/dash
vanilla extract	
6–8 drops Liquid Stevia, vanilla or plain	

Instructions
ONE. Warm the waffle maker while you weigh all ingredients in a small bowl. Mix well.

TWO. Grease the waffle maker and pour the batter onto the waffle maker. Cook until they are done. Note: Make sure the heat is on low or the apples won't have a chance to soften before the batter is over-cooked and dry.

Creative Alternatives
■ There are limitless possibilities to this recipe, which is why we named these waffles Wonder Waffles. Swap out the apples for virtually any fruit. Alter the consistency and flavor of the batter by using hazelnut flour, coconut flour, or any combination of flours. Add additional protein by

adding whey protein mix. Toss in a little cocoa for chocolate waffles. You can increase the ratio by pouring sweetened, melted butter over the waffles or by topping them with whipped cream, and you can lower the ratio by adding additional fruit or a side of bacon. Try cutting this recipe in half and serving the waffles with scrambled eggs or homemade yogurt.

Keto Bites

Blueberries are high in antioxidants.

Try a lime-flavored essence water to balance the sweetness of Polycitra-K when serving it as a drink.

SUMMER MUFFINS

KETO Facts	
Ratio 4:1	Protein 6.77 grams
Calories 398	Carbs 3.16 grams
Fat 39.68 grams	

The fresh basil in these flavorful muffins really tastes like summer. Since they are an all-in-one meal, they're perfect on the go, served hot or at room temperature.

fresh chopped basil	3 grams/1 Tbsp
raw zucchini	50 grams/⅓ cup
Fage Total Yogurt	20 grams/1¼ Tbsp
egg, mixed well	20 grams/1½ Tbsp
ground Macadamia nuts	15 grams/1¼ Tbsp
almond flour	5 grams/1½ tsp
olive oil	8 grams/½ tsp
Trader Joe's Mayonnaise	16 grams/1 Tbsp
pinch baking powder	
dash garlic powder	
salt and pepper	

Instructions

ONE. Place a large bowl on the scale and use a large cheese grater to grate the zucchini directly into the bowl. While you can use a Cuisinart or similar product to chop the zucchini, be careful not to overdo it. Zucchini can become watery.

TWO. Add all other ingredients to the zucchini bowl, either weighing them directly into the bowl or after weighing the ingredients in smaller bowls. Stir well.

THREE. Spoon the mix into greased silicone cupcake cups. The recipe makes three full-size muffins or six mini muffins. Place the muffin cups onto a baking sheet.

FOUR. Bake at 350 degrees until the muffins rise and are slightly golden on top, about 20–25 minutes.

FIVE. Allow them to cool just slightly before popping them out of the muffin cups.

Creative Alternatives

■ Swap out the zucchini for any colorful summer vegetable. Play around with seasonings to alter the flavor—a hint of jalapeno for kick or a dash of citrus zest. For lower ratios, add ground chicken or pork, or serve them with a pesto or Parmesan dipping sauce. You can also cut the recipe in half and serve these little muffins as a side to another Keto-friendly dish.

Keto Bites

For a heart-healthier mayonnaise look for one that's made with canola, safflower or olive oil.

Steaming vegetables retains the most nutrients.

SPANIKOPITA BITES

KETO Facts	
Ratio 4:1	Protein 7.21 grams
Calories 396	Carbs 2.67 grams
Fat 39.55 grams	

These super healthy spanakopita bites can be enjoyed as a muffin or as a fun, mouth-popping bite. They are loaded with calcium and protein, so they're delicious *and* they'll keep your warrior full.

raw spinach	35 grams/1 cup
fresh lemon juice	2 grams/splash
feta cheese	8 grams/1 Tbsp
egg, mixed well	17 grams/1¼ tsp
ground Macadamia nuts	10 grams/1 Tbsp, packed
almond flour	10 grams/1 Tbsp, packed
olive oil	8 grams/½ Tbsp
Trader Joe's Mayonnaise	18 grams/1¼ Tbsp
dash of garlic powder	
dash of onion powder	
salt and pepper	

Instructions

ONE. Chop the spinach finely and add it to a large bowl.

TWO. Add all other ingredients to the bowl with the chopped spinach, either weighing them directly into the bowl or after weighing the ingredients in smaller bowls. Stir well. The mixture will be very chunky.

THREE. Scoop out bite-size portions of the mixture and drop them onto a parchment paper-lined cookie sheet. You will need to use your fingers to shape the bites. If you are making muffins, spoon the mix into greased silicone cupcake cups. The recipe makes three full-size muffins or six mini muffins.

FOUR. Bake at 350 degrees for about 18–20 minutes for the bites and between 25 and 30 minutes for muffins.

FIVE. Allow the bites to rest on the parchment paper after you've taken them out of the oven so they can reabsorb some of the oil.

Creative Alternatives

■ Lower the ratio by adding less macadamia nuts and more almond flour, or add diced cooked chicken or lamb. A pinch of nutmeg will give these a unique flavor. Make your own cucumber yogurt sauce, or even try some olive oil infused with garlic for a way to add fat and flavor to the recipe.

Keto Bites

One cup of cooked spinach has more calcium than a 3/4 cup of skim milk.

Lime juice can be used as a salt substitute to boost flavor without increasing sodium.

ANYWHERE BARS

KETO Facts	
Ratio 4:1	Protein 6.77 grams
Calories 398	Carbs 3.16 grams
Fat 38.99 grams	

These Anywhere Bars are the perfect on-the-go snack. Make them as a meal or alter the recipe for fewer calories to use these as a convenient snack. You can use finely chopped nuts or you can use a variety of sizes for your nuts, giving this bar a lot of healthy crunch.

raw apple, diced finely	22 grams/2 Tbsp
raw egg whites	8 grams/½ Tbsp
sunflower seeds	7 grams/1 Tbsp
dry roasted macadamia nuts, chopped	24 grams/about ¼ cup, depending
flaxseed meal	3 grams/1 Tbsp + ¼ tsp
coconut oil	10 grams/½ Tbsp
dry roasted almonds	12 grams/2 Tbsp
3–5 drops of Liquid Stevia, any flavor	
dash of cinnamon	

Instructions

ONE. Weigh all dry ingredients and stir.

TWO. Add the egg whites, coconut oil, and Stevia. The mixture should be chunky and sticky.

THREE. Line a baking sheet with aluminum foil, folding up the edges to ensure no oil is lost during cooking. Grease the foil with non-stick cooking spray.

FOUR. Spread the batter to your desired thickness onto the foil. Using a rubber spatula, carefully divide the batter into bars.

FIVE. Bake at 275 degrees for about 35–45 minutes, or until the bars look and feel dry.

Creative Alternatives

■ Add some toasted coconut, Nestle mini chocolate chips, or any combination of nuts. To increase the ratio, use the higher fat nuts such as pecans or macadamia nuts. For more protein, toss in a few peanuts. Make a vanilla yogurt to dip these Anywhere Bars into and you have a snack that's healthy and fun.

Keto Bites

Try coconut oil for a Keto-friendly lotion or lip balm.

Use ground flaxseed instead of whole flaxseed to absorb the most nutrients.

CHOCOLATE HAZELNUT CUPCAKE WITH WHIPPED FROSTING

KETO Facts	
Ratio 4.01:1	Protein 8.1 grams
Calories 503	Carbs 4.46 grams
Fat 50.37 grams	

This cupcake is surprisingly light and fluffy, especially for a cupcake made of nut flour. The cocoa and hazelnut are perfect together, and the whipped frosting can withstand some party display time without melting, due to the cream cheese.

Cupcake
40% cream	20 grams/2 Tbsp
raw egg, mixed well	20 grams/2 Tbsp
butter	10 grams/1 tsp
flax meal	4 grams/2 level tsp
Bob's Red Mill hazelnut flour	16 grams/2½ Tbsp
Hershey's unsweetened cocoa	3 grams/3 tsp
splash vanilla extract	
6–8 drops Sweetleaf Vanilla Crème Stevia	

Frosting
40% cream, whipped	39 grams/¼ cup
cream cheese, Philadelphia	15 grams/1 Tsbp + 1 tsp
2–5 drops Sweetleaf Vanilla Crème Stevia	
splash of vanilla extract	

Instructions
ONE. Set the cream cheese out so that it becomes room temperature. Combine all dry cupcake ingredients in a medium-sized bowl and mix well. Add the wet ingredients, including the Stevia, and stir until the batter is well combined.

TWO. Spoon batter into a greased silicone cupcake cup. Bake at 350 degrees for about 18–20 minutes, until a toothpick comes out clean. Tip: Check the cupcake at the 15-minute point to ensure you don't overcook it or it will be dry.

THREE. While the cupcake is baking, whip the heavy cream. Weigh the cream after it has been whipped. Add the Stevia and vanilla, and then gently fold the room-temperature cream cheese into the whipped cream. Refrigerate the frosting while the cupcake cools.

FOUR. Once the cupcake is completely cool (about an hour later), frost it with the cooled frosting.

Creative Alternatives

- To lower the ratio of this fantastic cupcake, decrease the amount of cream in the cupcake recipe and try a combination of cream cheese with melted Nestle chocolate chips for the frosting. Don't stray from the hazelnut flour or this recipe loses its perfectly light texture. For another variation, try playing around with different Stevia flavors such as Valencia Orange or Chocolate Raspberry, or add a couple drops of a Bickford flavor such as cherry to complement the rich chocolate and hazelnut.

Keto Bites

To help stiffen whipping cream, add a few drops of lemon juice.

Replace your baking powder every four to six months.

BETCHA CAN'T TELL THESE ARE KETO CHOCOLATE CHIP COOKIES

KETO Facts	
Ratio 2.09:1	Protein 2.91 grams
Calories 159	Carbs 4.06 grams
Fat 13.79 grams	

Even non-Keto kids gave thumbs up to these quick and easy cookies. Because the fats come mainly from healthy sources, try making a big batch of these and serve them during a play date. When batching, weigh the chocolate chips last and sprinkle them onto each cookie to ensure the appropriate ratio.

egg, mixed well	7 grams/1 tsp
ground pecans	6 grams/1 Tbsp
almond flour	5 grams/1 Tbsp
butter, melted	7 grams/½ Tbsp
Nestle Tollhouse Mini	
Semi Sweet Chocolate Chips	5 grams/½ Tbsp
pinch baking powder	
3 drops Sweetleaf Vanilla Crème Stevia	
pinch of cinnamon (optional)	

Instructions

ONE. Weigh all ingredients except the chocolate chips into a medium-sized bowl. Mix well.

TWO. Spoon the batter into greased silicone cupcake cups, filling only about ⅓ of the cup. One recipe will use three silicone cups. Sprinkle the chocolate chips onto the cookies.

THREE. Bake at 350 degrees until the cookies have risen slightly and they are cooked through, about 7–9 minutes.

Creative Alternatives

■ To make this original recipe more fun, melt the chocolate chips and dip the cookie into the melted chocolate. Instead of chocolate chip cookies, try apple and peanut butter cookies. Swap out the chocolate chips for blueberries or raspberries. This recipe can also be converted into a cinnamon sugar cookie; by adding more pecans in lieu of the almond flour, you might even be able to sprinkle a little real sugar on the top.

Keto Bites

Buy butter in bulk if it's on sale—it freezes great!

Up the protein in a meal by adding a little natural whey protein powder.

TOASTED COCONUT TRAIL MIX

KETO Facts	
Ratio 3.99:1	Protein 4.29 grams
Calories 260	Carbs 2.22 grams
Fat 25.99 grams	

Spend some time on a weekend batching this recipe and you'll have on-the-go snacks all week. Full of healthy fats and packed with protein, this snack is the perfect power punch for an afternoon at school or at the park.

dry roasted almonds, sliced or slivered	12 grams/2 Tbsp
dry roasted Macadamia nuts	14 grams/2 Tbsp
dried, unsweetened flaked coconut	8 grams/2 Tbsp
coconut oil	4 grams/1 tsp
powdered Stevia	½ tsp

Instructions

ONE. Weigh all dry ingredients except the Stevia in a medium-sized bowl.

TWO. Melt the coconut oil in the microwave until liquid, and pour over the nut mixture. Sprinkle the powdered Stevia onto the nut mixture and stir with a spatula, scraping any oil that gathers on the side of the bowl.

THREE. Dump the mix onto a parchment-lined baking sheet. Scrape any remaining oil from the bowl and drizzle it on top of the nuts.

FOUR. Bake at 300 degrees until the coconut begins to turn light brown, around 10–15 minutes.

FIVE. Allow the trail mix to cool completely before bagging it.

Creative Alternatives

■ You can increase and decrease the ratio according to which nuts you choose. Macadamia nuts, pecans, or hazelnuts are great for higher ratios, though be forewarned that pecans have a tendency to be bitter in this recipe. Lower ratio nuts are peanuts, cashews, or pistachios. Serve the trail mix alone or sprinkle it on top of Greek yogurt, Keto ice cream, or even an avocado smoothie.

Keto Bites

Crunchy food helps to "trick" your brain into feeling full.

Macadamia nuts can help lower cholesterol.

Teens

CHEESY BREAD WITH DIPPING SAUCE

KETO Facts	
Ratio 1.07:1	Protein 19.97 grams
Calories 348	Carbs 5.46 grams
Fat 27.32 grams	

This golden brown, low-carb bread made of cauliflower and melted mozzarella is similar to the popular cheese bread sticks that American pizza chains are famous for. This versatile favorite makes a great side dish at dinner, travels well in school lunch boxes, can be frozen after baking for use later, and the dough can even be used as a base for low carb pizza.

Italian Cauliflower Strips

cooked cauliflower, riced or well mashed	80 grams/¾ cup
raw egg, mixed well	25 grams/2 Tbsp
mozzarella cheese	50 grams/½ cup
grated Parmesan cheese	1 0 grams/1 Tbsp + 1 tsp
parsley	½ tsp
oregano	½ tsp
dried basil	2 grams/½ tsp
dash garlic powder	
dash onion powder	
salt and black pepper to taste	

Dipping Sauce

olive oil	10 grams
Newman's Own Tomato and Roasted Garlic Sauce	25 grams

Instructions

ONE. For the cauliflower strips, mix all ingredients except the Parmesan cheese in a medium-sized bowl to form the dough.

TWO. Press the dough into a greased bread pan, so it is approximately ½-inch thick. Bake at 350 degrees for about 15 minutes. Let it cool in the pan for 10 minutes.

THREE. While the dough is cooling, mix together the Newman's Own tomato sauce and the olive oil to create the dipping sauce. Set it aside until ready to serve.

FOUR. Once the dough has cooled (the pan should be cool to the touch) loosen the dough around the edges with a flexible spatula, then carefully lift it and move it to a parchment-lined baking sheet.

SIX. Slice five 1-inch strips using a pizza cutter or knife. Separate each bread stick slightly. Dust with Parmesan cheese and an additional dash of garlic powder and salt. Bake at 450 degrees until the top of the bread sticks are golden brown and crisp, about 10–12 minutes.

SEVEN. Serve the bread sticks with the dipping sauce after it has been warmed in the microwave on low for about a minute.

Creative Alternatives

■ Use dough to make the base of a pizza. After you remove the square of dough from the oven on the first round, place it on a baking sheet and top with pizza sauce, grated mozzarella cheese, and toppings such as cooked ground meat, sausage, mushrooms, or olives. Bake again at 450 degrees until golden brown.

Keto Bites

Food labels can say "no carbohydrates" if the product contains less than 0.5 grams of carbs.

One portobello mushroom has more potassium than a banana.

CHINESE PORK AND ALMOND FLATBREAD

Keto Facts	
Ratio 2.03:1	Protein 18.17 grams
Calories 504	Carbs 4.36 grams
Fat 45.81 grams	

Savory flatbread pancakes in China are cooked on a griddle using lots of oil. This sizzling ground pork dish will entice the whole family into the kitchen. The flatbreads freeze well and can be microwaved for later use. Note: You will need an egg ring for this recipe.

Flatbread Batter

almond flour	31 grams/¼ cup packed
chopped raw green onion	10 grams/2 Tbsp
baking powder	1.5 grams/½ tsp
sesame or peanut oil	24 grams/2 Tbsp, divided
raw egg, mixed well	23 grams/2 Tbsp
water	1 Tbsp
basil	0.5 grams/½ tsp
garlic powder	¼ tsp
pinch of salt and pepper	

Filling

cooked ground pork	31 grams/¼ cup

Instructions

ONE. Cook ground pork with a pinch of salt and black pepper. Weigh it once cooked and set aside for later.

TWO. Mix the dry ingredients for the flatbread batter, including the basil and garlic powder. Add the eggs, water, 1 tbsp of the oil for MAD version or 18 grams of the oil for the Keto version. Add the green onion to the batter and stir until blended.

THREE. Oil a non-stick frying pan with the remaining oil (1 Tbsp for MAD and 6 grams for Keto).

FOUR. When the oil is hot, pour ½ of the batter into an egg ring.

FIVE. Press 1/2 of the cooked ground pork into the top of the flatbread, and let it cook. Turn, and cook the underside.

SIX. Using the same oil you fried the first flatbread in, repeat steps four and five for a total of two flatbreads.

Creative Alternatives

- Substitute ground beef, chicken, bacon, sausage, or sliced shrimp for the pork. Try a sprinkle of Parmesan cheese and oregano for an Italian flavor, spinach and feta for a Greek flavor, or give it a southwest flavor with a little cumin and chili powder. You can top the flatbreads with cheese, or you can swap out the green onions for any low-carb veggie or herb.

Keto Bites

Pork is high in iron, which can help fight off fatigue.

Meat from grass-fed animals has two to four times more Omega-3 fatty acids than meat from grain-fed animals.

CORN DOG POPPERS

KETO Facts	
Ratio 2:1	Protein 13.89 grams
Calories 399	Carbs 4.27 grams
Fat 36.3 grams	

This recipe was originally designed to be used with a mini corndog machine, but if you don't have one, this fun kid-friendly recipe will also work using mini silicone muffin cups. These mini corn dogs are compact and great for travel or school lunches.

40% cream	25 grams/1½ Tbsp
egg, mixed well	30 grams/2 Tbsp
almond flour	21 grams/¼ cup
Trader Joe's Uncured Hot Dogs	48 grams/nearly 1 hot dog
baking powder	1 grams/¼ tsp, packed
1–3 drops Sweetleaf Liquid Stevia	
dash salt	

Instructions

ONE. Weigh one hot dog and trim off the excess weight. Set aside.

TWO. In a medium-sized bowl, mix all the batter ingredients well.

THREE. If using silicone mini muffin cups, divide the hot dog into seven small pieces. Add a piece of hot dog to each mini silicone cup, the hot dog standing up, or vertically.

FOUR. Pour the batter over each hot dog slice until the batter is just shy of the top of the hot dog. The batter will rise above the hot dog, fully covering it and creating a cute little muffin.

FIVE. Place the mini muffin cups on a baking sheet and bake at 350 degrees for 15–18 minutes, or until just golden on top.

Creative Alternatives

■ Kids love to dip, so consider altering this recipe to add in a little ketchup combined with oil or mayonnaise, or try a natural high-fat ranch dressing. Swap out the hot dogs for any kind of sausage, or add a little cheese on top.

Keto Bites

Stevia was only approved by the FDA in 2008 but has been used across Europe for much longer.

You can save up to 90% by buying natural and organic foods—such as nuts—from bulk bins.

CHICKEN AND MACADAMIA STIR-FRY

KETO Facts	
Ratio 1.03:1	Protein 30.32 grams
Calories 505	Carbs 7.59 grams
Fat 39.12 grams	

Keep bags of chopped veggies in your fridge as a habit and you can have this exotic, flavorful meal in less than ten minutes. Alter this original recipe by sautéing the cabbage separately and serving the stir-fry on top of it, or serve the hot stir-fry on top of cold, chopped cabbage for an Asian salad.

broccoli, raw	25 grams/½ cup
white mushrooms, raw	35 grams/½ cup
onions, raw	25 grams/⅓ cup
chinese cabbage, raw	60 grams/1¼ cup
minced garlic	4 grams/½ Tbsp
raw chicken, diced	108 grams/½ cup
Kikkoman Naturally Brewed Soy Sauce	12 grams/1 Tbsp
chopped macadamia nuts	15 grams/1½ Tbsp
sesame oil	26 grams/2 Tbsp
2 dashes ginger powder	
crushed red pepper (optional)	

Instructions

ONE. Warm the oil, garlic, macadamia nuts, and onions in a wok or medium-sized frying pan until the macadamias begins to brown. Add the broccoli and chicken, letting them cook for a minute before adding the mushrooms and cabbage.

TWO. When the veggies are nearly cooked, add the soy sauce and ginger powder. Toss on high heat until the chicken is fully cooked and the veggies are cooked but still have their bright color.

THREE. Serve the stir-fry piping hot, or try it served as suggested above.

Allergy Options
■ Because Kikkoman soy sauce has gluten, try another gluten-free version.

Creative Alternatives
■ Swap out any of the vegetables of this stir-fry. Skip the soy sauce and add a little coconut milk or curry powder for a Thai taste or Chinese five-spice and peanuts for a Chinese flavor. You can also swap out the chicken for shrimp, scallops, beef or pork. To increase the ratio, use less chicken and more low-carb veggies, adding a cup of sweetened cream as a drink or as ice cream. Don't forget that you could serve this on top of Miracle Noodles, a carb-free specialty noodle.

Keto Bites

Mushrooms are not only low in carbs, they are also high in selenium.

MCT oil has a low flash point so use a low heat when cooking with it.

CHOCOLATE-COVERED STUFFED STRAWBERRIES

KETO Facts	
Ratio: 2.98:1	Protein 3.8 grams
Calories 262	Carbs 4.69 grams
Fat 25.31 grams	

These little lusties are about as good as it gets—sweet creamy filling, the tart contrast of strawberries and a topping that will satisfy your chocoholic cravings. This great finger food serves well as either a dessert or a party treat.

strawberries	50 grams/about 3 medium strawberries
cream cheese	25 grams/1½ Tbsp
butter	13 grams/1 Tbsp
cocoa powder	1 gram/½ tsp
Sweetleaf Vanilla Crème Liquid Stevia	

Instructions

ONE. Rinse the berries and cut around the top of each, removing the top and partially hollowing out the berry. Weigh the berries once they have been hollowed out. If the weight is too high, you can tweak it by further hollowing out each berry. Set aside.

TWO. Weigh the cream cheese in a small bowl and microwave on low heat for about 15–30 seconds. (Don't use high heat or the cream cheese will splatter.) Add the Stevia to taste—about 2–5 drops.

THREE. Fill the strawberries with the sweetened cream cheese. Refrigerate.

FOUR. Melt the butter in the microwave on a low heat and mix with the unsweetened cocoa powder and sweetener to taste. Because the cocoa is bitter, it will take about 8–10 drops of Stevia.

FIVE. Drizzle the chocolate mixture over the strawberries. You can either serve the strawberries with the warm chocolate on top or you can drizzle the chocolate on top and put the strawberries back into the fridge to cool so the chocolate hardens.

Creative Alternatives

- Cheesecake berries: Omit chocolate and instead mix ground almonds with cinnamon, then add sweetened melted butter and mix well. Press the mixture onto the top of each stuffed strawberry and refrigerate.

Keto Bites

Strawberries have more Vitamin C than oranges.

Cream cheese has the highest ratio of fat to protein of common cheeses.

Adults

AVOCADO AND BASIL PESTO WITH SHREDDED ZUCCHINI

KETO Facts	
Ratio 4:1	Protein 4.78 grams
Calories 498	Carbs 7.7 grams
Fat 49.86 grams	

This tart and creamy version of pesto provides a meal full of heart-healthy you'd-never-know-they-were-there fats tossed into shoestring zucchini in lieu of pasta. It's summer in a bowl!

avocado	140 grams/about ¾ of an avocado
olive oil	28 grams/2 Tbsp
fresh basil leaves	8 grams/⅓ cup
fresh lemon juice	12 grams/1 Tbsp
garlic, minced	4 grams/1½ tsp
raw zucchini	123 grams/1 small zucchini
dash of ground coriander	
salt and pepper	

Instructions

ONE. Julienne the raw zucchini by slicing it very thinly length-wise. The zucchini will act as your "spaghetti." It's easiest to weigh the zucchini after it has been sliced. Toss the zucchini into a steamer with a tiny bit of water and set aside for later.

TWO. Add all other ingredients to your Cuisinart or blender and pulse untill the pesto is creamy.

THREE. Steam the zucchini until it is soft but not too overdone or it will fall apart. Drain the water and transition the zucchini into a warmed pasta bowl or small warmed plate.

FOUR. Toss the pesto into the zucchini and serve immediately.

Creative Alternatives

■ To lower the ratio, add a little fresh tomato. It provides great color and vitamins. Reduce the avocado before lowering the olive oil when lowering the ratio. There are dozens of possible pesto creations that come together with olive oil, a blendable cheese, nuts and a carb or herb of your choice. Try ricotta and basil pesto, spinach and walnut pesto, macadamia nut pesto, goat cheese pesto, or a cheeseless version with lots of oil, basil, garlic, and any nut. Want to skip the nuts? Try sunflower, pumpkin, or sesame seeds instead. Swap out the zucchini for spaghetti and try Miracle Noodles, sliced eggplant, or spaghetti squash.

Keto Bites

Stick with Hass avocados over their Florida relative—they have more fat and less carbs.

The magnesium in nuts and seeds helps promote nerve function.

CHICKEN FLORENTINE

KETO Facts	
Ratio 2.01:1	Protein 21.19 grams
Calories 505	Carbs 1.67 grams
Fat 45.86 grams	

If you purchase ground chicken from your grocery store, this is a simple and high-protein meal that even picky eaters will enjoy. The spinach provides the perfect amount of color and vitamins, while the Parmesan cream sauce is reminiscent of a bowl of fettuccini alfredo.

Chicken Florentine

raw spinach, finely chopped	20 grams/½ cup
egg, mixed well	10 grams/1 Tbsp
ground Macadamia nuts	14 grams/1¼ Tbsp
Trader Joe's Mayonnaise	20 grams/1½ Tbsp
raw ground chicken breast	66 grams/⅓ cup
dash dried oregano	
dash onion powder	
salt and pepper	

Parmesan Cream Sauce

melted butter	11 grams/1 Tbsp
40% cream	13 grams/1 Tbsp
grated Parmesan cheese	7 grams/1 Tbsp and 1 tsp, packed

Instructions

ONE. In a medium-sized bowl, combine the ingredients for the Chicken Florentine. Using a rubber spatula, combine well.

TWO. Transfer the chicken Florentine into an ungreased non-stick frying pan, molding the chicken mixture into one large patty, about ½-inch thick. Cook on medium heat, turning it over once.

THREE. While the chicken is cooking, combine the cream, butter, and Parmesan cheese into a small microwaveable bowl. Heat in the microwave for one minute on 50% heat. Remove and stir well.

FOUR. Once the Chicken Florentine is cooked all the way through, place it on a plate and top it with the Parmesan Cream Sauce.

Creative Alternatives

■ Try finely diced mushrooms or green peppers and cilantro instead of the spinach, and top the chicken patty with a cheddar cheese sauce, spicing it up with a little cayenne pepper or jalapenos. A dash of cumin will also give it a punch of flavor. Or, try slicing the cooked chicken patty and serve it over a salad with a high-fat dressing and a sprinkle of shredded cheese.

Keto Bites

Try using a sweetened, dietitian-approved herbal tea as a "juice" replacement to serve with meals.

While spinach is high in vitamin C, kale is actually higher in fat and a better source of vitamin C than spinach.

TANGY WALDORF SALAD

KETO Facts	
Ratio 1.12:1	Protein 27.6 grams
Calories 500	Carbs 7.89 grams
Fat 39.72 grams	

The Waldorf salad is a classic that has been re-created time and again to suit a variety of tastes. Because the mayonnaise is the heavy hitter in this recipe, it's perfectly Keto—and perfect for a lunch while at work or school.

celery, diced	25 grams/¼ cup
apples, diced	60 grams/½ cup
cooked chicken breast, diced	83 grams/½ cup
Trader Joe's Mayonnaise	35 grams/2 Tbsp
walnuts, chopped	10 grams/1 Tbsp
5–7 drops Sweetleaf Liquid Stevia	

Instructions

ONE. Add all ingredients in a medium-sized bowl and stir until the apples, chicken, celery, and walnuts are completely coated in the mayonnaise.

TWO. Serve in a chilled bowl or factor in a couple leaves of lettuce for a sweet wrap.

Creative Alternatives

■ You can play around with the flavor of this recipe by using coconut milk and curry powder for an Asian feel, or try substituting some of the mayonnaise with full-fat Greek yogurt for a more tart taste. Lower the ratio by adding grapes or more chicken. Increase the ratio by eliminating the chicken and adding chopped roasted pecans or macadamia nuts, and cutting back on some of the apples and using more celery.

Keto Bites

Try a high fat Greek yogurt as the base of a salad dressing to punch up the protein of a simple salad.

Apples, oranges, pears and peaches are all low on the glycemic index.

ROSEMARY CHICKEN NUGGETS WITH DREAMY MASHED CAULIFLOWER

KETO Facts	
Ratio 1:1	Protein 33.19 grams
Calories 499	Carbs 5.4 grams
Fat 38.4 grams	

The joy of eating a chicken nugget just never seems to go away, no matter our age. These Rosemary Chicken Nuggets are a sophisticated and flavorful twist on the classic fun food, and when paired with the creamy Dreamy Mashed Cauliflower you'll be smiling with every bite.

Chicken Nuggets

raw chicken breast, chunked	95 grams/½ cup
almond flour	12 grams/2 Tbsp
1 large garlic clove, minced	4 grams
Trader Joe's Mayonnaise	11 grams/2 tsp
safflower oil	5 grams/1 tsp
1–2 dashes of dried rosemary	
dash onion powder	
salt and pepper	

Dreamy Mashed Cauliflower

soft, cooked cauliflower	100 grams/⅔ cup
whole milk ricotta cheese	20 grams/1 Tbsp, packed
grated Parmesan cheese	11 grams/3 tsp
butter	13 grams/1 Tbsp

Instructions

ONE. For the chicken nuggets, weigh the mayonnaise into a medium-sized bowl. Add the garlic and stir well.

TWO. In a separate bowl, weigh the almond flour and add the rosemary, salt, pepper, and the onion powder. Stir all with a fork until all ingredients are well combined.

THREE. Rinse the chicken breast, chop it into 1-inch chunks, pat it dry, and weigh it. Add the chicken to the mayonnaise mixture, stirring with a rubber spatula to ensure all the chicken is well coated.

FOUR. Pour the almond flour on top of the chicken mixture and stir until the almond flour and the mayonnaise have formed a batter over the chicken.

FIVE. Using the spatula, drop the chicken pieces into a pan that has already been warmed with the safflower oil. Scrape off any remaining batter from the bowl and press it onto the chicken. Cook the chicken until golden brown, flipping once—about 5 minutes.

SIX. While the chicken is cooking, weigh out the cauliflower (make sure it is well cooked for easy mashing), ricotta, Parmesan, and butter into a small microwaveable bowl or baking dish. Cook in the microwave on 50% power for about three minutes. When the contents are heated through, mash the cauliflower with a masher or pulse it in a Cuisinart. If you want, broil the Dreamy Mashed Cauliflower for a couple minutes to get a crispy top.

SEVEN. Serve the Rosemary Chicken Nuggets and the Dreamy Mashed Cauliflower together.

Creative Alternatives

■ Instead of chicken, try chunks of pork or turkey, and for a higher ratio, switch out the almond flour for macadamia nut flour. You can add additional fat to this meal by making a rosemary-seasoned mayonnaise or a goat cheese and olive oil sauce to dip the nuggets in. If you're not a fan of garlic and rosemary, switch both out for finely-flaked coconut and a little Jamaican seasoning. Cauliflower might be the perfect Keto food because of its low carb content, but it's not for everyone; try smashed broccoli, spaghetti squash, or turnips instead.

Keto Bites

One clove of garlic has about 1 gram of carbs.

Due to its fat content, you should only freeze meat for two to three months.

KALE CHIPS WITH LEMON MAYO

KETO Facts	
Ratio 4.04:1	Protein 1.36 grams
Calories 201	Carbs 3.61 grams
Fat 20.07 grams	

Loaded with vitamin C, kale chips are easy, whole-food treats that are gaining popularity with healthy eaters. Dipped in lemon mayo, it's the perfect combination of crispy, salty, and tangy.

raw kale leaves, torn	48 grams/About 4 cups
Trader Joe's Mayonnaise	23 grams/2 Tbsp
fresh lemon juice	5 grams/1 tsp

Instructions

ONE. Remove the stem and the large vein from the raw kale leaves, tear into chip-size pieces and then weigh. Put the kale on a piece of parchment paper on a large baking sheet, making sure they don't overlap. Spray them with an olive oil or canola oil spray to help them crisp up.

TWO. Bake the kale at 350 degrees for about 10–15 minutes. The kale leaves should be crunchy and slightly browned on the edges.

THREE. While kale is baking, weigh out the fresh lemon juice and mayonnaise in a small bowl. Add salt and pepper to taste and stir. Serve the mayo as a dip for the kale.

Allergy Options

■ For those allergic to eggs, try kale chips dipped in a homemade macadamia hummus made with olive oil and macadamia nuts, with either lemon or garlic.

Creative Alternatives

■ For those on lower ratios, try making carrot chips or sweet potato chips and using a little dill weed to season the mayonnaise. Try adding a little sour cream to the mayonnaise and some onion powder for your own onion dip.

Keto Bites

Increase calcium naturally with kale.

For a fiber-rich smoothie, try blending spinach or kale into your creamy concoction—your child will never taste it.

AVOCADO AND GOAT CHEESE DIP WITH CRISP TORTILLAS

KETO Facts	
Ratio 2.51:1	Protein 10.4 grams
Calories 494	Carbs 8.19 grams
Fat 46.7 grams	

This cool dip is so delicious that it flew off the counter when we tested the recipe. The avocado fortifies this dip with vitamins, protein, and healthy fat, and the goat cheese adds a sophisticated flavor that will make you second-guess that this is a Keto meal.

The Dip
chunked avocado	85 grams/½ cup, firmly packed
cream cheese, Philadelphia	40 grams/½ Tbsp
olive oil	14 grams/1 Tbsp
goat cheese, Trader Joe's	20 grams/1½ Tbsp
fresh lime juice	4 grams/1 tsp
garlic	2 grams/1 tsp
dash cumin	
dash of salt and pepper	

The Crunch
Mission Carb Balance Tortillas	27 grams/almost ½ a tortilla
celery spears	30 grams/about ½ a celery stalk

Instructions

ONE. Cut the low-carb tortilla into triangles. Place them on a parchment-lined baking sheet and drizzle a small amount of olive oil on them. Dust with salt. Bake in the oven at 350 degrees until crisp and slightly toasted, about 10–12 minutes. Keep an eye on them while they bake, as they will need to be rotated to ensure they are equally crisp. Set aside to cool.

TWO. While the tortillas are baking, combine all other ingredients, except the celery, together in a bowl, mash, and stir well. You can use a hand mixer or a Cuisinart to blend everything together if you want. Add additional seasonings to taste.

THREE. Slice celery—or any other low carb vegetable—length-wise for dipping spears.

FOUR. Serve the celery spears and the tortillas with the dip.

Allergy Options

■ The Mission Low Carb Tortillas contain gluten, sucralose, caramel color, and other ingredients. This element of this recipe is best saved for when seizure control has been achieved and there are no other food sensitivities; instead opt for the Almond Crackers recipe from the Charlie Foundation (www.charliefoundation.org) or veggies spears.

Creative Alternatives

■ Skip the goat cheese and cream cheese and add oil with chopped fresh veggies and cilantro for a chunky guacamole, or add full fat Greek yogurt instead of the goat cheese for a tart version. You can also try homemade cheese crisps to dip: just place tiny pieces of cheddar cheese on parchment paper in the microwave for about 60–120 seconds, or until they are firm and crunchy.

Keto Bites

Microwave any cheese on parchment paper in the microwave for 60 to 120 seconds and get a perfect cheese cracker for dipping.

Ground low-carb tortillas make a delicious alternative to bread crumbs.

Bibliography

About.com. "Low Carb Guide to Chain Restaurants A-D, E-M, N-R, S-Z." 2012, http://lowcarbdiets.about.com/od/chainrestaurantsad/LowCarb_Guide_to_Chain_Restaurants_AD.htm

Access STEM. "What is the Difference Between an IEP and a 504 Plan?" last modified November 30, 2011. Accessed July 9, 2012, from http://www.washington.edu/doit/Stem/articles?52

American Academy of Neurology. "Working with Your Doctor." http://patients.aan.com/go/workingwithyourdoctor

Aragon, Alan, *Girth Control: The Science of Fat Loss & Muscle Gain*. Los Angeles, CA: Author, 2009.

Balk E, M Chung, P Chew, S Ip, G Raman, B Kupelnick, A Tatsioni, Y Sun, D Devine, and J Lau. "Effects of Soy on Health Outcomes: Summary." *Agency for Healthcare Research and Quality*, 2005. http://www.ncbi.nlm.nih.gov/books/NBK11870/

Bender, Mary, Jeanne Rader, and Foster McClure. "Guidance for Industry: Nutrition Labeling Manual—A Guide for Developing and Using Data Bases." U.S. Food and Drug Administration, last modified November 10, 2011. http://www.fda.gov/Food/GuidanceComplianceRegulatoryInformation/GuidanceDocuments/FoodLabelingNutrition/ucm063113.htm

Berry-Kravis E, G Booth, A Sanchez, and J Woodbury-Kolb. "Carnitine Levels and the Ketogenic Diet." *Epilepsia 42*, no. 22 (2001): 1445–51. http://www.ncbi.nlm.nih.gov/pubmed/11879348

Bortfeld, Holly. "Tips for Including Dietary Restrictions in Your Child's IEP." *Talking About Curing Autism*, last modified February 6, 2011.

http://www.tacanow.org/family-resources/tips-for-including-dietary-restrictions-in-your-child%E2%80%99s-iep/

Bower, Sylvia Llewelyn, Mary Kay Sharrett, and Steve Plogsted. *Celiac Disease: A Guide to Living with Gluten Intolerance.* New York: Demos Medical Publishing, 2006.

Bulk is Green. "2012 Bulk Foods Study." http://www.bulkisgreen.org/Docs/2012-PSU-BIGStudy.pdf

Camfield, Carol, and Robert S. Fisher. "What is Epilepsy?" Epilepsy Therapy Project, last modified November 2, 2008. http://www.epilepsy.com/101/Ep101_EPILEPSY

Carpender, Dana. *1,001 Low-Carb Recipes: Hundreds of Delicious Recipes from Dinner to Dessert That Let You Live Your Low-Carb Lifestyle and Never Look Back.* Beverly, MA: Fair Winds Press, 2010.

Coppola, Giangennaro, Giuseppina Epifanio, Gianfranca Auricchio, Rosario Romualdo Federico, Gianluca Resicato, and Antonio Pascotto. "Plasma Free Carnitine in Epilepsy Children, Adolescents and Young Adults Treated with Old and New Antiepileptic Drugs with or without Ketogenic Diet." *Brain and Development 28*, no. 6 (2006): 358–65. http://www.sciencedirect.com/science/article/pii/S038776040500238X

Devinsky, Orrin. "Absence Seizures." Epilepsy Therapy Project, last modified February 1, 2004. Accessed July 8, 2012, http://www.epilepsy.com/epilepsy/seizure_absence.

Devinsky, Orrin. "Myoclonic Seizures." Epilepsy Therapy Project, last modified February 11, 2004. Accessed July 8, 2012, http://www.epilepsy.com/EPILEPSY/seizure_myoclonic

Devinsky, Orrin. "Tonic-Clonic Seizures." Epilepsy Therapy Project, last modified February 11, 2004. http://www.epilepsy.com/epilepsy/SEIZURE_TONICCLONIC.

Devinsky, Orrin. "Tonic Seizures." Epilepsy Therapy Project, last modified February 11, 2004. Accessed July 8, 2012, http://www.epilepsy.com/EPILEPSY/SEIZURE_TONIC

Diabetes UK. "The Glycaemic Index." http://www.diabetes.org.uk/Guide-to-diabetes/Food_and_recipes/The-Glycaemic-Index/.

Diasability Rights Network of Pennsylvania. "How to Resolve Special Education Disputes." http://www.drnpa.org/File/publications/how-to-resolve- special-education-disputes.pdf.

Doose Syndrome Epilepsy Alliance. "The Syndrome." *Doose Syndrome Epilepsy Alliance.* http://doosesyndrome.org/mae-explained/syndrome

Douglas, Lisa. *25 Quick & Easy Low Carb Breakfast Recipes: Delicious Food That Helps You Stick to Your Diet.* Amazon Digital Services, Inc., 2012.

Dravet. "What is SMEI or Dravet syndrome?" http://dravet.org/about-dravet/smei

Drislane, FW. "Status Epilepticus." http://professionals.epilepsy.com/page/seizclass_epilepticus.html

Eat Wild. "Health Benefits of Grass Fed Products." http://eatwild.com/healthbenefits.htm

Emmons, Robert. "Gratitude and Well Being Summary of Findings." UC Davis, University of California, November 23, 2011. http://psychology.ucdavis.edu/Labs/emmons/PWT/index.cfm?Section=4

Epilepsy Foundation. "Getting Started." http://www.epilepsyfoundation.org/aboutepilepsy/treatment/ketogenicdiet/gettingstarted.cfm

Epilepsy Foundation. "Ketogenic Diet." http://www.epilepsyfoundation.org/aboutepilepsy/treatment/ketogenicdiet/index.cfm

Epilepsy Therapy Project. "Find a Doctor." http://www.aesnet.org/find-a-dr/find-a-doctor-epilepsy-com

Epilepsy Therapy Project. "Ketogenic Physicians—Middle East." Last modified December 22, 2009. http://www.epilepsy.com/epilepsy/keto_physicians_mideast

Harvard School of Public Health. "The Nutrition Source – Carbohydrates: Good Carbs Guide the Way." http://www.hsph.harvard.edu/nutrition-source/what-should-you-eat/carbohydrates-full-story/index.html

Harvey A, L. Peleg-Weiss, R. Cohen, and A. Shaper. "An Update on the Ketogenic Diet." *RMMJ 3*, no. 1 (2012): e0005, doi:10.5041/RMMJ.1—72.

Hatloy, Inger. "Making Sense of Cognitive Behavioral Therapy." *Mind,* 2012. http://www.mind.org.uk/help/medical_and_alternative_care/making_sense_of_cognitive_behaviour_therapy

Health Canada. "Food Allergies and Intolerances." Last modified August 26, 2011, http://www.hc-sc.gc.ca/fn-an/securit/allerg/index-eng.php

Henneman, Alice. "NUTS for Nutrition." *Food Reflections,* March 2004. http://lancaster.unl.edu/food/ftmar04.htm

Hitti, Miranda. "Tips on Flight Safety Rules and Airport Security in the US." WebMD, last modified July 2, 2007. http://www.webmd.com/a-to-z-guides/features/flying-latest-carry-on-rules

Jewish Virtual Library. "Kashrut: Jewish Dietary Laws." Last modified 2012. http://www.jewishvirtuallibrary.org/jsource/Judaism/kashrut.html

Kossoff, Eric, and Beth Zupec-Kania. "Diet Therapy for Epilepsy in the Mideast." *Epilepsy Therapy Project*, last modified June 2009. http://www.epilepsy.com/epilepsy/keto_news_jun09

Kossoff, Eric, John Freeman, Zahava Turner, and James Rubenstein. *Ketogenic Diets: Treatments for Epilepsy and Other Disorders*. New York: Demos Medical Publishing, 2011.

Kossoff, Eric H., Roberto H. Carabollo, Tuschka du Toit, Heung Dong Kim, Mark T. MacKay, Janak K. Nathan, and Sunny G. Philip. "Dietary Therapies: A Worldwide Phenomenon." *Epilepsy Research* (2011). doi 10.1016/j.eplepsyres.2011.05.024.

Kossoff, Eric H., Sarah S. Doerrer, and Zahava Turner. "How do Parents Find Out about the Ketogenic Diet?" *Epilepsy and Behavior* 24, no. 4 (2012): 445–48. http://www.ncbi.nlm.nih.gov/pubmed/22677375

Kübler-Ross, Elizabeth. "The Kübler-Ross Grief Cycle." ChangingMinds .org. http://changingminds.org/disciplines/change_management/kubler_ross/kubler_ross.htm

LDOnline. "IDEA 2004." http://www.ldonline.org/features/idea2004

Li, James T. C. "Food Allergy – What's the Difference Between a Food Intolerance and a Food Allergy." Mayo Clinic, last modified June 3, 2011, https://www.mayoclinic.com/health/food-allergy/AN01109

Liao, J, Li Y, Z Xiao, Z. "Effect of Ketocal on childhood intractable epilepsy in China." Poster presentation at the 28th International Epilepsy Congress, Budapest, Hungary, June 28–July 2, 2009.

Lieberman, Phil, and Hugh Sampson. "Potential Cross-Reactivity between Peanut, Coconut, and Sesame." American Academy of Allergy, Asthma, and Immunology. http://www.aaaai.org/ask-the-expert/potential-cross-reactivity-between-peanut-coconut.aspx

Matthew's Friends. "About Our Founder." http://site.matthewsfriends.org/uploads/OurFounder.pdf

MedlinePlus. "Feeding Tube Insertion – Gastronomy." Last modified June 28, 2012. http://www.nlm.nih.gov/medlineplus/ency/article/002937.htm

Mittan, Robert A. "S.E.E. Program Parent's Manual, How to Raise a Kid with Epilepsy, Part 1: Coping with Fear," *Exceptional Parent Magazine*, October 2005.

National Heart Lung and Blood Institute. "What Is Cholesterol." last modified July, 01, 2011. http://www.nhlbi.nih.gov/health/health-topics/topics/hbc/

Nelson, Jennifer. "Plant Palette: Winter Squash." University of Illinois Extension, last modified November 14, 2010. http://web.extension.illinois .edu/dmp/palette/101114.html

Office of Dietary Supplements: National Institute of Health. "Dietary Supplement Fact Sheet: Carnitine." Last modified June 15, 2006. http:// ods .od.nih.gov/factsheets/Carnitine-HealthProfessional/

Office of Dietary Supplements: National Institute of Health. "Dietary Supplement Fact Sheet: Magnesium." Last modified July 13, 2009, http://ods.od.nih.gov/factsheets/Magnesium-HealthProfessional/

Pfeifer, Heidi. "The Low Glycemic Index Treatment and the Ketogenic Diet." Epilepsy Therapy Project, last modified April 25, 2007. http:// www.epilepsy.com/epilepsy/keto_news_may07

Pfeifer, Heidi H., and Elizabeth A Thiele. "Low-Glycemic-Index Treatment: A Liberalized Ketogenic Diet for Treatment of Intractable Epilepsy." *Neurology 65*, no. 11 (2005). http://www.ncbi.nlm.nih.gov/ pubmed/16344529

Queensland Health. "What is a Dietitian?" November 2010. http://www .health.qld.gov.au/workforus/careers/Dietitian.pdf

Quotegarden.com. "Quotes about Worrying." http://www.quotegarden .com/worry.html

Rewega, Alicia, editor. *The Best of Clean Eating: Improving Your Life One Meal at a Time*. Toronto, Ontario: Robert Kennedy Publishing, 2010.

Rewega, Alicia, editor. *The Best of Clean Eating 2: Improving Your Life One Meal at a Time*. Mississauga, Ontario: Robert Kennedy Publishing, 2011.

Roberts, Seth. "General Medicine Community; the Ketogenic Diet." *Wellsphere*, last modified July 1, 2008. http://www.wellsphere.com/ general-medicine-article/the-ketogenic-diet-continued/16092

Schachter, Steven C. "What is a Seizure?" *Epilepsy Therapy Project*, last modified November 20, 2006, http://www.epilepsy.com/101/ep101_seizure.

Schneider, Karen. "Director Jim Abrahams Says a Controversial Diet Saved His Epileptic Son." *People*, April 17, 1995. http://www.people.com/ people/archive/article/0,,20105525,00.html

Science Daily. "Anticonvulsant." http://www.sciencedaily.com/articles/a/ anticonvulsant.htm

Smith, Art. *Kitchen Life: Real Food for Real Families-Even Yours!* New York: Hyperion Books, 2004.

Stephensen, Charles B. "Vitamin A, Infection, and Immune Function." *Annual Review of Nutrition 21,* (2001): 167–92. http://www.ncbi.nlm .nih.gov/pubmed/11375434.

The Charlie Foundation. "Epilepsy Terminology." http://charliefoundation .org/resources/epilepsy-terminology.html

The Charlie Foundation. "Ketogenic Diet." http://charliefoundation.org/faq/ ketogenic-diet.html

The Disney .Food Blog, "Dining with a Special Diet in Disney World and Disney Land." http://www.disneyfoodblog.com/special-diets-resources/

The New York Times. "Miss Jean Clemen Found Dead in Bath," December 25, 1909. http://www.twainquotes.com/19091225.html

Transportation Security Administration, U. S. Department of Homeland Security. "Travelers with Disabilities and Medical Conditions." http:// www.tsa.gov/travelers/airtravel/disabilityandmedicalneeds/index .shtm

Trix, Victoria. "The Differences Between an IEP, a 504 Plan and Title 1." Bright Hub Education, last modified April 12, 2012. http://www.bright-hubeducation.com/parents-and-special-ed/24249-brief-overview-of-iep-plans-504-and-title-1/

United States Department of Agriculture. "Super Tracker: Food-A-Pedia." www.choosemyplate.gov/supertracker/foodapedia

Walt Disney World. "Guest Assistance Cards (GAC's) Who Should Get Them and How to Use Them." http://www.diz-abled.com/Disney-Resources/ Articles/Disney-Guest-Assistance-Cards.htm

Walt Disney World. "Special Dietary Requests." http://disneyworld.disney .go.com/guest-services/special-dietary-requests/

Web MD. "20 Common Foods with the Most Antioxidants." *Web MD,* last modified April 1, 2005. http://www.webmd.com/food-recipes/ 20-common-foods-most-antioxidants

Worden, Lilia T., Zahava Turner, Paula L. Pyzik, James E. Rubenstein, and Eric H. Kossoff. "Is There an Ideal Way to Discontinue a Ketogenic Diet?" *Epilepsy Research 95,* no. 3 (2011): 232–36.

World's Healthiest Foods. "Blueberries." http://www.whfoods.com/genpage .php?tname=foodspice&dbid=8

Wright, Peter W.D, and Pamela Darr Wright. "Your Child's IEP: Practical and Legal Advice for Parents." *LDOnline,* last modified 2003. http:// www.ldonline.org/article/6078/

Index